D0212823

HISTORY OF 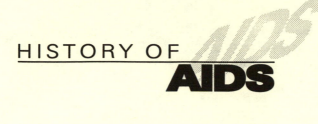 AIDS

HISTORY OF AIDS

EMERGENCE AND ORIGIN OF A MODERN PANDEMIC

Mirko D. Grmek

Translated by

Russell C. Maulitz

and

Jacalyn Duffin

Princeton University Press, Princeton New Jersey

Originally published as
Histoire du sida: Début et ori-
gine d'une pandémie actuelle
by Éditions Payot (c) 1989

Library of Congress Cataloging-in-Publication Data

Copyright © 1990
by Princeton University Press
Published by
Princeton University Press,
41 William Street
Princeton, New Jersey 08540
In the United Kingdom:
Princeton University Press,
Chichester, West Sussex
All Rights Reserved

Grmek, Mirko Dražen.
[Histoire du SIDA. English]
   History of AIDS : emergence and origin of a modern
pandemic /
Mirko D. Grmek ; translated by Russell C. Maulitz and
Jacalyn Duffin.
   p.   cm.
Translation of: Histoire du SIDA.
Includes bibliographical references.
ISBN 0-691-08552-8 (alk. paper)
   1. AIDS (Disease)—History.   2. AIDS (Disease)—
Epidemiology—History.   I. Title.
[DNLM: 1. Acquired Immunodeficiency Syndrome—
history.   WD 308 G525h]
RA644.A25G7613   1990
614.5'993—dc20
DNLM/DLC
for Library of Congress   90-32514

This book has been composed in Times Roman and
Helvetica typefaces

Princeton University Press books are printed on acid-free
paper, and meet the guidelines for permanence and
durability of the Committee on Production Guidelines for
Book Longevity of the Council on Library Resources

Printed in the United States of America

10   9   8   7

Contents

vi CONTENTS

Translators' Preface

IN SPITE OF the burgeoning mass of literature on the Acquired Immunodeficiency Syndrome (AIDS), this is the first international history of both the disease and the research that has tracked it across the globe. It is difficult to imagine anyone other than Mirko Grmek having written it. Physician, philologist, and historian of science, he has spent more than a generation moving across many different boundaries, from medical practice to disease in antiquity, to studies of nineteenth- and twentieth-century science. Crossing borders can be a complicated business, yet traversing and communicating across borders is intrinsic to the story of AIDS and, of course, to the task of translation itself.

Consider the twin frontiers explored in these pages: the one, that of a sinister "new" disease; the other, that of scientists' efforts to grapple with it. AIDS itself has demonstrated a remarkable ability to breach the natural barriers of geography. Those who seek to block its progress also encounter barriers: between the patient's bedside and the laboratory; or in the nearly always murky zone between health science and health policy.

Often enough, the medical scientist is thrust into the multifaceted role as translator for several different groups: those who are themselves afflicted with a disease, struggling to surmount it; those who care for patients, seeking to learn how to cure (or at least modify) it; those who see it as a scientific problem they long to understand; and those, in government and industry, who want to determine how best to distribute resources both public and private to each of these first three groups. These four interested parties have claims that are at times congruent, and at times most emphatically not so; yet, they are not mutually exclusive.

Like the medical scientist, the historian of AIDS becomes an interlocutor in still other dimensions. Because of AIDS, new borders have been uncovered, and others newly erected, between cultural, national, social, and linguistic groups. Historians must find the intellectual links, in terms of our current understanding, and they must also translate between the official chronology—the guild account so easily passed off as "history"—and the "reality" as the lone writer can best discern it peering between the facts, between the lines, and between the theories. The priority dispute over the discovery of the AIDS virus, discussed in Chapter 7, illustrates the problem. Most often an official, triumphal history emerges as a sort of gradual extrusion of historical retrospect, generated over a long time, from eyewitness accounts and the detritus of official scribes. In this case, an unusual reification of this process took place. As national borders were crossed—by the virus, by the theories about it, by the people studying it—the "official chronology" explicitly became something like an out-of-court settlement. It was drafted treatylike, in appropriate elliptical phrases to mask the painful, the unresolvable, the untranslatable.

In our efforts to translate the author's own "translation" of the events, we join with him in attesting to the poignant spectacle of AIDS as it stalks across and around the world. It is a story of dimension and moment, demanding dialogue between elements of our society often seemingly ill prepared and little equipped to understand one another. This book attempts to redress that circumstance. Many debts have been incurred along the way. Special thanks are owed to Elizabeth Severino, Edward Tenner, and Robert Wolfe for their criticism, comments, and support on the many drafts. But our greatest debt is to the author himself, who took more than an active interest in the task, becoming a de facto third member of our small team. We hope that our efforts have done justice to his thoughts and to his words.

May 1990   RUSSELL C. MAULITZ
                    JACALYN DUFFIN

Introduction

Un mal qui répand la terreur . . . les tourterelles se fuyoient: plus d'amour, partant plus de joie.

—Jean de La Fontaine, fabulist

I AM NOT SO NAIVE, in the middle of an epidemic still in full advance, as to believe its history can be written with the serenity and knowledge afforded only by distance from the events. But I am bold enough to think that, even at this early date, a look back by a physician trained in historical method might be of benefit. Chronological distance and subjective detachment may, on the one hand, be lacking. But on the other hand, direct experience and passion can serve as more than mere epistemological obstacles.

The time has come, I think, to take stock—not to predict the outcome but to better understand what is taking place. In recounting the beginnings of this pandemic, in probing behind the scenes of official science, in explaining current research strategy and the vicissitudes of the struggle against an unexpected plague, and in reflecting on its biological and social causes, I hope not only to shed light on this problem for the contemporary reader, but to provide a testimony for the future historian.

Without yet being able to write the "official biography" of AIDS, I offer in these pages two interwoven stories: that of the reality of an unprecedented epidemic event, and that of the growth of our ideas about it. The historical narrative, to some extent more positivist and factual, is coupled with an attempt at a causal explanation, which, though necessarily hypothetical, is not arbitrary. I have applied the same method to the study of this contemporary disease as I used in my work on *Diseases in the Ancient Greek World*. Past and present clarify each other.

No doubt historical inquiry can illuminate the present. But it should not be used to make predictions. Historians are poor prophets. Thus in 1977, for example, in the very year in which AIDS was already lapping on American shores, the eminent historian of diseases, William Beveridge, published a book called *Influenza, the Last Great Plague*. Influenza was the last of the classic pestilences; AIDS, both unpredicted and unpredictable within the framework of the old nosology, is the first of the postmodern plagues.

Is AIDS really a new disease? Formulated in this way, without nuance or qualification, the question summons answers that seem equivocal and contradictory. Yes, AIDS is necessarily new in the sense that it was inconceivable until the 1970s. A disease was either defined by its symptoms or by its associated anatomical lesions. Neither sort of definition characterized AIDS: a disorder without its own specific symptoms; marked only by invisible, subcellular lesions; and induced by an agent undetectable before the most recent analytical methods. Yes, AIDS is also a new disease with respect to the extent of its current epidemic spread. And at the same time, no, AIDS is not a truly new disease, in the sense that its virus has been around for a long time: in the shadow of other infectious states, it has been there, triggering various pathological conditions that, whether isolated or sometimes even collective, were highly confined in time and space.

This book is written in four parts, each with four chapters. Part One explores the beginnings of an epidemic that was felt to be unprecedented. The events are described as they appeared to contemporaries. Part Two contains an analysis of scientists' progress in the attempt to understand this disease and identify its causative agent. Step by step I trace scientific research in this domain, going behind the scenes to examine the efforts of biologists and doctors absorbed in a relentless race where success was the only judge. Part Three delves into the remote past of hidden AIDS, using the latest investigative techniques to probe the origins of the present epidemic. Finally, in Part Four, I go on to seek the biological and social causes of AIDS. The emergence of this scourge, though unexpected, is in no way inexplicable.

On closer look, this book seems to follow a classical structure, the four parts corresponding to the progressive use of the four key concepts of historical inquiry: *prophasis, crisis, arché*, and *aitia*. I noticed this, with some surprise and a certain intellectual satisfaction, only after the work was complete: isn't it the goal of history, as Thucydides once taught, to proceed from the description of first appearances to a revelation of the ultimate cause?

In considering the initial appearance of this epidemic, its prophase, one might be disturbed, or at least astonished, by a series of chronological coincidences. In 1978 for the first time in history the conceptual and technical means were available for identifying and isolating a human retrovirus. And it was just then that AIDS began to spread. Is it not asking too much of chance to assume that the AIDS virus appeared through a sudden mutation at that very moment? Can we postulate such an improbable conjunction of events? The discovery of a second AIDS virus put an end to all hesitation on the subject: it was impossible to sustain the hypothesis that two accidental, parallel, and independent mutations could take place at the exact moment in all human history when it first became possible to identify them. Another coincidence was soon added: the eradication, announced in 1977, of smallpox, one of the greatest killers of all time. The last naturally infected smallpox patient was an

African from Somalia. And out of Africa may have come the virus that took its place.

These coincidences intrigued me. On the one hand, I found it hard to accept that these events could be totally independent, that their congruence was pure chance. On the other hand, it is difficult to find any direct causal link between them.

The insight came to me on the shores of Lake Annecy after a symposium organized by Charles Mérieux in the summer of 1987. All these events were not causally related among themselves, but instead flowed from a common source: from progress in medicine, or more generally speaking from the technological upheaval of the modern world. Scientific and technological advances conquered smallpox, gave us the means to identify the retrovirus, and then opened the way to the ravages of a virus with which they had previously lived in peaceful coexistence. Medicine contributed to the epidemic as much by rupturing the fragile pathocenosis, that is, by suppressing competing diseases, as it did by facilitating the transmission of the infection, notably through new means of direct blood contact. Moreover, modern technology contributed to the intermingling of peoples and the liberalization of social mores, both important factors in the emergence and dissemination of AIDS. The present epidemic is the other side of the medal of progress, the unexpected cost of having tampered radically with the ecological equilibria of the ages.

The AIDS virus is extremely variable. It had once been controlled by natural selection favoring less virulent strains. Social factors enlarged its routes of transmission and allowed it to break through a sort of critical threshold that had previously limited its expansion. A profound analogy exists between the process by which the AIDS epidemic came into being and one which, by exceeding a critical mass, touches off an atom bomb; or one which, on an individual level, causes a cancer to break through the equilibrium between the forces of immunological control and those of inevitable, incessant cellular errors.

Another analogy, drawn from informatics—the science of information— relates AIDS to a "computer disease." This is an insidious dysfunction of computers, propagated through electronic channels from machine to machine after the introduction of a sequence of instructions which, when executed, disrupt and disorganize normal function. Only in the last five years have computer specialists recognized the existence of this kind of sabotage. Is it not significant that they gave it the name "computer virus" and, to explain events taking place in the artificial world, made use of models forged by biologists to explain natural events?

This diabolical AIDS virus, malignant in every sense, first disrupts the organism's immune defenses, disorganizes its internal regulation. It then ricochets outward to disturb sexual relations and finally, dangerously, to poison social habits in a new way, more subtle and more insidious than medieval leprosy, Renaissance syphilis, or machine-age tuberculosis. Susan Sontag, in her *Illness as Metaphor*, also published in 1977, has shown how the sensitivities of each era favor a certain disease—not necessarily the most common or the most deadly. In 1977 cancer had replaced pulmonary consumption and captured the mid-twentieth century imagination to become a horrible taboo. But cancer lacked certain elements to qualify it as the ideal metaphor for a society that, at least since the late 1960s, had spawned major social convulsions.

We now have that metaphor: with its links to sex, drugs, blood, and informatics, and with the sophistication of its evolution and of its strategy for spreading itself, AIDS expresses our era.

PART ONE

A CALAMITY FOR OUR TIMES

CHAPTER 1

Proclaim a New Disease

This is a very,

very dramatic illness.

I think we can say

quite assuredly that

it is new.

—James Curran,

epidemiologist

AROUND 1980, suddenly and much to their own great astonishment, physicians detected the existence of an illness that seemed "new." New because they thought they had never seen it before. New because to understand it they were forced to resort to explanatory models unknown in classical pathology and epidemiology.

That first surprise grew from the discovery of a category of diseases scarcely foreseen by medical theory. It was rapidly followed by other findings, unexpected and increasingly disquieting: a new "plague" had just struck mankind, an intractable infection was spreading inexorably, and those struck down by it died in spite of optimal therapy. Mass hysteria greeted the disclosure that this disease was linked to sex, blood, and drugs. The disease was felt to be not only "strange," because of its singular clinical and epidemiologic characteristics, but also "foreign," coming from "strangers." It seemed to have burst into one's orderly world from another world entirely, a world that was underdeveloped and peopled by marginal and morally reprehensible classes. As the title of one of the first books on AIDS neatly stated, its cause could only be "[a] strange virus from beyond."[1]

Los Angeles (1980–June 1981): The First Warning

Since the end of 1979, Joel Weisman, a Los Angeles physician known for his sympathy with homosexuals, noticed among his patients an increase in cases of a mononucleosis-like syndrome, marked by hectic fever, weight loss, and swollen lymph nodes. The patients were young. And they were from the growing California gay community. They improved fitfully, without real recovery. At first the diagnosis of cytomegalic disease seemed to fit the clinical picture. Since 1956 cytomegalic disease had been linked causally with the cytomegalovirus (CMV). This widespread virus belonging to the herpes virus family could cause fatal lesions in the immunologically impaired newborn, but seemed to present no danger to adults. Serologic tests showed that most American homosexuals had been infected by it. Occasional instances of a febrile mononucleosislike syndrome were attributed to it. There was no effective treatment, but patients ordinarily recovered spontaneously.

Weisman's patients also suffered from diarrhea and from oral and anal thrush. This clinical picture suggested some deficiency in the immune system. Two patients, treated since fall 1980, went from bad to worse. One lost weight and had respiratory distress. He was hospitalized in February 1981 in the immunology division of the University of California at Los Angeles (UCLA) hospital. It reminded physician Michael Gottlieb of a case he had seen there in December 1980: the blood of a patient with similar symptoms had shown a reduction in the population of lymphocytes, due to the almost complete disappearance of the helper T subgroup. They found the same phenomenon in Weisman's patient. In both cases microscopic examination of bronchial brushings revealed *Pneumocystis carinii* pneumonia (PCP). Both patients shared another characteristic: they were gay.

Weisman's initial hypothesis was a combined attack on the immune system by CMV and another virus, the Epstein-Barr virus (EBV). For Gottlieb the difficulty consisted of explaining why a virus as widespread as CMV—94 percent of the California homosexual community had been infected—led to these disastrous immunosuppressive effects no more often than it did. The causal chain had to be reversed. Unless, as Weisman suggested, a strain of CMV had become virulent by mutation, or through some synergy with another, unknown virus.

Gottlieb spoke with Wayne Shandera, a physician with the Los Angeles County Department of Public Health, who found a similar case in his files. By May 1981 the number of such patients hospitalized in Los Angeles, examined with careful scientific precision, grew to five. Soberly and discreetly, California physicians issued the alarm signal.

The first official announcement was published on June 5, 1981, by the Centers for Disease Control (CDC), the federal epidemiology agency in Atlanta. Its weekly bulletin, the *Morbidity and Mortality Weekly Report (MMWR)*, described the five severe pneumonia cases observed between October 1980 and May 1981 in the three Los Angeles hospitals.[2] Two unusual facts justified their warning: all the patients were young men (twenty-nine to thirty-six years old) whose sexual preference was homosexual, and all had pneumonia attributable to *Pneumocystis carinii*. This protozoan is nearly ubiquitous. It parasitizes numerous animals. It is found often enough in the human body, but it causes serious illness only when fostered by a deficit in the immune system, either in newborns or in adults receiving immunosuppressive drugs. The diagnosis of PCP had been confirmed by lung biopsy samples obtained either by the bronchoscopic or surgical approach.

The five patients also suffered from candidiasis, a benign fungal disorder of the mucous membranes. Serologic tests had confirmed CMV infection. All five used "poppers" (amyl or butyl nitrite inhalers, so named for the noise their ampules made when broken); one was also an intravenous drug abuser. In three, the T-lymphocyte population was markedly diminished; in the two others it had not been studied. The severity of the disease was impressive: despite intensive treatment, directed mainly against the PCP and certain viral agents, two patients rapidly succumbed, and none of the other three showed signs of recovery.[3]

The first died in March 1981. In 1978 this patient had been given the diagnosis of Hodgkin's disease. He was treated successfully by radiotherapy alone. But when no trace of Hodgkin's was found at autopsy, the validity of the antemortem diagnosis was called into question. Could this patient have been suffering from AIDS in 1978?

According to the CDC report, "the occurrence of pneumocystosis in these five previously healthy individuals without a clinically apparent underlying immunodeficiency is unusual." Infection by CMV had been singled out as a possible, indeed probable, etiologic cofactor whose precise role in the pathogenesis of pneumocystosis remains unknown. The homosexuality of all the patients was noted and even emphasized. This fact suggested "an association between some aspects of homosexual lifestyle or disease acquired through sexual contacts and *Pneumocystis* pneumonia in this population."

The American experts' conclusion was at once prudent and prophetic: "All the above observations suggest the possibility of a cellular-immune dysfunction related to a common exposure that predisposes individuals to opportunistic infections such as pneumocystosis and candidiasis."[4] If this document was not the birth certificate of AIDS, it was certainly the witness to its civil birth registration.[5]

East Coast Alert

A year before, several cases of an unusual form of acquired immune deficiency were observed in New York City. Their nosological similarity had not been recognized at first, and, at the beginning, no one had dreamed of making a connection with the California mini-epidemic.

Paradoxically, as Weisman explained, Los Angeles had the advantage of having only two medical schools, whereas New York had several. For New York physicians is was thus more difficult to discern the common character, the particular pattern in different cases of sudden immunosuppression among young, previously healthy, adults.

In March 1980 a young New York City homosexual nicknamed Nick began to experience a debilitating illness that left his doctors perplexed—lassitude, weight loss, spiking fevers, and slow consumption of the whole body, but without specific signs. The patient and his lover traveled the nation's cities looking for a remedy, unwittingly spreading their pathogenic sperm, the seed of destruction. An infectious agent began to be suspected when one of their New York friends became ill with similar symptoms. In a sudden turn for the worse Nick lost consciousness. A brain scan showed cerebral lesions. Surgical exploration revealed a precise diagnosis: *Toxoplasma gondii* infection. *Toxoplasma* infection was not uncommon but almost always benign, especially in adults, often indeed going unnoticed. In Nick, who died January 15, 1981, the cerebral toxoplasmosis was a fatal complication. The severity of his case gave rise to the notion that some strange and enigmatic calamity in the immune system must have preceded the other pathological events.[6]

Beginning in 1980 a series of severe cases of PCP were found in New York City. The Atlanta federal agency noticed them because of the increase in demand for a particular drug, pentamidine. This drug was being used for antibiotic-resistant cases of PCP. Because it was used infrequently, it was distributed by the government outside of usual commercial channels. During the twelve years between 1967 and 1979, they had supplied the drug in only two cases of PCP infection among adults with neither cancer nor recent immunosuppressive therapy. In April 1981 Sandra Ford, a technician responsible for nonroutine drug orders, informed her superior, the deputy director of parasitic diseases at CDC, that nine orders had come from New York City since February, and that rumors were circulating there about the unusual appearance of certain rare sarcomas.[7]

New York City and San Francisco (1979–August 1981): "Gay Cancer"

Indeed, rumors were spreading that a rare malignant disease had appeared in the New York gay community. In the hematology division at New York University Medical Center, Linda Laubenstein had in fall 1979 examined a man with Kaposi's sarcoma. Soon after, a colleague alerted her to a similar case at the Brooklyn Veterans Administration (VA) Medical Center. Both patients were young, homosexual, and—an important coincidence—had friends in common. By March 1981 at least eight cases of an especially aggressive form of this sarcoma had been identified in three New York hospitals.[8]

Kaposi's sarcoma is a serious skin disease, a sort of multicentric tumor. It is rather rare, but not to the extent that the simultaneous appearance of several cases in a huge city of diverse population should draw particular attention from epidemiologists. But there was more. The general profile of these eight patients did not correspond to those of a usual Kaposi's victim. In medical textbooks Kaposi's sarcoma was described as a chronic disorder, relatively benign and limited to older individuals, 90 percent male and of well-defined ethnicity: Jews, or at least of eastern European descent; dark-skinned men from the northern shores of the Mediterranean; and certain black African tribes, notably the Bantu.

The New York patients displayed none of these "racial" characteristics and, moreover, were young. Their disorder was acutely malignant, departing from the traditional prognosis. Of the first eight New York homosexuals struck by the sarcoma, four were already dead by March 1981.

The textbooks also failed to mention a behavioral characteristic common to all the New York Kaposi's sarcoma victims: they were homosexual. Hence around the beginning of 1981 some New York physicians, for example Donna Mildwan and Daniel William, advanced the suspicion that a new disease had begun killing homosexuals and destroying their immune systems.[9]

In San Francisco, the first diagnosis of Kaposi's sarcoma was made in April 1981, in a patient who had skin symptoms since December 1980 but whose signs of immune depression went back to 1978. He also had PCP. On April 24, 1981, John Gullett reported the case to the CDC, but the information was not exploited right away. In the course of that year dermatologist Marc Conant studied other cases of Kaposi's sarcoma in San Francisco's gay community.[10]

It was rather to Alvin Friedman-Kien, a New York University professor specializing in herpesvirus infections, that the credit went for establishing systematic research on the New York and San Francisco situations, and synthesizing them for the CDC. In the Atlanta centers, the sexually transmitted diseases were the province of James Curran, then chief of the Venereal Disease branch. Scarcely a week after the publication of the June 5, 1981, communique, he made his way to New York to see whether he could establish a link between the observations made on the two coasts. A Kaposi Sarcoma and Opportunistic Infections (KSOI) Task Force was formed under his direction, with the object of clarifying the story of this enigmatic illness that was killing gay men.

The reports of Gottlieb and Friedman-Kien were recalled. The different forms of Kaposi's sarcoma, as well as PCP, thrush, and toxoplasmosis were surely clinical expressions of a single disorder, a collapse of the immune system that struck almost exclusively homosexuals.

The second report of this strange epidemic was published in the *MMWR* on July 4, 1981. Its title: "Kaposi's sarcoma and *Pneumocystis* pneumonia among homosexual men—New York City and California." In a measured dry style the CDC informed the medical community that, during the preceding thirty months (since early 1979), Kaposi's sarcoma had been diagnosed in twenty-six men, twenty in New York and six in California. Eight had died, all in less than two years. Only one was nonwhite. None was more than fifty-one years old; the mean age was thirty-nine. All were homosexual. Six suffered also from pneumonia (PCP in at least four), four from toxoplasmosis of the central nervous system, and one from cryptococcal meningitis. Twelve were seropositive for CMV, and none were negative (fourteen had not been tested).[11]

Moreover, the report stressed that, a month after the PCP report from California, ten new cases—four in Los Angeles and six in the San Francisco Bay Area—had been added to the five initial ones. Four New York homosexuals had been described with advanced perianal herpes infections.[12]

Commenting on these data, the CDC epidemiologists recalled the extreme rarity, especially in New York between 1960 and 1979, of Kaposi's sarcoma among individuals under fifty years of age. Normally this disease was found only in the elderly; median survival was eight to thirteen years. Two key exceptions were known to this rule: inhabitants of an endemic belt across equatorial Africa, and patients receiving immunosuppressive treatment. The occurrence of this number of Kaposi's sarcoma cases during a thirty-month period among young homosexuals qualified as "highly unusual."

The CDC commentary ended with the advice, "Although it is not certain that the increases in Kaposi's sarcoma and *Pneumocystis carinii* pneumonia is restricted to homosexual men, the vast majority of recent cases have been reported from this group. Physicians should be alert for Kaposi's sarcoma, *Pneumocystis carinii* pneumonia, and other opportunistic infections associated with immunosuppression in homosexual men."[13]

The day before this report, on July 3, 1981, Lawrence Altman, the medical correspondent of the *New York Times*, under the title "Rare Cancer Seen in 41 Homosexuals," published a summary of the official report as well as the interviews with Friedman-Kien and Curran. It was thus that the nonprofessional public was informed for the first time about the appearance of the curious pathological phenomenon that had intrigued the specialists and begun to frighten the gays of New York. Altman's report took up a single column on page 20 of the *Times*, eclipsed by a huge bank advertisement. No one could yet have suspected that this "rare cancer" represented the malady of the late twentieth century or that this seemingly esoteric subject would come to occupy millions of pages in the newspapers of the world.

Though the official CDC report took into account only twenty-six registered cases of Kaposi's sarcoma, the journalist cited Friedman-Kien, who spoke of forty-one patients. The great majority lived in New York. Several California patients had reported that they had been in New York before the onset of symptoms. According to Friedman-Kien, the physicians were looking with particular interest at two cases diagnosed in Copenhagen. One of the Danish victims had previously visited New York.

"The cause of the outbreak is unknown and there is as yet no evidence of contagion." Friedman-Kien had demonstrated severe malfunctions of B- and T-lymphocytes in nine patients. Were these immunological defects primary, or were they induced by infection or drug use? Malignant disorders were not thought to be infectious, but perhaps they could be facilitated by a virus or by addiction to drugs. That might explain the appearance of a specific cancer in a particular social group. Perhaps there was a special linkage between CMV infection and Kaposi's sarcoma. Friedman-Kien was already leaning toward the viral hypothesis. James Curran was skeptical. According to him, "The best evidence against contagion is that no cases have been reported to date outside the homosexual community or in women." That seemed most reassuring. If there was a danger, it seemed confined to a marginal group. The article in question underlined that "the sudden appearance of the cancer, called Kaposi's sarcoma, has prompted a medical investigation that experts say could have as much scientific as public health importance because of what it may teach about determining the causes of the more common types of cancer."[14]

In that summer of 1981, the gay and liberal press of New York, San Francisco, and Los Angeles entertained illusions: that the "gay cancer" was the invention of "homophobic" physicians, or, more exactly, the effect of some noncontagious environmental factor unrelated to anal intercourse. They hoped to be able to show that these poor young men had died because they had eaten, drunk, or inhaled a specific substance ("poppers" of some particular chemical composition or natural food with spoiled ingredients?); adopted some unusual practices ("fist-fucking"?); or had otherwise frequented unsanitary places.

Friedman-Kien made a connection with the endemic occurrence in Africa of Kaposi's sarcoma. Some American homosexuals in their own way might have reproduced, in their "back rooms" and with inadequate hygiene, the sanitary conditions of equatorial Africa. In the heart of the great American cities there may have been a "sexual third world." Returning to a more civilized lifestyle and a little more propriety should suffice to nip this epidemic of poor people in the bud.[15]

Unfortunately the facts were stubborn. They confounded not just these optimistic elucubrations, but even the most pessimistic predictions. On August 28, 1981, the CDC announced that it had registered 108 patients. The patients were mostly young men, the great majority homosexual or bisexual (94 percent). Few blacks and one woman. The mortality was terrible: 40 percent of these patients were already dead at the time of the third report, and the others lurched inexorably toward the same end.[16]

The first scientific articles now appeared in the medical literature. To begin with, G. J. Gottlieb (not to be confused with M. S. Gottlieb) and his colleagues published a preliminary communication in the *American Journal of Dermatopathology* on the histological peculiarities of disseminated Kaposi's sarcoma in American homosexuals.[17] Published in a specialty journal and emphasizing technical aspects, this article went almost unnoticed. Another publication, in the September 19, 1981, issue of the English medical journal, *Lancet*, made more of a splash. Its authors, Kenneth Hymes, Linda Laubenstein, and six other New York physicians, wanted to avoid any furor and hence dared not openly invoke the possibility of a "new" disease. They sought only to "describe the clinical findings in eight homosexual men in New York with Kaposi's sarcoma showing some unusual features." Seven of these eight patients, treated in three New York hospitals between March 1979 and March 1981, had generalized lymphadenopathy, and one suffered from the fungal disease cryptococcosis. Prudently, the authors of this article limited themselves to the following conclusion: "This unusual occurrence of Kaposi's sarcoma in a population much exposed to sexually transmissible diseases suggests that such exposure may play a role in its pathogenesis.[18]

Continued Spread (September–December 1981)

By November 1981, American public health officials already counted 159 registered cases. Inclusion of suspected cases brought the figure closer to 180. At the beginning of 1982, the number of recognized cases had passed 200. The disease no longer confined itself to the homosexual enclaves of three large cities: fifteen states were now reporting cases. The cases were not emerging in an autochthonous manner, but rather presenting as though a single pathogenic agent were spreading from three initial centers: New York, Los Angeles, and San Francisco. Epidemiologic research outside these centers established a chain of contacts linking them with homosexual communities in the original cities.

In New York, some rapidly fatal cases of *Pneumocystis* pneumonia were found in heterosexuals. Almost all exhibited a particular feature: they were drug addicts. Among them was a woman, until then the only officially recognized female case of acquired immune deficiency. More than any other drug, heroin posed the risk of dying from *Pneumocystis* infection. No such complication of heroin addiction had been known before. But, as physician Mary Guinan pointed out, there was an instructive precedent: could it not be analogous to hepatitis-B virus infection, already understood to be transmitted both by contaminated needles and by sexual activity?[19]

Before the end of 1981, the CDC investigators reached the conviction that the causal agent was infectious and that it was spread by sexual contact. They were convinced of it, but could not furnish irrefutable evidence.

The disease still lacked a scientific name. The newspapers spoke of "gay cancer," or of "gay pneumonia," even of "gay plague." Some started to use an acronym that had a more scholarly ring: GRID (Gay-Related Immune Deficiency). The *Lancet* correspondents proposed to call it the "gay compromise syndrome."[20] The medical press still avoided these terms in favor of long, cumbersome circumlocutions.

Despite the absence of a convenient and generally accepted term, the clinical profile of this immune deficiency syndrome was clarified in the course of

1981. In its December 10, 1981, issue, the *New England Journal of Medicine*, a journal known for its conservatism, prudence, and outstanding scientific reputation, published several articles concerning this new scourge.

Included in one of them were the results of an epidemiologic investigation directed in the hospitals of New York by Henry Masur, a physician from Cornell University Medical College. Clearly, *Pneumocystis* pneumonia had begun to blaze its way through New York earlier than the CDC report had suggested. The earliest case Masur recalled went back to July 1979. Between then and April 1981, fourteen cases of *Pneumosystis* pneumonia had been observed in nine different New York hospitals. Masur and his colleagues published epidemiologic and clinical data on eleven of these patients, of whom eight died before December 1981. They were young men, twenty-seven to forty years old, without important antecedent conditions. In one case Kaposi's sarcoma had been associated with *Pneumosystis* pneumonia. In all these cases laboratory testing had demonstrated a profound lymphopenia, that is, a reduction of the number of lymphocytes in the blood. Particularly affected were the T-lymphocytes. Humoral immunity was not impaired. All this correlated well with the California physicians' findings. But there was also an important difference: six of the eleven patients were overtly homosexual, the other five declared themselves to be heterosexual. All of them, according to Masur, were acknowledged drug addicts. In the light of our more recent knowledge, it is disturbing that Masur's team should have included alcoholics among the "drug users."[21]

Among Masur's eleven patients it was thought a factor could be discerned that was related not only to the patients' particular sexual comportment but also to their membership in a marginal social subgroup. The syndrome thus became "community-acquired" and not simply "gay."

Frederick Siegal, a physician at Mount Sinai Medical Center in New York City, and thirteen of his coauthors described, in the *New England Journal of Medicine*, the clinical history of four cases of particularly severe herpes seen in New York between July 1979 and July 1981. Three of these patients had died rapidly, and one had Kaposi's sarcoma with an unquestionably gloomy prognosis. These patients were young homosexuals. Siegal related their cases to those of the immune deficiency syndrome reported in the July 1981 CDC paper. Laboratory examinations revealed lymphopenia and depression in the so-called "natural killer" cell activity directed against herpes-infected cells. Various cutaneous tests for delayed hypersensitivity demonstrated skin anergy.[22]

In the same issue of the prestigious Boston journal, Michael Gottlieb and his colleagues described the clinical picture of four patients suffering from *Pneumosystis* pneumonia and candidiasis—three cases already reported in *MMWR* plus a new one—and, aided by sophisticated techniques, analyzed the patients' immune systems. In one of Weisman's and Gottlieb's very first pneumocystosis patients from the *MMWR* series, Kaposi's sarcoma had supervened. A marked lymphopenia was found in all four. By monoclonal antibody analysis Gottlieb could specify which subpopulation of T-lymphocytes was affected, namely the helper T-cells identifiable by a surface antigen or marker dubbed OKT4 (now also known as CD4). These white blood cells are indispensable for the proper induction of cell-mediated immune defenses. Gottlieb also showed that the T-lymphocytes with suppressor function, which carry the OKT8 surface marker (a marker which also identifies the so-called killer T-lymphocytes), were relatively increased. In all the patients studied, the helper-to-suppressor T-cell ratio was reversed.[23]

That the disease seemed confined to homosexuals suggested that its cause was a sexually transmitted agent. In a postscript revision added in proof, Gottlieb and his colleagues acknowledged having encountered the syndrome more recently in two exclusively heterosexual males. In one, cytomegalovirus had been found in the sperm. Gottlieb strongly suspected an etiologic role for this virus. Repeated reinfection with massive CMV inocula could at first overstimulate and finally overwhelm and wipe out the immune defenses. While admitting this was unproven, the article's authors nonetheless insisted on the implication of an infectious factor. Even if CMV was not the cause, several lines of evidence seemed to permit the conclusion that "this syndrome represents a potentially transmissible immune deficiency."[24]

CHAPTER 2

Epidemiologic Research in the American Homosexual Community

From a drop of water a logician could infer the possibility of an Atlantic or a Niagara without having seen or heard of one or the other.

—Sherlock Holmes,

detective (by way of

Sir Arthur Conan Doyle,

physician and novelist)

O NCE RECOGNIZED, this strange disorder seemed to expand as though it were a young, growing, living being. Its prevalence increased exponentially. Already in 1981 the New York physician Alvin Friedman-Kien warned that recognized cases represented merely the tip of the iceberg. But the Cassandras went unheeded. And who, looking forward from that moment, could have imagined that behind each patient was a column of marked men, bearers of what would later become the cross of seropositivity?

After a prelude of uncertain duration, and a brief prologue filled with dramatic events whose meaning would be fully understood only later, AIDS sprang onto the scene in June 1981. The first act would last scarcely a year. It was, in fact, in summer 1982 that the disease was finally named, that incontrovertible proof of its viral etiology was available and, alas, that its beachhead could be found on every continent.

Medical Detectives at Work

The recognition of AIDS, identification of the etiologic agent, and the struggle against this scourge all essentially owed to four institutions—two American, one French, and one international: the Centers for Disease Control (CDC), the NIH (U.S. National Institutes of Health), the Pasteur Institute, and the WHO (World Health Organization).

In the first phase, that of clinically identifying and epidemiologically characterizing the disorder, the CDC deserves most of the credit. The key American establishment for disease surveillance, it is a formidable epidemiological tool in the service of not just the United States but the entire world. As the journalist Joseph Carey has said of them, the federal medical sleuths track the most powerful killer diseases, from influenza and Lassa fever to AIDS.[1]

This institution originated in a federal agency created in Atlanta in 1942 to control exposure to malaria among military personnel and to prevent its introduction into the United States from Far East battlefields. In 1946 the Atlanta agency had run out of missions, but instead of dismantling it the American government had the fortunate idea of transforming it into the CDC, the acronym then denoting the Communicable Disease Center. The new federal institution took as its mandate the collaboration with the individual states within the United States in order to combat the principal transmissible diseases. Little by little its activities extended also to noninfectious disorders, especially to malignant and occupational diseases. Beginning in 1951, a basic research division, the Epidemic Intelligence Service (EIS), operated within the CDC framework. Under the direction of Dr. Alexander Langmuir, the EIS acquired a worldwide reputation. Several striking successes, coming notably between 1955 (the antipolio compaign) and 1976 (investigations on hemorrhagic fever due to the Ebola virus, and on Legionnaire's disease) assured the institution's renown well beyond public health specialists. Its weekly report, published since 1961 under the title *Morbidity and Mortality Weekly Report* (*MMWR*), increasingly became the mirror of American public health. Admired and feared, the CDC, renamed the NCDC (with the addition of the "National" qualifier), enjoyed the sobriquet "FBI of medicine."[2]

In 1980, on the eve of the AIDS research effort, the NCDC was transformed back to the CDC, this time the acronym denoting the plural Centers for Disease Control. This change was a result of the victory thought to have been won over infectious diseases. It seemed appropriate now to enlarge its initial mandate and to commit the institution to research, surveillance, and prevention of all causes of morbidity and mortality.[3]

The Centers were compartmentalized. From the start AIDS was considered a problem for the CID (Center for Infectious Diseases), a vestige of the earlier structure. But it was impossible to know whether in fact another department, such as the CEH (Center for Environmental Health), should not have spearheaded the task. For such cases it was possible, however, to form ad hoc interdepartmental task forces. Such was the case with AIDS, where it was recognized as a nationwide phenomenon encompassing a malignancy enmeshed in an infectious pathological process.

At the moment when the medical furor over a supposedly homosexual disease broke, the CDC needed to refurbish a transiently tarnished image. To prevent an epidemic portended by the swine flu virus in 1976, the Center had recommended a national program for the development, distribution, and administration of a specific vaccine. With great effort, and much to the profit of the pharmaceutical industry, something on the order of fifty million Americans were vaccinated. The flu had a minimal impact, but the vaccination campaign led to more than five hundred cases of Guillain-Barré syndrome. To forestall a hypothetical risk, the CDC had thus triggered a certain one, a serious iatrogenic disorder of the nervous system. The director resigned, but for years the institution bore the bitter memory.[4]

In the AIDS episode the CDC's response was exemplary. Even those, such as David Black and Randy Shilts, who criticized the behavior of the American authorities, addressed their barbs only to the high-placed politicians and the "big boys" of the NIH. There was general recognition of the responsibility, the competence, and the rapidity which the CDC had responded since the onset of the epidemic. In the case of Toxic Shock Syndrome (TSS), eighteen months had elapsed between the first case reports and the official publication in *MMWR*, and another month was necessary before a team could be formed to begin the real epidemiologic research. Matters proceeded more rapidly with the Legionnaire's outbreak, since behind the research lay the pressure of strong public opinion. The personnel and financial assets were then immeasurably greater than at the outset of the AIDS epidemic. But we should admire American public health officials for their diligence in studying the phenomenon epidemiologically: the first *MMWR* report was published the same month Gottlieb sounded the first alarm. Scarcely three months later a detailed investigation followed.[5]

The First Etiologic Hypotheses

From the beginning Michael Gottlieb favored the hypothesis postulating the cytomegalovirus (CMV) as the causative agent. This explanation was insufficient, however, in that almost all homosexuals were known to have been infected by the virus, yet only a few fell seriously ill. There had to be a cofactor which, in a given epidemiologic situation, became the veritable "cause."

In December 1981, in a *New England Journal of Medicine* editorial accompanying the three fundamental articles on the new syndrome, David Durack synthesized dominant opinion as follows:

> In our present state of ignorance, some frank speculation seems permissible. Let us postulate that the combined effects of persistent viral infection plus an adjuvant drug cause immunosuppression in some genetically predisposed men. During the early stages, patients may have only a nonspecific illness and minor infections such as thrush. Then Kaposi's sarcoma may develop as an opportunistic tumor (perhaps cytomegalovirus-induced) which is set free by a failure of immune surveillance. Finally, as the defect in cellular immunity becomes progressively more severe, serious opportunistic infections develop.[6]

In other words, a multifactorial hypothesis giving roughly equal weight to infection, to drug effects, and to genetic predisposition.

Unfortunately, physicians at this time were in total ignorance on all three groups of factors. What sort of chemical substance were American homosexuals exposed to more than others? One such material was quickly found in "poppers," the vials of rapidly evaporating liquid (amyl or butyl nitrite), smelling of banana. They were powerful dilators of blood vessels, supposed to enhance orgasm.[7]

But while many homosexuals used and abused "poppers," in fact no pharmacologic data could justify the hypothesis that the substance had such a devastating action on the immune system. And should one have accused amyl nitrite or butyl nitrite, rather than some contaminant present in the commercial products?[8] Experiments on rodents at the CDC led to negative results. And the epidemiologic data condemned the hypothesis in any case. There were too many patients who had never so much as sniffed the pleasurable vapors. That did not prevent "the odor of the AIDS popper," as Jacques Leibowitch put it, "from lasting a long time."[9]

In similar fashion accusations were directed at the corticosteroid creams used so abundantly by American homosexuals in treating their skin conditions and hemorrhoids.[10] Alvin Friedman-Kien hailed an idea that seemed seductive at first view: repeated assaults overwhelmed the immune system, which then ceased to function.[11] According to him, "a large number of exposures adds insult to injury, so the immune system is overtaxed and ceases to perform." Other authors also spoke of an "antigenic overload."[12] This explanation was but a metaphor, as unscientific as that of "mental overload" in certain psychiatric disorders. Often in the past, human populations had sustained a much greater challenge to their immune system than this recent group of American homosexuals.

Given the difficulty conceding how the immune system could be exhausted by infectious agents, G. Shearer, Steve Witkin, and other physicians thought of sperm, which, instilled into the rectum, might act as a "natural" immunosuppressant.[13] Experiments were conducted to pursue the idea, but here, too, a historical objection immediately comes to mind. If true, why was this effect not noticed earlier?

As for the genetic factor, certain authors made vague reference to the notion of "racial preference" in Kaposi's sarcoma. More precisely, but without confirmation in follow-up studies, other scientists noted in some of these immunosuppressed patients the prevalence of the HLA-DR5 histocompatibility group.[14]

The First Statistically Significant Cohort

Once launched on the trail of the disease, the CDC was able to proceed systematically, since experience accumulated over three decades had dictated a particular protocol. The problem was attacked on two fronts: biological and biochemical research on serum and tissue specimens, as well as careful interrogation of patients and their physicians.

The first tack was initially deceptive. Laboratory-based research confirmed lymphopenia, notably the spectacular drop-off in helper T-cells, leading to a reversal in the helper-suppressor cell ratios. It further confirmed a drop in antibodies to the varicella virus, and an increase in antibodies to the CMV, Epstein-Barr, and hepatitis-B viruses, as well as the treponeme of syphilis. But the investigators could find neither a specific chemical substance, nor a new infectious agent.[15]

The second tack was more productive. It consisted of a series of case control studies, incorporating field research, the collation and registration of all individual patient data that might have epidemiological significance, and their subsequent statistical analysis. The Task Force assembled for this purpose included Harold Jaffe, William Darrow, Mary Guinan, Dennis Juranek, Harry Haverkos, and others. James Curran was the coordinator. Team members questioned every practicing physician and two-thirds of their known patients. They established a control group and pored attentively over a wide range of circumstances of the patients and their matched healthy controls. Their report, based on an analysis of every case detected by the CDC between June and October 1981, appeared in January 1982.[16] Later this was followed by an even deeper analysis of fify representative cases, published only in August 1983 but concerning the same patients registered in 1981.[17]

In retrospect, early cases could be traced back to 1978. But only from January 1981 did the disease spread in an observable way. Though it had already been detected in fifteen states and two foreign countries (Denmark and Haiti) at the time of this investigation, more than two-thirds of the then known AIDS patients lived in three large cities: New York, Los Angeles, and San Francisco. More than half of all the diagnosed cases in the epidemic's earliest days came from a single urban cluster (the New York City area). The investigation was limited to the homosexual community—that is, by definition, to men having had sex with a male partner within a year before the onset of the disease—for the number of heterosexuals seemed negligible. The patients were divided among "whites" (70 percent), "Hispanic" (16 percent), and "blacks" (14 percent). Among the three groups no difference could be discerned in the pathology. Their age varied between fifteen and fifty-seven years, with a median of thirty-seven years old.

The full-blown presentation of the syndrome was often preceded by certain nonspecific or relatively mild symptoms: fever, night sweats, weight loss, and chronic diarrhea. One particular sign seemed to bear special importance for early diagnosis: a persistent, generalized enlargement of the lymph nodes. On May 12, 1982, a CDC report had drawn practitioners' attention to this aspect of the syndrome.[18] But it was not yet possible to know with assurance if this unexplained persistent lymphadenopathy was merely an initial phase of the more serious illness, a mild form of the disease, or indeed, at least in some cases, a separate disorder *sui generis*.

Inhaled nitrite exposure had no effect on initiating the disease. Indeed the only risk factor revealed in this investigation was homosexual promiscuity: "The variables most strongly associated with Kaposi's sarcoma or pneumocystis pneumonia were those related to number of male sex partners and to meeting such partners in bathhouses."[19]

The same disease was also diagnosed, though, in a woman and in several heterosexual men (8 percent).[20] This favored the infectious hypothesis. Observations on these "atypical" patients suggested a role for blood in transmitting the agent. But in accepting the hypothesis of a specific microbial agent, the route of infection in homosexuals had to be intimate contact, probably through anal intercourse. Its transmission thus came to look more and more like that of the hepatitis-B virus. Favoring this supposition at the time was the epidemiological analysis of a cluster of lovers in southern California. The development of an epidemic focus in Orange County was paradigmatic.[21]

In Search of "Patient Zero"

David Auerbach, William Darrow, and other investigators at the CDC discovered that nine out of thirteen homosexual patients they questioned in Los Angeles and Orange counties, out of a total of nineteen tallied, formed a sort of sexual network.[22] Over the last five years each of these nine patients had had sex with at least one other member of the group. In most cases their sexual relations went back to the period before the partner's symptoms had appeared. Hence apparently healthy individuals could transmit the disease. A history of relations was established between members of the California network and a similar group in New York. At the center of this diagram of homosexual contacts was a young man, Gaetan Dugas. He was nicknamed "Patient Zero."[23]

Dugas, an Air Canada flight attendant, was both an active and receptive homosexual. Directly or indirectly through intermediate contacts, he had infected at least forty of the 248 American patients diagnosed before April 1982. He was found to have been a sexual partner of nine of the nineteen first Los Angeles cases, twenty-two of the New York patients, and nine cases in eight other cities (Miami, Chicago, etc.). As an airline steward, Dugas, on vacation, could fly free. A great traveler, handsome and generous with his charms, he had sown the disease and death all along his route, at the rate of about 250 partners per year. The investigators confirmed to their own horror that he had been contagious before experiencing the slightest sympton. According to their analysis, the incubation period for this new disease exceeded ten months.

The Dugas case formed both an example and a caricature. The epidemiological demonstration of his role as the central link, the "point of intersection'' in a network of sexual contacts, ''established the reality of intimate transmission, the activism of some individuals, the danger of contagion.'' In this context the word ''activism'' indicated promiscuity and in no way prejudged the importance of the active or passive role in the sex act, since—as Leibowitch remarked in 1984—the quantitative data were lacking with respect to this important point.[24]

Afflicted in June 1980 with Kaposi's sarcoma, identified in November 1982 as a carrier and warned of the risk he could pose for his partners, Dugas refused to change his lifestyle. Until his death on March 30, 1984, at the age of thirty-two, he carried on his sex life with no protective measures. Sometimes he informed his partners, but only after the act. He had thus adopted the habit of saying to them, ''I've got gay cancer; I'm going to die and so are you.'' A kind of deaf rage against fate had seized him, a desire for vengeance. In a medical interview, he had shamelessly declared, ''I've got it; they can get it too.''[25] Every historian of disease knows that such an attitude of vengeance, or at least of recklessness, had contributed in other times to the spread of tuberculosis and syphilis.

The Dugas case illustrates certain initial errors committed as much by those responsible for public health as by the homosexual organizations. There was a hesitancy to place any limits on the free expression of the ''right to sexuality.'' Later, beginning in 1985, several authors underscored this hesitancy (they called it ''irresponsibility'') among both the politicians and the leaders of the homosexual community in the face of the early signs of the epidemic's spread. The statesmen had not immediately made adequate financial means available, nor had they known how to impose legal constraints. The spokesmen of homosexual organizations had not pleaded for moderation of some customs, nor had they yielded to the ''medicalization'' of the group's sexuality.

Confronted by this scourge, almost all politically and socially responsible parties had reacted at first with incredulity. They simply hoped the disease was not contagious. Reluctantly, in finally admitting its contagiousness they found it inconceivable that such a strange disorder was not also foreign, an invader from beyond. Who had introduced it to the United States, at what point in time, and from what foreign quarter? Answers could be found which at first seemed satisfactory enough, but which later came to seem insufficient and arbitrary.

Gaetan Dugas, a French-Canadian, was not an American citizen, which made him a convenient scapegoat. But there was no plausible reason to say that the disease had come from Canada. If, at the beginning of the epidemic, Dugas was an outstanding ''promoter'' of the contagion, that still did not prove that he should have functioned effectively as ''Patient Zero'' in the strong sense of the term. He had certainly imparted the fatal agent to a goodly number of his American partners, but in no way did that exclude the possibility that he had received it from an American himself. It is worth noting that some of his partners manifested the symptoms of AIDS before he did.[26]

The initial concentration of patients in the New York region made that city the epicenter of the epidemic. Was it not also therefore its port of entry? The true ''Patient Zero'': might we find him among the sailors from the four corners of the world who arrived in New York on July 4, 1976, to celebrate the bicentennial of American independence?[27] A possible hypothesis, but vague and ungrounded in the facts.

CHAPTER 3

First Stirrings in Europe

Poca favilla gran

fiamma seconda.

—Dante,

poet who visited

the inferno

THESE DAYS even viruses travel by airplane. In antiquity Hesiod indulged in a play on words in which he juxtaposed "plague" (in Greek *loimos*) with "famine" (*limos*) thus expounding a profound epidemiologic truth of his time. In modern times we might try another comparison: "plague" (in French *peste*) lines up with "postal" (*poste*). Pathogenic organisms benefit from the perfecting of all our means of transportation: their spread depends on a network of communications; the rapidity of their expansion coincides with that of our postal services. Carriers of bacteria and viruses who in another day may have taken the stagecoach, the long haul trains, and ships now take to the skies: in a single day infectious diseases can now cross continents, or jump between them.

"Dangerous Liaisons" between America and Western Europe

Scarcely a month after the CDC's first report was published, the American investigators found out about two Danish cases that brought to mind the syndrome seen in California and New York.[1] At that moment, and for several months thereafter, they were the only cases identified outside the United States.

The first of these European patients died in September 1980 at the Copenhagen Rigshospitalet after suffering from interstitial pneumonia and progressive deterioration. He was a thirty-seven-year-old agricultural engineer without any striking antecedent pathology. Jan Gerstoft and his colleagues had recognized this man's *Pneumocystis* pneumonia and a failure of the immune system, for which they had found no explanation. But this was happening in Copenhagen, the most tolerant city in Europe when it came to matters sexual. The patient's homosexual lifestyle had escaped his physicians' attention. At the end of June 1981 they became retrospectively interested in his sexual habits, however, since the clinical characteristics of the

case matched those of the gay Americans. They then learned that the dead
Dane had in fact had direct contact with the latter, especially in 1977, during
a New York stopover. They also recalled how he had mentioned a strange
disease of one of his partners.[2]

The partner had had Kaposi's sarcoma. Right after the second CDC report
came out, two more cases were diagnosed in young Copenhagen homosexuals. In one the disease was rapidly fatal and an autopsy disclosed concomitant
Pneumocystis pneumonia. The other had a slowly progressive skin disorder
associated with chronic amebiasis. Then, between August 1980 and December 1981, four homosexuals were hospitalized in Copenhagen with symptoms
corresponding to the American definition of the "gay syndrome." Three of
them had never visited the United States but had had sexual contact, either
directly or through intermediate partners, with New York homosexuals. Of
the two who had had contact with each other, one had *Pneumocystis* pneumonia, the other Kaposi's sarcoma. These Danish observations thus advanced
the arguments of those favoring the identity of the underlying pathological
process, as well as its infectious origin.[3]

This appearance of Kaposi's sarcoma was curious. Was it really a new
phenomenon, or was it a false novelty borne of physicians' recent sensitiza-
tion through their reading of the American medical press? Polemics ensued.
The statistical data, drawn from the Danish national cancer registry, weighed
in favor of a real novelty. But Johannes Clemmesen, formerly head of the
registry, observed pertinently that the previous way of classifying Kaposi's
sarcoma could lead to a false underestimation of its earlier incidence.[4]

After Copenhagen, the merry-go-round of organized group homosexuality
in other capitals of European gay life signaled the presence of this strange
disease. In December 1981 physicians at the Brompton Hospital in London
published the first observation of an English case of *Pneumocystis* pneumonia
and of cytomegalic inclusion disease in a previously healthy man without any
history of immunosuppressive therapy. The patient, a forty-nine-year-old
man, endured three months of weight loss and several weeks of respiratory
distress before dying at the end of ten days in hospital. The autopsy confirmed
the diagnosis, proposed antemortem by transbronchial biopsy. An avid homosexual, this patient had vacationed each year in Miami. The last of his American sojourns went back nine months before the fatal onset.[5]

In Spain, a young Barcelona homosexual, hospitalized in October 1981,
died from Kaposi's sarcoma associated with cytomegalovirus infection and
candidiasis. He had had homosexual contacts in New York in 1974, and in
Turkey in 1980.[6] Then, beginning in 1981, several cases were confirmed in
Switzerland. The first three Swiss patients were homosexuals, one having
sojourned in the United States, the two others in Haiti.[7]

In the German Federal Republic, two cases could be diagnosed retrospectively from 1976 and 1979, but none from the 1980–1981 period. How, for
example, did the city of Hamburg come to be spared? In effect this was no

more than an illusion. With the seven new cases that appeared in 1982, West Germany found itself in the vanguard of most-affected European nations.[8] At the head of this vanguard stood France and Belgium. But in the case of these two countries certain additional factors came into play, factors not dependent on the international gay network.

According to the official statistics of the member nations of the World Health Organization, at the end of 1981 there were thirty-six recognized cases of this nameless syndrome in Europe: France, 17; Belgium, 6; Switzerland, 5; Denmark, 3; United Kingdom, 2; West Germany, 2; and Spain, 1. The European cases described above seemed to confirm fully the initial American conception of a disease limited to homosexuals. In fact, there was a sort of self-confirming circularity at work, since homosexuality was from the start regarded as an essential diagnostic criterion. Thus, for example, in the case of a woman who died in Copenhagen in December 1977 and whose clinical picture corresponded to that of the gay Americans, no one dared make the connection until 1983—that is, until well after the publication of American observations on heterosexual patients. The Danish patient exhibited neither lesbianism, drug addiction, nor any history of American travel. But she had worked as a surgeon in central Africa. Her case, having first been excluded by definition, actually went on to bolster quite another interpretation of the origin of AIDS.

The Italian situation furnished a good example of the insidious way in which the epidemic was introduced into most European countries. In 1981 American physicians diagnosed the disorder in two Italian homosexuals traveling in the United States. No case was identified on Italian soil in either 1981 or in the first ten months of 1982. The Ministry of Health stated in September 1984 that there was still no epidemic in Italy and that no native cases were known.[9] Yet retrospective serologic tests show that there were persons already infected here as early as February 1979, and that their numbers were growing exponentially by 1981.

In a series of 716 serum specimens, taken in the course of a study of viral hepatitis in patients hospitalized between 1978 and 1985 in the University Clinic for infectious diseases at Milan, none of 15 specimens from 1978 were positive. They were, however, all taken from addicts who "skin-popped." Seropositivity to HIV-1 appeared in February 1979. Two sera of 28 specimens collected that year were already positive, 5 of 79 in 1980, 10 of 121 in 1981, and 28 of 123 in 1982. The incidence climbed spectacularly thereafter and, by 1985, two thirds of Milanese addicts were infected. None presented at that time with clinical signs of immune depression.[10] Statistics on these patients' sexual habits are hard to come by, but one has good reason to suppose that while some youths among them occasionally resorted to prostitution, the majority did not participate in homosexual activities. This Milanese study and others done in 1986 in a province with a U.S. military base leave the clear impression that the infection was introduced into Italy by tourists and by gay

American soldiers, and that it then spread through the use of contaminated syringes as well as by bisexual and heterosexual contacts.[11]

Meanwhile in France

It was July 1981, scarcely a month after the publication of the first CDC report from Atlanta on the appearance of an unusual form of opportunistic pneumonia among homosexuals. At the Claude Bernard Hospital in Paris, a thirty-eight-year-old man, V. M., himself a well-known French homosexual, had just been hospitalized in the department of infectious and tropical diseases. His symptoms were hardly characteristic: cyclical fever evolving over a month, refractory diarrhea, asthenia, weight loss, dry cough. On physical exam he exhibited only some localized enlargement of his lymph nodes. He was quickly discharged, without a diagnosis, but was readmitted in August 1981 for an exacerbation of these symptoms. One side of his body became paralyzed. Chest X-ray and bronchoalveolar lavage now disclosed the presence of *Pneumocystis* pneumonia. At the same time tomography of the skull revealed a cerebral abscess. Chemotherapy improved his condition, and he was discharged, only to be readmitted in November 1981 with a new lung disorder, this time tuberculosis. He also had mucocutaneous candidiasis and anal herpes. Skin tests for delayed hypersensitivity to tuberculin and candida were negative. Cytomegalovirus was recovered from his blood and urine. And he had a discrete drop in his lymphocyte count with a particularly conspicuous fall in his helper T-cells.

Once *Pneumocystis* pneumonia was diagnosed in this patient, Willy Rozenbaum made the connection with the immunosuppressive syndrome of the American homosexuals. The Parisian case was typical as much by virtue of the clinical picture as by the history. The patient was an airline flight attendant; he had traveled in a number of American and African countries. Given to promiscuity, he had slept with about forty occasional partners per year and had already had syphilis. At the time of his last New York stay, in February 1980, he had had homosexual sex and had used nitrite inhalants.[12]

The December 1981 articles from the *New England Journal of Medicine* and *Lancet* immediately aroused the attention of certain French physicians, notably of the immunologist Jacques Leibowitch.[13] Memories of "problematic" early cases were evoked. Physicians in the Léon M'Ba Institute of medicine and epidemiology at the Claude Bernard Hospital then decided to alert the homosexual community and the lay press. In January 1982, the French daily newspapers began writing about the "mysterious cancer among American homosexuals," and indicated there was "a patient under observation in Paris." In February, Leibowitch noted, a deputy of the right-wing Gaullist party in Parliament hurled a treacherous question at the health minister, then a Communist, on the subject of "how to protect our young people against the rise of homosexuality, flowering now like a rose'' (symbol of the French left).[14]

In the first quarter of 1982 one could already find five suspected cases in Paris hospitals. All the data suggested that this was but the visible part of a problem that was much larger and still growing. A coordinating group was therefore constituted in Paris, made up of voluntary hospital staff (Willy Rozenbaum, Jacques Leibowitch, Serge Kernbaum, Jean-Claude Gluckman, David Klatzmann, Odile Picard, Charles Mayaud, and others); an epidemiologist, Jean-Baptiste Brunet; and a member of the Gay Physicians' Association, Claude Villalonga. This French AIDS Task Force (Groupe de travail français sur le SIDA) took as its goal the collection of information; notification of physicians; alerting groups at risk (notably homosexuals in the French-American jet set); uncovering of all French cases; and verification of whether those patients had experienced homosexual behavior, American travel, or the use of particular chemical products.[15]

On the one hand, these European physicians could have been seduced just then by the hypothesis that the outbreak of this small epidemic could be explained via the use of ''poppers,'' for this had already been the case with the toxic Spanish syndrome. A year earlier, more than two hundred people had tragically died from consuming contaminated olive oil. It was thus tempting to think that this new syndrome could also result not so much from the amyl nitrite itself but perhaps from its contamination. Investigations and analyses were undertaken, without positive results.

On the other hand, European observers were better placed than their American colleagues to confirm the infectious nature of the disease. In order to act at such a distance in both time and place, the ''self-perpetuating American contaminant'' necessarily had to be a living organism. Straight away two etiologic hypotheses drew the French physicians' attention: cytomegalovirus under still poorly elucidated conditions, or infection by a virus that was either new or at least heretofore wholly unknown.

Increasingly, one thought preoccupied public health officials: if the disease was infectious, it could escape the homosexual milieu. *Le Figaro* of July 24, 1982, pointed out ''eleven cases in France of a disease to which no name has yet been given, and which one might in fact dub the gay syndrome.'' The eleven cases tallied in France (three with *Pneumocystis* pneumonia and eight with Kaposi's sarcoma) were all homosexuals. But the Task Force warned the journalists that from now on the menace would spread into the masses of heterosexual men and even women.

The First French Patients' Characteristics

Between March 31 and December 19, 1982, the French AIDS Task Force counted twenty-nine cases in whom the clinical picture corresponded to the

CDC definition. With perhaps two exceptions, these cases were picked up in Paris. In nine cases, the diagnosis had been made retrospectively, referring back to observations made between 1974 and June 1981. The majority of the patients presenting only with Kaposi's sarcoma, and all those who had Kaposi's sarcoma associated with an opportunistic infection, were homosexuals. But eight of the thirteen patients suffering only from opportunistic infections were either heterosexual men or women.[16]

These twenty-nine early French cases could then be subdivided into six groups:

1. Some patients solely with Kaposi's sarcoma, observed before June 1981, relatively old and with survival periods of several years. Retrospectively, these cases had to be considered doubtful, probably of the "classical" type of Kaposi's sarcoma.

2. Eight gay patients with opportunistic infections alone (5), or associated with Kaposi's sarcoma (1), or with Kaposi's sarcoma alone (2), observed between July 1981 and December 1982. These patients had visited the United States in the course of the five years before the onset of their illnesses. The four most typical cases, treated at the Claude Bernard, Pitié, and Tenon hospitals, became the subject of a detailed scientific study.[17] Among these four cases was one mentioned earlier in this chapter, the first to have been actually diagnosed in France. These patients' histories corresponded perfectly to the American descriptions. The origin of their infection was not in doubt: their illnesses resulted from homosexual contacts in the United States, notably in New York, in 1980 or 1981.

3. Five heterosexual patients with opportunistic infections either alone or in association with Kaposi's sarcoma had either traveled to the Caribbean or were of Haitian nationality. A Haitian couple fell into this group. The wife had lived in Paris since August 1979. She sojourned in the United States in 1980 and engaged in an extramarital affair with a Haitian who himself was to become ill with AIDS in 1982. Back in Paris, she had been hospitalized in August 1981 and died six months later with cerebral toxoplasmosis. The husband came to Paris in October 1981, having previously never been in the United States. A year later he died of disseminated tuberculosis associated with Kaposi's sarcoma.[18]

In September 1978 a thirty-one-year-old French geologist, M.D., had a road accident in Haiti. Critically ill, he was moved to the Port-au-Prince Hospital and had an emergency operation. They amputated his left arm and gave him transfusions of fresh blood donated by eight Haitian volunteers. In September 1981 M.D. began to experience debilitating chronic diarrhea and vomiting. He lost weight. Treated since April 1982 at the Saint-Lazare Hospital in Paris, he presented with all the clinical and hematologic signs of acquired immune deficiency and died in October of intestinal cryptosporidiosis together with cerebral toxoplasmosis.[19] He was neither gay nor an addict. His young wife and their daughter, who accompanied him to Haiti, remained without major health problems. This patient's lymphocytes, retained and frozen after his death, were later sent to Bethesda, Maryland. There Robert Gallo's NCI team cultivated them and isolated an "exotic" HTLV virus that was supposed to be the key etiologic agent of this disease. If they had really isolated a strain of HTLV, then it was there only as an accompanying infection. Four years after the transfusion in the Port-au-Prince Hospital the eight donors were relocated; all remained in apparent good health.[20] Their serologic status at the time is unknown.

The patient designated "M.D." in scientific publications was in fact Claude Chardon. His real name was revealed by the American press and merits preserving for posterity, since his blood played a key role in the debates over the cause of the new disease. In restrospect, it seems highly probable that certain fallacious conclusions suggested by his case may have resulted from confusion over simultaneous infection by two different viral agents.

Another French scientist, M.C., forty years old, had left France in 1978 to live in Haiti with a young woman islander. Four years later he returned to France, where he fell ill "in the grip, it was said, of the evil spell his companion had cast on him." He died in Paris of cerebral toxoplasmosis in December 1982.[21]

4. Four homosexual patients had Kaposi's sarcoma by itself (two cases) or in association with an opportunistic infection (two). These patients, observed in 1982, had never traveled outside Europe. They could only have been infected in France. Their pattern of homosexual activity, however, made probable their link with the carriers of the American virus.[22]

5. Two problematical cases, a woman (Kaposi's sarcoma in 1980) and a heterosexual man (thirty years old, opportunistic infection in 1982) had not traveled outside France. In the second case there was the possibility of parenteral drug abuse. Noteworthy was the low incidence of intravenous drug use among the first French victims.

6. Four heterosexual patients with opportunistic infections, observed in 1976, 1978, and 1982, who had spent time in equatorial Africa. These patients had never been to the United States. Two of them, diagnosed retrospectively, showed that for Europeans the African infection preceded that with an American source.

The African Source

Jacques Leibowitch, reading the American press in December 1981, recalled a case from 1979 that had stumped several renowned Parisian physicians. A Portuguese taxi driver, M. Fel. . ., had lived in Paris since 1976. Between 1977 and 1979 he had regularly consulted the department for infectious and tropical diseases of the Claude Bernard Hospital complaining of various recur-

rent infections. He was discovered to have *Pneumocystis* pneumonia, oropharyngeal candidiasis, enormous papovavirus warts and, finally, multiple
cerebral abscesses. His lymphocytes were decreased, and their function profoundly impaired. Near the end of 1979, this patient had left Paris for Portugal
and died there, probably of complications of cerebral toxoplasmosis. Clearly
his disorder was immunological in nature, and Leibowitch had hypothesized
"a serious infection, still unknown, of African origin." Did not long-standing
experience teach us that the dark continent was the cradle of strange microbes? In fact the young Portuguese man had served in the colonial navy at
the beginning of the 1970s and, after serving in the Angolan war, had remained in Africa as a truck driver. He was not gay. His livelihood placed him
in contact with native women. Between 1973 and 1976 he had frequently
plied the route between Angola and Mozambique, passing through Zaire. Ten
years later the frozen serum of this patient would test positive for antibody to
the HIV-2 virus.[23]

Also recalled were three adults, admitted to the Tenon Hospital in 1976,
1978, and 1980 with *Pneumocystis* pneumonia. These patients had died of the
complications of an undefined immunodeficiency state. All had previously
lived in equatorial Africa.[24] Three other patients, hospitalized with undeniable
symptoms of acquired immune deficiency, gave histories of African links;
they mentioned neither homosexual practices nor prior stays in America. Two
of these three patients were, moreover, female. The man was a Zairian, aged
twenty-five. One of the two women was African, a resident of the Cape Verde
islands off the Senegalese sea coast. The other was a Frenchwoman who,
having married a Zairian native, had lived there for a long time, only to return
to Paris and become ill.[25]

In the course of 1982, physicians from the French Task Force reported this
African pattern to the CDC in Atlanta and apprised James Curran of a similar
case in West Germany in an African originally from Zaire. There was also talk
of a Danish case, but it was not made public officially until March 1983.

Margrethe P. Rask, a woman of forty-seven at the time of her death in
Copenhagen on December 12, 1977, had returned from Africa with *Pneumocystis* pneumonia, the severity of which surprised her colleagues, notably a
physician friend, Ib Bjygberg, who was familiar with tropical diseases. Rask
was a physician herself, having worked from 1972 to 1975 as a surgeon in a
rural north Zairian hospital, at Abumombazi (not far away was the spot where
the Ebola virus epidemic erupted), then, from 1975 to 1977, in a larger hospital in Kinshasa. During her stay in Africa she had been ill with recurrent bouts
of diarrhea, which had responded to metronidazole. But beginning in 1976 her
diarrhea became chronic and refractory to treatment, and was accompanied by
fatigue, weight loss, and, a bit later, generalized lymphadenopathy. In July
1977, recuperating in South Africa, she was overcome by respiratory distress
and returned to Denmark. The *Pneumocystis carinii* infection was recognized.

Despite vigorous treatment, her condition worsened. The *Pneumocystis* pneumonia was complicated by further infections with oropharyngeal candida and with *Staphylococcus albus* septicemia. She had never traveled in the United States and was not an addict. But during her work in Zaire she had been exposed to African patients' secretions and blood.[26]

The "African hypothesis," formulated by the French AIDS Task Force, was presented in the United States first by Jacques Leibowitch in a seminar held in Boston (February 1983) and then by Jean Baptiste Brunet and Odile Picard in a symposium in New York (March 1983): two successive waves of a new infectious disease had washed ashore in Europe; the first came from Africa and struck without regard to sex. The second came from the United States and was preferentially transmitted by means of sexual contact between male homosexuals.[27]

The importance of an African reservoir was only really revealed, however, in the wake of the observations from a group of Belgian physicians, first in their own country and then in Africa. Belgium still had connections with some of its former colonies. Zairian and Rwandan nationals who had the means still preferred to obtain their health care in Belgium. It was thus that a thirty-four-year-old Kinshasa woman, working as a secretary for an airline, came to Louvain in 1977 to have her infant examined for a case of oral thrush, present since the child was born three months earlier. In her first marriage the woman had borne three healthy children. But in her second she had already delivered two infants, both of whom had died quickly following "respiratory infections" and "septicemia." The two previous infants, like the third, had had thrush since birth. During the third and last child's hospitalization, the Zairian patient herself felt ill and had herself examined. Her physicians were surprised to find a series of microbes in her blood, including *Cryptococcus neoformans*, *Candida albicans*, *Staphylococcus aureus*, and several subspecies of *Enterococcus*. She also had enteritis due to *Salmonella montevideo* and herpes affecting the genital and perianal area. As her condition continued to worsen, she decided to return to Kinshasa, where she died in February 1978.[28]

Another Zairian woman, aged twenty-three, turned up in Belgium in June 1981. Eight days after she arrived she had to be hospitalized for fever. A series of opportunistic infections followed during several hospitalizations: a bout of *Pneumocystis* pneumonia was followed by tuberculous lymphadenitis, then, as the coup de grâce, *Salmonella typhimurium* septicemia. At autopsy in March 1982, she was found to have generalized cryptococcosis as well.[29]

In 1982 at the Saint-Pierre University Hospital in Brussels, Nathan Clumeck and his colleagues treated five middle-class central African patients who were neither homosexual nor parenteral drug abusers, and who nonetheless came down with an immune deficiency syndrome.[30]

Among these early African patients first observed in Europe, the clinical picture conformed to that already noted in the American homosexuals, except for certain details, especially with the respect to the frequency of opportunistic infections. They tended to exhibit more diarrhea, cryptococcosis, and tuberculosis, but less Kaposi's sarcoma.

By all evidence, the European observations gave but the palest reflection of the clinical reality in Africa. In Zaire, physicians had already confirmed a clear-cut increase in the incidence of cryptococcosis. Over an eighteen-month period in 1980–1981, fifteen new cases of cryptococcal meningitis appeared at the Mama Yemo Hospital in Kinshasa, a much higher incidence than the previous rate of about one case per year.[31] European doctors had the impression that a virus, heretofore either nonexistent or at least dormant, had begun by the late 1970s to spread in Zaire, Rwanda, Chad, and Uganda. Retrospectively, certain Belgian physicians posed the clinical diagnosis of AIDS in several Zairian and Burundian patients whose first manifestations occurred before 1976. They now think they can date the beginning of the disease in a Congolese patient even as far back as 1962.[32] But until the end of 1982 no one outside Africa had direct information on the epidemiological situation concerning AIDS on that continent.

CHAPTER 4

AIDS/SIDA: The "Four-H" Disease

Blut ist ein ganz

besondrer Saft.

—Mephistopheles,

genius of evil

(by way of Goethe)

IN THE COURSE of 1982, the clinical characteristics of the new disease were defined. It was ready to be given a name. The earliest investigations had already demonstrated its transmissibility. But it was only toward the end of that summer of 1982 that the infection among hemophiliacs who had received filtered blood products established the viral nature of the etiologic agent. From the moment it was believed to be infectious, inevitably fears arose that it would jump beyond the restricted circle of the gay community. Still, the rapidity and, above all, the extent of its spread into heterosexuals detonated not only a sense of surprise but a veritable social explosion.

In America the lay press gave broad coverage to the subject in late 1982. In Europe the call to arms did not come until the summer of 1983. The tone was at once reassuring and alarming: a new scourge has descended on humanity, but not in blind or wholesale fashion. Journalists avoided the term "epidemic" and emphasized the paucity of victims and the fact that they were confined within certain "risk groups" or "target populations." Since it was no longer certain that homosexuals alone were at risk, commentators strove to insinuate that all the risk groups were in some way "marginal." "Honest individuals" such as you or me were not in danger—only people stigmatized in advance either by their behavior, by their ethnic origin, or by some inborn defect.

American epidemiologists, in an exquisite twist of black humor, called the most exposed groups the "Four-H Club": homosexuals, Haitians, heroin addicts, and hemophiliacs. Some replaced the last group with hookers, bringing in fact the fateful club membership to five. To reassure the public, two "innocent" groups were omitted from this club of the damned: recipients of blood transfusions, and newborns infected in utero.

Readers of the lay press were told that the disease was inevitably fatal, but only provisionally so, since science was toiling away with its proven know-how to find the right antibiotic as well as the protective vaccine.

The virus was isolated in 1983. But its etiologic role was only truly admitted beginning in April 1984, whereupon it became necessary to redefine the pathologic states caused by this virus. Its isolation made possible serologic screening tests, routinely available beginning in the summer of 1985. The notion of seropositivity radically changed the epidemiology of this disorder and opened a new chapter in its history.

Naming the Disease

Much as with syphilis in other times, the earliest names of the newly conceptualized disease were not appropriated. They were too restrictive: "Neapolitan disease" or "morbus Gallicus" (French disease) in the former example; "gay pneumonia," "GRID" (Gay-Related Immune Deficiency), or "gay compromise syndrome" in the more recent case. For historians these names are interesting precisely to the extent that they reveal medical error and either national or moral prejudice.

Once the universality of these two diseases was recognized, they were given names that were neutral and of more general validity. But while the definitive name of syphilis, thanks to the poetic inspiration of Girolamo Fracastoro (1530), came from the shepherd Syphilus ("pig lover"), the new venereal disorder was baptized, in a much more prosaic way, by an acronym: A.I.D.S. At the very first, this set of initials signified Acquired Immune Deficiency Syndrome; now it is generally interpreted as the abbreviation of Acquired Immunodeficiency Syndrome. It was further simplified by eliminating the periods after each letter, and some people started to write it as a normal noun: Aids, or even aids.

Official use of the acronym began in the summer of 1982 and, owing to its use in the CDC reports, rapidly expanded thereafter.[1] It was actually fashioned during a CDC meeting in Atlanta. Those attending, unaware of its future importance, took no notice of precisely who among them created the word. The witnesses are still alive: some believe they can recall Don Armstrong, a New York epidemiologist, inventing the moniker.[2] Still others recall it being proposed by Bruce Voeller, at the time a Rockefeller Institute biochemist.[3]

Unfortunately, the name AIDS was not phonetically adapted outside of the English language and was not linguistically malleable in languages with declension, thus posing problems for those outside the anglophone scientific community. Thus another term seemed preferable for use in Slavic as well as in French or Spanish. In France an analogous acronym, SIDA, an anagram of AIDS, was created, signifying Syndrome d'Immuno-Déficience Acquise (or Syndrome d'Immuno-Dépression Acquise).[4] The Russians adopted the acronym SPID. In China, it appears, the English name gave way by a curious convergence to the ideographic transliteration ''ai zi,'' these two words meaning literally ''[disease] spread by love''.

Various sensitivities and sensibilities also had an impact when it became necessary to create an adjective and from that a substantive form to designate affected patients. In English patients were dubbed, in a term as neutral as it was obscure, PWA, ''People With AIDS.'' In France the term *sidaïque*, used by ultraconservative Jean-Marie Le Pen and carrying with it obvious anti-Semitic connotations, elicited a sharp social reaction and was rejected.

In 1983 the expression ''acquired immunodeficiency syndrome (AIDS)'' entered the *Cumulated Index Medicus* of the National Library of Medicine. Only then did the bibliographers and documentary experts finally register the birth of a new disease entity, rendering the name henceforth definitive. But perhaps it was premature to make it immutable. Both terms, AIDS and SIDA, pointed expressly to a *syndrome*, that is, a constellation of symptoms constituting a clinical entity but not an etiological unity. Applied to a disease in the strong sense of the term, the name is no longer pertinent. When it was created, uncertainty reigned about the specificity of a causal agent in this strange illness. According to the definition imposed by the CDC at the beginning of 1983, and adopted by the World Health Organization, AIDS is characterized by the onset of a syndrome of either malignancy or infectious manifestations from opportunistic organisms, or by the two together, in adults under sixty years old, and with no previous underlying pathology or immunosuppressive therapy.[5]

The name thus suggested a clinical, not a pathologic, concept. It was chosen in order to prejudge neither the unity of the syndrome's cause nor the unity of its pathogenesis. It was for this reason, moreover, that it became necessary to invent other appellations to specify some clinical states in which the causal link with AIDS was suspected but the description did not correspond to the official clinical definition of AIDS. To these forms various names were given, including ARC (AIDS-Related Complex), LAS (Lymphadenopathy Syndrome), PGL (Persistent Generalized Lymphadenopathy), pre-AIDS, and so forth. The situation changed radically once it was demonstrated that AIDS as a clinical condition resulted from the action of a specific virus. According to the new definition, AIDS is a pathologic state emanating from infection with the HIV virus, exactly like tuberculosis is a pathologic state resulting from infection by Koch's bacillus.[6] AIDS thus becomes not so much a syndrome as a retroviral infectious disease.[7] There are latent forms of tuberculosis but no one would think of calling them TRC (Tuberculosis-Related Complex) or pre-tuberculosis. The former notion of AIDS is no more than a particular stage of an etiologically defined disease. HIV infection can manifest itself in a broad spectrum of clinical states, ranging from asymptomatic and minor forms all the way to overt AIDS.

A Group at "Racial Risk": The Haitians

From the beginning of 1982, Arthur Pitchenik and his colleagues at the University of Miami noticed that several Miami-Dade residents were presenting with undeniable symptoms of AIDS. They were not, however, homosexual, nor were they I.V. drug abusers. They shared one trait: all were Haitians.

These investigators undertook a prospective study of all Haitians admitted to Miami's Jackson Memorial Hospital between January and June 1982, as well as a retrospective analysis of the records of those treated between April 1980 and December 1981. The result was startling: at least twenty Haitian immigrants living in Florida (seventeen men, three women) had been stricken by the new disease. They suffered not only from the entire gamut of opportunistic infections but also Kaposi's sarcoma, with a high incidence of tuberculosis and cerebral toxoplasmosis. Half died before the end of the study. In nine cases, the onset of the illness was certainly before 1982. Only three AIDS patients hospitalized in Miami before June 1982 were not Haitians. One was a drug addict, two others were gay.[8] The physicians were confused by the fact that virtually none of the Haitians were homosexual or addicts. Other similar cases in Haitians were observed in New York, Canada, and elsewhere. By the summer of 1982 their ranks reached 6 percent of the total number of AIDS patients in the United States.[9]

Why Haitians? Why were they alone affected outside those groups of individuals who practiced anal intercourse or intravenous injection? Certainly the early, "classical" observations on Kaposi's sarcoma made one consider a sort of "racial determinism" in such diseases, but they accorded poorly with an exclusively infectious etiology. The ideological convictions of one part of the medical community, as well as of the public, created resentment toward any racist interpretation of the new plague. The political and nationalist sensibilities of another highly important group made them more receptive. The Haitians were declared a "risk group," and official reports began to array this geopolitical group alongside the more definite categories by a particular way of life. The Haitians were stigmatized as potential carriers of the contamination, some among them even coming under suspicion for being the importers, veritably the original source of AIDS. A scapegoat had been found.

In three Haitians hospitalized in Miami, symptoms had begun to appear before they left their native land. Alerted by their American colleagues, Haitian physicians confirmed that the disease was indeed present on their island. B. Liautaud, a dermatologist, and his colleagues described eight cases of aggressive Kaposi's sarcoma observed in Port-au-Prince.[10] Other physicians drew attention to the frequency of enteric forms of AIDS among the inhabitants of Haiti.[11] But in going over earlier patient records as well as their own personal recollections they also felt confident that the Haitian AIDS was a recent epidemiological phenomenon and not some long-standing but poorly known endemic. Its appearance dated back only to the end of the 1970s and hence was strictly contemporary with the onset of the American epidemic. The history of the unfortunate French geologist, infected by blood from Haitian donors, proved that AIDS certainly existed in Port-au-Prince in 1978.[12]

Some Americans thus accused the Haitians, especially its illegal immigrants into the United States, of importing the new plague from a native setting with disastrous hygienic conditions into a clean and well-policed country. An attitude consonant with traditional epidemiologic teaching, it became in the event a vehicle for scientific and moral bias. Speculations abounded on the germ-bred misery, on the filthy water, on the intestinal and skin parasites, on the alcoholism of the Haitians, on their use of marijuana and all sorts of other privations and deprivations. Two authors went almost so far as to say that the origin of AIDS, or at least its transmission, could be explained by the bloody practices of voodoo.[13]

Throughout 1983 the most highly reputed American and French specialists could still claim that the mode of transmission of AIDS in the Caribbean remained unexplained, "mysterious." Today this blindness astonishes, for the truth was so simple. It was, moreover, clearly proclaimed at the May 1983 conference organized by the Haitian Physicians' Association. Interrogated by local physicians, 30 percent of the Haitian AIDS patients admitted homosexual contacts, notably with foreigners. This was economic necessity rather than personal preference. They did not consider themselves homosexuals, a shameful label in that culture. They were, in fact, bisexual. Mainly male prostitutes, they continued for their own pleasure to engage in heterosexual relations. Thus they transmitted the disease in two different social settings. Most American epidemiologists at that time denied the possibility of heterosexual transmission. Based on the epidemiological facts as they were then understood as much as on sociological considerations and irrational fears, this negation constituted a powerful epistemological obstacle.[14]

Until the beginning of the 1980s Port-au-Prince was a high point for "sexual tourism," a center for bordellos, some of them welcoming pedophiles. American and European gays came in droves. It is possible, perhaps even probable, that among them there were carriers of the AIDS virus. Until 1984 practically all the AIDS patients tallied in Haiti were inhabitants of the tourist areas. If the disease was endemic on the island, why were there no patients in the Dominican Republic?

Once introduced into Port-au-Prince, the AIDS agent found conditions propitious for expanding beyond its initial circle. The gay communities in California and New York had formed relatively closed groups, from which the passage of the infection into the general population was more difficult than from the bisexual brothels of Haiti. To this other factors were added, notably the practice of the *piqûristes*. This group of medically untrained practitioners treated patients by injecting various substances, using old syringes and needles without properly sterilizing them. As in Africa, this grafting of certain elements of modern medicine onto ancestral customs was to have catastrophic effects.

In our present state of understanding, we can take as proven the notion that AIDS was introduced to the Caribbean after 1972. The virus probably came from the United States but we cannot exclude a possible African origin. Subsequently, the Haitians greatly contributed to the worldwide spread of the epidemic, first through the commercialization of sex at home, and later through emigration. The political and socioeconomic conditions of the island led a considerable number of its people to become refugees in the United States, Canada, South America, and Western Europe. By September 1983 there were at least 250 people in this Haitian diaspora with overt AIDS, as well as several thousand carriers who appeared to be in good health.

Hemophilia Patients: Bad Luck

Once it was established that AIDS affected not only homosexuals but also heterosexual parenteral drug abusers, it seemed necessary to consider the danger of infection by blood and blood products. The appropriate analogy was that of posttransfusion hepatitis, which offered a similar epidemiologic profile. Confirmation was not long in coming. In January 1982 the first case of an opportunistic infection in a hemophiliac was reported at the Atlanta surveillance center. Monitoring controls on requests for pentamidine allowed two more cases to be discerned at the beginning of that summer. The CDC hence reported in July 1982 three cases of AIDS in heterosexual hemophiliacs who had received massive amounts of concentrated blood factor VIII.[15] In the course of 1982, the number of infected hemophiliacs increased to eight, reaching a total of twenty-one American and eight European cases in 1983.[16]

One of the original three cases was a twenty-seven-year-old man with hemophilia-A who had been treated since 1974 with between two and four monthly injections of a commercial blood product. In the summer of 1981 he began to have disturbances of the immune system—first oral thrush and then disseminated infection with *Mycobacterium avium intracellulare*.[17] From the epidemiologic point of view, this case was especially important in that the patient lived in Canton, Ohio. Ohio until then had been spared the disease even among its homosexual and addict communities. The two other patients also had hemophilia-A and had been treated with blood products. One lived in Westchester County, New York, the other in Denver, Colorado. Both succumbed to *Pneumocystis carinii* pneumonia.

The Denver patient, aged fifty-nine, had been treated since 1974 with concentrated factor VIII. The first clinical evidence of immune depression emerged in May 1980, but he did not have to be hospitalized until April 1982. He was then diagnosed with chronic *Pneumocystis carinii* pneumonia, confirmed by open lung biopsy.[18] A group of Alabama physicians went on to demonstrate a fourth hemophilia patient with several opportunistic infections.[19]

The earliest of the known cases of hemophilia infected with the AIDS virus was a young eighteen-year-old Pittsburgh youth who in 1978–1979 received several infusions of factor VIII. Beginning in December 1979, the lymph nodes of his neck became swollen. But when his case was first published in 1983 he had not yet suffered any serious clinical disturbance.[20]

Lymphadenopathy and minor immune problems had already been reported in a number of hemophiliacs. The magnitude of the problem, however, seemed to be a novelty. Hence the anguish felt by hematologists and hemophilia patients over the burning question: did the AIDS cases identified so far merely represent the visible tip of a tragically massive iceberg?[21]

Among the twenty-one hemophiliac AIDS patients identified in the United States by the end of 1983, nineteen suffered from hemophilia-A and two from hemophilia-B. In Europe there were eight patients, of whom seven had hemophilia-A. All had received units of concentrated commercial factors VIII and IX. When blood derivatives of this sort were prepared, plasma specimens from thousands of donors were pooled, markedly increasing the risk of infection.

The Blood of Others Can Be Dangerous

As late as September 1982, no publication had yet reported the possibility that AIDS could be transmitted by the transfusion of blood or its products in nonhemophiliac recipients. People recoiled before the social, economic, and psychological consequences of this hypothesis. Harry Haverkos, one of the most highly respected specialists on the subject, still maintained that under normal conditions there was no proof that AIDS could be transmitted by blood. Hemophiliacs were an exception because they received massive quantities of foreign organic substances in a manner that was not comparable to ordinary transfusion.[22]

It was still possible to quibble about the first case of posttransfusion AIDS outside of hemophilia, since this was a newborn baby, delivered by caesarian section, who received six complete exchange transfusions in the first six days of life. This radical treatment, carried out in March 1981 in a San Francisco hospital, was necessary to treat the Rh-incompatibility that existed between the infant and mother. Beginning in the fourth month the child came down with a multitude of opportunistic infections leading ineluctably to death. In December of the following year, retrospective studies showed that one of the blood donors whose platelets had been given to this infant had died later with a clinical picture consistent with AIDS, though at the time of the donation and for seven months thereafter he had appeared to be in good health.[23]

One could, in fact, still quibble about this case even now, since the relative quantity of infused materials had been enormous and the infant presented from the outset with the signs of erythroblastosis fetalis, in which the immunologic implications are hard to evaluate. But it was under ordinary conditions in November 1980 that a medical team at the Mayo Clinic in Rochester, Minnesota, during open heart surgery, transfused six units of whole blood, a unit of packed red blood cells, six units of platelets, and four units of fresh frozen plasma to a man of fifty-three suffering from angina pectoris. Twenty-nine months later, the patient had AIDS. He was neither homosexual, an addict, nor Haitian.[24]

The publication of the Mayo case in November 1983 had the effect of a bombshell. An act of mercy, a triumph of modern medicine, had become a mortal menace. Similar cases were disclosed in Paris (with a transfusion performed in Haiti), at Stanford, in Tel Aviv, and in Dallas.[25] In the course of 1983 the CDC in Atlanta registered thirty-nine cases reported in adults in whom the only factor able to explain the onset of AIDS was a blood transfusion during the preceding five years. Until 1986 the number of these cases grew exponentially, with a doubling time of about eight months.[26]

"Normals" Are Not Safe

Only at a relatively late date, in the course of 1983, was the possibility of heterosexual transmission demonstrated. The first reliable observations concerned the onset of the disease among the companions of bisexual and addicted AIDS patients. In some instances the disease was found in both members of a heterosexual couple in which only the man carried a known risk factor.[27] In June 1983 AIDS was diagnosed in the wife of a hemophiliac. Despite their advanced age (the husband was seventy-four, the wife seventy-one), this couple continued to have sexual intercourse.[28]

Once passage from man to woman by vaginal intercourse had been established, infection in reverse remained an unresolved and controversial issue.[29] There was a curious paradox: the women were more easily infected by heterosexual intercourse than the men, and yet the number of women patients was relatively small. This situation arose because of the preponderant role of male homosexuality in triggering the recent epidemic in the United States and Western Europe. The African example shows that women are not protected from AIDS by their gender but essentially by certain social conditions involved in transmitting the agent.

By 1984 observers recognized the importance of the role played by female prostitution in the explosive propagation of AIDS in equatorial Africa.[30] In North America as well as Europe, several women prostitutes had become ill rather early with the disease; but all told, they exerted only a minor effect on the initial expansion of the epidemic.

Between 1981 and 1984 the proportion of women with AIDS increased in the United States from 3 percent to 6.5 percent. For the most part they were intravenous drug abusers. But the category of women infected by a heterosexual contact also increased consistently.[31]

Infected women played a principal epidemiological role in transmitting AIDS to the newborn and the fetus. In 1982 the onset of AIDS was confirmed in four infants between two months and two years of age. Three were born to AIDS-infected mothers, while the fourth was delivered by an apparently healthy mother of Haitian origin. Soon the number of such children began increasing at a distressing rate. The immediate conclusion was that the route of infection was transplacental passage of the virus in utero.[32] The contamination was doubtless vertical, from mother to child. But no one yet knew with certitude whether it occurred during pregnancy, at the time of birth, or later, in the nursing process or even in the course of the close physical contact with the mother at a time of particular vulnerability.

Ancestral Fears Reawaken

Routine lavatory activities, contacts between skin and bodily membranes, a simple kiss, or the sharing of crockery—could these things not cause AIDS? A terrible suspicion had just loomed up, fueled by the analogy with hepatitis, which public health personnel had such great difficulty preventing. Even the prestigious *Journal of the American Medical Association* echoed these fears. According to James Oleski, infants with AIDS might have become infected through routine contacts in an unwholesome family environment.[33]

Amplified by the print and broadcast media, physicians' fears fed a wave of collective hysteria that seized some Americans, especially in the urban middle classes. Medical experts and politicians denied the possibility of viral transmission by simple cohabitation or by simple daily social contact other than sexual intercourse. But the public only half believed them. Timeworn principles of the struggle against infectious disease were resurrected, and vigorously (if at times incorrectly) applied to this new danger. Heightened consciousness of the possibility of contamination by heterosexual activity and by blood transfusion, moreover, fanned the hatred of certain minorities. This unexpected plague, divine retribution, placed the mark of infamy on homosexuals, drug addicts, Haitians, and in general the "marginals" and the "criminals."

News of the relatively increased incidence of AIDS in prison threw kerosene on the fire. The links between AIDS and criminality were certainly indirect: the imprisonment of numerous drug addicts and the fact of homosexual practice in prisons.[34] But that did not prevent the majority of the good citizens from finding confirmation for their own prejudices about the moralistic aspects of this illness, which was so different from all the rest.

"This disease," said a woman interviewed at the time, "affects homosexual men, drug users, Haitians, and hemophiliacs—thank goodness it hasn't spread to human beings yet." A man added, "If it spreads to the general public, it would be a medical crisis, demanding immediate government response." And when the journalist asked him how he would see the situation if the illness could be kept hemmed in, he replied, "It's God punishing homos." Another respondent declared that he hoped scientists would discover a cure soon, and added maliciously, "but not too soon."[35]

Margaret Heckler, Secretary of Health and Human Services, denounced the "unjustified panic," and James Curran spoke of "hysteria."[36] Homosexuals were the first target of a terrified public. The sexual revolution and liberalization of customs must, some said, be revised. Many gathering spots were closed. Within the gay community, the blow of the epidemic elicited contradictory reactions. At the beginning it was minimized: they did not want to believe what the doctors were saying, and accused them of exploiting an imaginary danger to "revive their symbolic power." They refused to play with the adversary in a game whose rules required accepting arguments that might lead to "moral repression." Then they panicked, demanding that public authorities provide the financial means to struggle against the disease.

A year after the Americans, the French homosexuals followed the same trajectory. First, indignation over the publicity surrounding a medical problem: "They would chatter about this less if the disease attacked a group of Chilean truck drivers." Then they came up with the opposite: "In the struggle against this disease, they would surely be making more of an effort if it hit the tennis players." Claude Lejeune, president of the Association of Gay Physicians in Paris and columnist for the magazine *Gai-Pied*, wrote in April 1982: "Fucking is dangerous? Then so is crossing the street!" In July 1983 he complained of the "permanent exaggeration of a quantitatively minor fact," but the following summer he published a tract admitting the gravity of the situation and urging French homosexuals to adopt voluntary preventive measures.

The social rejection of the Haitians in the United States was especially hard and effective. It was easier to find them than other risk groups: they were black, poor, and spoke French. They were shunned, evicted, and registered. In Haiti, the American reaction took on the case of a national catastrophe, since the island nation's budget depended largely on tourism.[37]

The first AIDS patients, wrote English virologist Robin Weiss, triggered fear and prejudice disproportionate to their numbers.[38] Accidental road deaths were much more common, yet society considered those odds as the penalty, an entirely acceptable price, to pay for access to modern transportation. AIDS, said this savant, by all rights must preoccupy us because it is a new ailment and because it is spreading. I might add that AIDS fascinates also because it concerns sex and blood: an extraordinary outlet for phantasms. AIDS is fatal in its overt form. We had forgotten that such plagues existed.

The AIDS epidemic caught us unaware and aroused the return of irrational fears because it exposed the impotence of modern medicine just when we had begun to believe that the infectious diseases had been vanquished for good.

Some Statistical Facts (1982–1984)

After 1982 the AIDS epidemic spread like wildfire.[39] In the United States the number of cases reported to surveillance centers grew regularly; its incidence (number of new cases) grew exponentially.[40] There were ten new cases each week in 1982, one hundred in 1984. The cumulative number doubled roughly every six months. Among heterosexuals the doubling time was less rapid: roughly every nine to ten months.[41]

The total number of patients registered by the CDC had passed 200 by the end of 1981; 450 by mid-1982; 750 at the end of 1982; 1,800 in mid-1983; and 3,000 by the end of 1983. It attained 5,000 by mid-1984 and 8,000 at the end of that year. None of the American patients diagnosed before 1983 is alive today. The rate of lethality (ratio of yearly deaths to diagnosed cases) was around 40 percent.[42] These figures have been rounded off to underscore the epidemic's expansion.

At a 1983 conference Michael Gottlieb predicted that by 1985 roughly 20,000 Americans would have AIDS.[43] He was not in the least mistaken. This figure, which seemed incredible as an estimate of the total burden of cases, merely accounted for the annual incidence in 1987. Although reported by the end of 1983 in forty-four states, the distribution of AIDS cases remained quite unequal. New York, California, Florida, and New Jersey accounted for about 80 percent of all cases, and New York City alone for about half of those.[44]

The distribution of cases by risk group also evolved in important ways: the percentage of male homosexuals, who represented 92 percent of all cases reported until 1982, decreased to 75 percent in January 1983, and about 72 percent toward the end of 1984. The majority of these patients were white, aged thirty to forty, well educated and well heeled. Their principal risk factor was pronounced sexual promiscuity. The relative number of drug-abusing patients constantly increased, meanwhile, moving from some 3 to 4 percent in 1981 to 17 percent in 1984. This group was mainly black and Hispanic, young, heterosexual, and mostly heroin addicts. In 1983–1984 about 6 percent of American AIDS patients were Haitians who conceded neither homosexuality nor addiction. Hemophiliacs constituted about one percent of the total. Constantly increasing in number were the heterosexual partners of members of the risk groups. And, tragically, every month more and more babies were gravely stricken.[45]

The distribution of cases by diagnostic category showed a clear predominance of opportunistic infections: of 2,000 patients reported until the end of August 1983, slightly more than half had *Pneumocystis carinii* pneumonia, about five hundred had Kaposi's sarcoma, and roughly one hundred fifty had both. Improved diagnosis certainly augmented the relative number of recognized cases of cerebral toxoplasmosis[46] and cryptosporidiosis.[47] Disseminated tuberculosis became more frequent because of the spread of the AIDS virus among the Haitians and other medically underserved groups in New York and California.

In Europe the epidemic lagged behind the United States, and the exponential growth was less pronounced at the start: between 1982 and 1984, the total number of patients doubled roughly every eight to nine months.[48] The regional office of the World Health Organization (WHO) took on the task of epidemiologic surveillance in Europe. By the time this office organized a meeting in Denmark in October 1983, AIDS cases could be confirmed in fifteen member countries of the WHO European region, for a total of 267 cases. In decreasing order of absolute numbers of reported cases, they were France, West Germany, Belgium, United Kingdom, Switzerland, Denmark, the Netherlands, Austria, Spain, Sweden, Norway, Finland, Czechoslovakia, Italy, and Ireland.[49]

The few dozen cases diagnosed at the end of 1981 had increased to over one hundred by the end of 1982. A year later they reached three hundred and, by the end of 1984, eight hundred. The relative frequency was highest in Denmark and Switzerland. But one feature in particular was different than the North American case: about 22 percent of the European cases were of African origin. In fact, two epidemics were superimposed on European soil. The epidemiologic characteristics combed from the non-African cases corresponded to those observed in the United States: about 80 percent of these were male urban homosexuals; more than half were thirty to forty years old. The drug addicts were a second risk group but their proportion was clearly less (1.5 percent) than in America.[50]

Epidemiologic AIDS surveillance began in France in March 1982. The cumulative number of cases increased from 17 in 1981 to 47 in 1982, then 107 in 1983, reaching 180 (including 74 deaths) by the June 1984 count. At that time homosexuals formed the great majority (90 percent) of French patients. As yet no cases of nonhomosexual drug addicts had been reported.[51] A multifactorial case-controlled analysis of male French homosexuals showed the risk factors to include the high level of promiscuity with casual sexual partners, a history of syphilis, and the use of local steroids.[52]

In Italy the first diagnosis of AIDS was made in November 1982 by Ferdinando Aiuti in a Roman homosexual. By September 1983 the presence of ARC—AIDS-related complex—had been recognized not only in Latium but in Lombardy as well. The number of overt AIDS cases officially recognized in Italy swelled from two at the end of 1982 to ten by June 1984. Italian political authorities were not yet ready to admit the presence of indigenous cases, and denied the possibility of a budding epidemic.[53] In 1983 AIDS was also diagnosed in Japan and Australia. Africa was already severely affected,[54] yet public health authorities on that continent denied the fact. Worldwide, the number of cases reported to WHO increased from 408 at the beginning of 1982, to 1,573 in December 1982, then to 5,077 in 1983, and 12,174 at the end of 1984. All such numbers underestimated the real situation. Only after the serologic findings fully emerged could the real measure of the catastrophe be taken.

PART TWO

THE ORACLES OF SCIENCE

CHAPTER 5

Stalking
the Virus

Nature is never truly

conquered. The human

retroviruses and their

intricate relationship with

the human cell are but

one example of that fact.

Indeed, perhaps conquest

is the wrong metaphor

to describe our relation-

ship to nature, which not

only surrounds but in the

deepest sense also

constitutes our being.

—Robert Gallo,

discoverer of the first

human retrovirus

I N A TYPEWRITTEN "protocol" dated May 25, 1982, for the Centers for Disease Control, John Bennett claimed that the new disease was a sexually transmitted viral infection and that the causative agent could be either a common virus producing new effects as a result of certain environmental factors, or one of several "novel agents, e.g., mutant or recombinant strains of human or animal pathogens."[1] At the time, this was merely a hypothesis, but by the end of that summer, the appearance of AIDS in hemophiliacs who had received filtered blood products proved that the cause of the disease was indeed a virus.[2] Blood components were not sterilized through ordinary procedures because of the risk of destroying some useful molecules, but they were filtered to remove bacteria, fungi, and protozoa. Since the infectious agent had obviously passed through a filter, it had to be a virus.[3]

The First Suspects

From the very beginning, suspicion fell on cytomegalovirus (CMV). Early in the AIDS epidemic, some signs of a possible relationship between this pathogen and Kaposi's sarcoma had been identified.[4] Almost all the original patients had elevated titers of antibodies against this virus, and CMV itself had been found in their urine, blood, and even pulmonary tissue.[5] Yet CMV infection had been recognized for years prior to the new epidemic and had been found in many individuals with none of the manifestations of the immunodeficiency syndrome. How could it be known whether or not a pathogen found in immunosuppressed persons was cause or consequence of their condition?[6]

The urine of one patient contained an adenovirus, while the blood of several others contained antibodies against hepatitis-B virus. Nevertheless, these findings were not sufficient evidence to attribute a decisive role in the etiology of the new syndrome to either of these viruses.[7] A special place in the lineup of first suspects was accorded the Epstein-Barr virus, causative agent of infectious mononucleosis and, in Africa, of Burkitt's lymphoma, a malignancy of lymph nodes that had been found to occur in a geographic distribution largely resembling that of Kaposi's sarcoma. But here too was the same problem. Why would a complete change take place in the pathological manifestations of a well-established virus? Such a profound mutation would be virtually equivalent to the birth of a completely new virus.[8]

More convincing was the hypothesis that an animal virus had suddenly become pathogenic for humans. Historical analogies lent plausibility to this idea. Jane Teas, a Boston epidemiologist, suggested that the AIDS virus could be a particular strain of the causative agent of swine fever. Since the turn of this century, this epizootic raged throughout Africa. By 1975 it had spread to Cuba, and around 1978 it began to kill pigs in Haiti. Some blamed Cubans for having brought the disease from Angola, and others saw it as the disastrous result of some sort of biological warfare waged by the CIA.[9]

Known strains of swine fever virus were not pathogenic for humans, and the first serological tests done on AIDS patients were negative for these agents.[10] Nevertheless, Jane Teas clung to her hypothesis, modifying it to place more emphasis on cofactors than on the virus itself, and trying to confirm it by the demonstration of trace amounts of antibodies to swine fever in nine out of twenty-one AIDS patients.[11]

Animal analogies were not devoid of relevance, and oncogenic retroviruses first isolated in animals pointed to the right direction. The Atlanta virologist, Donald Francis, and his former mentor, Myron Essex of Boston, have been credited with having realized that there was an analogy between the new human syndrome and feline leukemia as early as the summer of 1981. They noticed that the AIDS pathogen combined characteristics of the feline leukemia retrovirus with those of the agent of human hepatitis-B.[12] The transmission of AIDS was similar to that of hepatitis-B, and it seemed reasonable to suspect the latter of being an associated factor in AIDS pathogenesis. But what did cancer in cats have to do with AIDS?

A look at the history of virology will help answer this question. Even a brief examination of these events will emphasize to what extent the intellectual and technical tools needed to identify and explain the mechanism of action of the AIDS virus are recent acquisitions.

What Is a Virus?

The term "virus," which in Latin can mean "juice," "humor," or more commonly "poison," was used in the nineteenth century to describe any substance capable of multiplying within an organism and making it sick. It was applied indiscriminately to all pathogens. Pasteur spoke both of the "anthrax virus," knowing perfectly well it was a bacillus, and of the "rabies virus," knowing next to nothing about it at all. He knew that rabies virus was contained in saliva and brain tissue of patients and sick dogs, that he could heighten or reduce its virulence, and that he was able to vaccinate against it with matter containing attenuated viral strains, but he was never able to isolate it or examine it under the microscope. Throughout the second half of the nineteenth century, scientists tried in vain to visualize the causative agents of some of the most serious human diseases, such as smallpox and rabies, or the most common, such as influenza and the cold. These germs were thought to be extremely small, beyond the power of the microscope, but in all other ways similar to bacteria.

In 1891 Dmitri I. Ivanovski, a Russian botanist, was able to demonstrate that a pathogen could indeed be "inframicroscopic." He passed liquid, containing infected material derived from a plant diseased with tobacco mosaic, through a porcelain filter and demonstrated that it did not lose its virulence. Seven years later, his Dutch colleague, Martinus Willem Beijerinck, confirmed these findings and announced that the agent, which he called *contagium vivum fluidum*, retained its virulence after drying, but lost it on heating to 72°C. In the same year, 1898, Friedrich Löffler and Paul Frosch discovered that the virus of aphthous fever was also filtrable. Following these discoveries, filtrability was demonstrated for the causative agents of several other human diseases, including yellow fever (Walter Reed and James Carroll, 1901) and rabies (Paul Remlinger, 1903). When in 1903 Emile Roux published a review of the "so-called invisible microbes," only nine such pathogens were known. One year later, his colleagues at the Pasteur Institute, Henri Vallée and Henri Carré, identified the filtrable virus of equine infectious anemia and thereby isolated the first lentivirus, later to be called EIAV, a cousin of the AIDS virus.[13] Yet no one really understood the peculiar properties and significance of these tiny beings. For Roux, they were no more than "small bacteria."[14]

Before the term "virus" was applied exclusively to this category of living beings, they were given other names, such as "filtrable virus" and "ultravirus." I have just referred to them as "living beings," but whether or not viruses are actually alive is a problem that has been around since 1935. In that year California scientist Wendell M. Stanley showed that purified tobacco mosaic virus formed a crystal of nucleoprotein. Could a crystalline substance be alive? In order to allow viruses to "live," it would be necessary to redefine life. Twenty years later, the dilemma was revived. In 1955 Heinz Fraenkel-Conrat and Robley Williams reconstituted an active tobacco mosaic virus from inactive protein and ribonucleic acid. At the same time, Frederick Schaffer and Carlton Schwerdt crystallized poliomyelitis virus. After much study, it seemed clear that while isolated viruses were incapable of independent vital functions, including metabolism, movement, growth, and multiplication, they could reproduce like other life forms, as long as they were in contact with appropriate living cells. Viruses may have no autonomous life, but they are nonetheless "alive" because they can control and accomplish their own reproduction through the use of a foreign cellular apparatus. Viruses are absolute parasites, fundamentally different from bacteria. Pathogenic bacteria are only relative parasites. They live off their host, but they use their own metabolic and reproductive machinery.

It was easy to conceive of different microbes competing with each other as they parasitized the same prey, but it was with some astonishment, if not incredulity, that biologists and physicians greeted the discovery of the bacteriophage, a parasite of parasites. During the First World War, both Frederick Twort of London (1915) and Canadian-born Félix d'Hérelle of Paris (1917), working independently, observed and described the phenomenon of bacteriophagy: a filtrable factor, thus a virus, was capable of reproducing in a bacterial milieu and destroying bacteria. Then came the recognition of "lysogenic" bacteria, in which the bacteriophage could suddenly appear without evidence of prior infection (Jules Bordet and Mihai Ciuca, 1921). Bacteriophages were found to be made half of proteins and half of nucleic acids (Max Schlesinger, 1934). The significance of these discoveries was not fully understood until twenty years later, when the fundamental role of nucleic acid in heredity and cell regulation was established. In 1957 Heinz Fraenkel-Conrat showed that destruction of the viral proteins did not affect the virulence, thereby demonstrating that infection was due to the nucleic acid portion of the virus.

The "infra-microbes" became visible in 1940–1942, after the invention of electron microscopy. Viruses were first cultured in living chick embryos, then, in vitro, in tissue cultures, and finally, when the cells could be separated by the digestive action of trypsin, in cell cultures. The development of continuous or permanent cell lines, a major contribution to cell biology, was the result of a kind of "cancerization" of cells, which made them capable of surviving by division through countless generations. This "immortality" could be induced either by viral infection, as was the case for the well-known cell line 293, a product of human embryonic kidney cells, or by a previous malignant transformation, such as the HeLa cell line, derived in 1952 from a human cancer of the cervix.

Since the 1950s virology has experienced extraordinary progress, inextricably linked to the development of molecular biology. Bacteriophages, or as they are now called, "phages," the viruses of bacteria, became the favorite model for molecular biologists, among them Max Delbrück, Alfred Hershey, Renato Dulbecco, Eugène Wollman, and André Lwoff.

A bacterium is a complete living cell; a virus is not. Most phages and pathogenic viruses are made up of protein and a long nucleic acid molecule. This molecule is a biological program that in some cases may be inserted into the chromosomal material of the infected cell. When it has been so inserted, the viral genes act like the genetic material of the host. Study of this phenomenon has contributed as much to our understanding of heredity as it has to our understanding of viral infection. A pathogenic virus attacks a target cell, taking over its genetic controls and using its synthethic apparatus to accomplish its own reproduction.[15]

Slow and Latent Viral Infections

The hunt for the causative agent of AIDS would have met with failure without concepts derived from research done since 1950 on slow viruses, latent infection, oncogenic viruses, and reverse transcription of genetic information.

Scarcely thirty years ago it was thought that all viral infections were acute: brief incubation, abrupt onset, and rapid progression. As the virus invades and begins to take over, the host organism mounts an immune response. The process results in either rout of the viral onslaught or death of the host. Measles and influenza were the classic examples.

The notion of slow virus infection came from veterinary science and gradually infiltrated human medicine, over a period of decades. B. Sigurdsson coined the expression "slow virus" in 1954, during his studies of four diseases: three of sheep and one of goats. From a historical point of view, the most interesting of these is visna, a word meaning "fatigue" in Iceland, where this epizootic decimated the sheep population. Visna is an insidious disease, with a very long incubation period and a duration that can last ten or more years, a significant proportion of a sheep's life. The pathological effects are characterized by plaques of demyelination in the central nervous system, similar to those observed in human multiple sclerosis. The peculiar viral pathogen is now known to be related to the AIDS virus.

Visna was first introduced to Iceland in 1933, in sheep imported from Germany, but because of the insidious nature of the infection, the epizootic was not recognized until 1939, when a high percentage of livestock had already been lost. The disease was eradicated through a vigorous campaign of systematic slaughter of infected flocks. Sporadic outbreaks of visna have occurred elsewhere in the world, but there have been no other serious epizootics. It is not known why this virus, which in all likelihood has been around for a long time, provoked the Icelandic epizootic.[16]

In 1957 a bizarre human disease was described by D. Carleton Gajdusek and Vincent Zigas. Many members of the Fore tribe, isolated natives of the eastern New Guinea highlands, were afflicted with a peculiar illness, which they called *kuru*, meaning "shivering" or "trembling with fear." This central nervous system disorder begins with a disturbance in coordinated movements and progresses slowly but relentlessly to paralysis, dementia, and miserable death in a state of complete prostration. Patients do not have fever or any other signs suggestive of an infection. Autopsy reveals widespread decrease in brain cells.[17]

Two years later, W. Hadlow first drew attention to the clinical and pathological relationship between kuru and scrapie, the latter already known to be a particular slow virus disease of sheep. It took several more years of failed attempts, however, before Clarence Gibbs and D. Carleton Gajdusek managed to transmit kuru to chimpanzees by inoculation of brain tissue taken from victims. The appearance of this disease in the Fore people, at the turn of the century, coincided with the introduction of ritual cannibalism, which included consuming the brain of the deceased. Since this practice was abandoned, around 1960, the incidence of kuru has steadily declined. New cases still appear in individuals born before this date, suggesting that the incubation period is very long. Kuru exemplifies the fact that an infectious disease can be strictly limited and demonstrates the importance of behavior in the origin and persistence of a viral infection.[18]

The term "slow virus infection" is reserved for those diseases, which, like visna, progress slowly but steadily with no intervals of apparent health. Brain tissue is the usual target of these so-called unconventional viruses, including the agents for kuru and Creutzfeldt-Jakob disease.[19]

Latent viruses are different from slow viruses. They are "quiescent." After an initial or primary infection, they cause occasional and varied clinical manifestations over a relatively long time. Herpes simplex infection, chicken pox, and cytomegalovirus inclusion disease all display latency with possible periodic reactivations and remissions. Study of the lysogenic bacteria, which carry quiescent viral genes on their chromosomes, has facilitated the understanding of the seeming appearances and disappearances of viruses in these diseases.[20]

Oncogenic Viruses

Do viruses cause cancer? Until the middle of the twentieth century, this might have been a strange question, because explanatory theories of neoplasia excluded the notion of infection. At most, microbes were thought to favor carcinogenesis by a nonspecific irritation of tissues. Yet in 1908, long before virology came into its own, Vilhelm Ellermann and O. Bang of Denmark claimed that chicken leukemia was an infectious disease transmissible by inoculation of ground and filtered malignant cells.

In 1910 Francis Peyton Rous, physician-virologist at The Rockefeller Institute (now The Rockefeller University) created a stir when he announced the successful transmission of chicken sarcoma with an inoculum of ground and filtered tumor. Twenty-six years later, John Joseph Bittner demonstrated that murine breast cancer was passed, mother to offspring, through milk.[21] Despite these isolated observations, little change was made in the reigning theories of cancer causation. In retrospect, knowing what we know now, not much could be done before the revolutionary discoveries in molecular biology elucidated the structure of DNA and RNA and their role in cellular control.

Armed with new ideas and advanced technology, scientists returned to the notion of viral etiology of cancer many years later. Ludwik Gross, a New

York biologist, demonstrated the viral origin of mouse leukemia in an elegant series of experiments in 1951. His success depended partly on the happy accident that he selected, as recipients, newborn mice now known to have undeveloped immune systems.[22]

The first human malignancy to be associated with a virus was a jaw tumor that occurred in Ugandan children. Denis Burkitt, during his British overseas service in 1958, noticed that aside from its peculiar course, which was unlike that of any other malignancy, this lymphoma had a striking geographic distribution, which seemed to depend on climatic factors. In 1961 Burkitt traveled through East Africa and confirmed his initial impression: the lymphoma affected large numbers of children, but only those who lived in regions displaying a specific range of temperature, humidity, and elevation. The geographic distribution of Burkitt's lymphoma, as it is now called, could be superimposed on that of certain mosquitos. Burkitt concluded that the disease was caused by a virus carried by an arthropod vector.[23]

For three years, researchers tried in vain to identify the virus in Burkitt's lymphoma with the electron microscope and to isolate it from cancerous tissue using standard techniques. Finally, in late 1963, an English oncologist, Michael Anthony Epstein, and his Australian colleague, Yvonne Barr, established a continuous line of Burkitt's lymphoma cells and identified the virus, a close cousin of the herpes simplex virus.[24]

However, instead of unraveling the etiological knot of Burkitt's lymphoma, events following this finding made it more tangled than ever. Quite inadvertently, the Epstein-Barr virus was found to be the cause of infectious mononucleosis. This unexpected discovery was made through a series of extraordinary circumstances, which included the accidental infection of a technician working in the Philadelphia lab of Gertrude and Werner Henle. Subsequent work showed that the virus was ubiquitous: 80 to 90 percent of North American adults have been infected at one time or another; in Africa, close to 100 percent. When the infection occurs after infancy, it results in a fairly innocuous flulike illness, the "kissing disease" of adolescents. When it occurs in infancy, as is the case in Africa, the viral genetic material can be integrated into the host genome where it usually resides, as a potential oncogenic operator, without producing any illness. Occasionally, however, the virus can be activated by as yet poorly understood factors, possibly including malaria, to induce malignant transformation of B-lymphocytes. The virus has also been shown to be the cause of a cancer of the nose and throat common in south China.

Guy de Thé, who conducted a vast prospective study on Ugandan children in 1978, has referred to Burkitt's lymphoma as the "Rosetta stone of oncology."[25] This historical comparison better applies to the discovery of the *sarc* (sarcoma) gene, responsible for the production of Rous' sarcoma yet present regularly in the normal cells of chickens.

Since the 1960s, experimental results have hinted at the existence of genes innate to a cell and capable of triggering its malignant transformation when exposed to particular external stimuli. It was thought that those oncogenes innate to a cell might be even more important than those introduced by viral infection. These ideas culminated in the hypothesis of Robert Huebner and George Todaro, who suggested that all cancers are the result of activation of the normally silent gene sequences by the effect of carcinogens or radiation.[26] In the early 1970s several researchers managed to identify the gene of the Rous virus that is responsible for malignant transformation of cell cultures. In 1976 a French-American team, including Dominique Stehelin of Paris and Michael Bishop and Harold Varmus of San Francisco, discovered that this gene, called *sarc*, is a homologue of another found in healthy chicken cells. The cancer-causing gene comes from an apparently normal cellular gene after recombination with another carried by a virus. Viruses and cellular genomes interact in extremely complex ways. Retroviruses borrow genes from cells and modify them; cells integrate part, or sometimes all, of the retrovirus into their genome, to be passed on to future generations as a Mendelian trait.

Speculations about innate cellular oncogenes opened up a new direction in cancer research, but nearly closed the door on another, one which ultimately led to identification of the human retroviruses. The exact significance of endogenous viruses is still not clear. They seem to be epidemiological "scars," evidence of prior, possibly very ancient infections, and they may play a role in biological evolution.

In 1966, after a telling delay, Francis Peyton Rous was awarded the Nobel Prize in Medicine. An appropriate year, as it turned out, because at the same time, William Jarrett, veterinary scientist at the University of Glasgow, discovered the feline leukemia virus (FeLV). This virus provokes a malignant transformation of some blood cells, prevents other infected cells from developing normally, and induces an immune suppression similar to that which would later be observed in AIDS. William Jarrett and his brother Oswald, in collaboration with Myron Essex of Harvard and William Hardy of the Sloan-Kettering Institute, examined the properties of this virus and concluded that feline leukemia, unlike other known viral cancers, could be passed under natural (i.e., nonlaboratory) conditions between nonconsanguinous cats. This finding silenced all remaining critics of the idea of infectious viral oncogenes.[27]

Reverse Transcriptase

Newly acquired genetic knowledge has provided an elegantly simple explanation for the malignant transformation of infected cells: the viral genome, once inserted in the genome of the host, constitutes an oncogenic sequence, which provokes cell division rather than viral reproduction. Instead of killing the infected cell, oncogenic viruses enter into a state of symbiosis with it. This brilliant hypothesis ran up against a major difficulty in the 1960s: neither Rous' avian sarcoma virus, nor Jarrett's feline leukemia virus contained DNA. The place of DNA in these viruses was filled by RNA; yet takeover of the cell's genetic mechanisms can be accomplished only with DNA. According to one of the fundamental tenets of molecular biology, DNA makes RNA and RNA makes protein. It was thought not possible for the mechanism to operate in the opposite direction. Francis Crick, one of the founders of molecular biology, called this tenet its "central dogma." [28] This heuristic hypothesis qualified as "dogma" precisely because it was unproven and, in its generalized formulation, largely unprovable. [29]

The dogma was overturned by Howard Temin (who first proposed the hypothesis in 1964) and Satoshi Mizutani, biologists at the University of Wisconsin, and David Baltimore of Massachusetts Institute of Technology. In 1970 they demonstrated the possibility of transcription of RNA into DNA. The impact of this "heresy" was very fruitful, and a short five years later, the two Americans were awarded the Nobel Prize. It is still accepted that a virus can integrate into the cellular genome only in the form of DNA, but certain RNA viruses can accomplish this task with the help of a specific enzyme, known as reverse transcriptase, which is supplied by the virus and allows the elaboration of a complementary strand of DNA from the chain of viral RNA. This DNA can penetrate the nucleus of the cell. One family of RNA viruses possesses reverse transcriptase and makes use of it to traverse part of the biological cycle in reverse gear; hence the family name, "retrovirus." [30]

Discovery of the Human Retroviruses

Having identified the reverse transcriptase, Temin and Baltimore removed an epistemological obstacle to the understanding of how viral genes could cause cancerous transformation and, at the same time, provided scientists with an extremely useful tool. This enzyme would be used in the pursuit of retroviruses and from 1975 on, in the development of molecular cloning techniques.

The causal explanation and the treatment of cancer were the main concerns of a great many scientific institutions around the world, particularly in the United States. The American government gave top priority to cancer in its funding of biomedical research. The most important federal cancer research center, the National Cancer Institute (NCI) is part of the National Institutes of Health (NIH), located in Bethesda, Maryland. Just as Temin and Baltimore were announcing their discovery of reverse transcriptase, another young researcher, Robert Gallo, was working at the NCI on a group of the related enzymes, DNA polymerases of blood cells. Lively and imaginative, Gallo understood right away that reverse transcriptase could add a new dimension of tremendous theoretical and practical importance to his own research. At that time, only the retroviruses causing cancer in animals were known, and all ambitious oncologists dreamed of finding a human oncogenic retrovirus. To date, elaborate experiments in viral culture had failed, just as had the most painstaking scrutiny with the electron microscope. New hope was offered by the possibility of using reverse transcriptase as a specific marker whose presence would betray that of its invisible virus.

"Under the influence of Temin's ideas," Gallo recalled, "I decided to search for reverse transcriptase in human leukemic cells, hoping to find a retrovirus there. In doing so I was gainsaying accepted wisdom. . . . Careful electron microscopy of human leukemic cells had yielded no such images, leading most investigators to conclude no human retrovirus exists."[31]

Disappointment followed disappointment, for five years, as Gallo and Sol Spiegelman refined their tests for reverse transcriptase, finally giving it a sensitivity superior to that of the electron microscope. In order to obtain sufficient quantities of virus, the malignant cells had to be grown in culture, but the leukemia cells refused to cooperate. The plant derivative, phytohemagglutinin (PHA), had been identified as a stimulus to white cell division by Peter Nowell of the University of Pennsylvania several years before. In 1976 Doris Morgan and Francis Ruscetti, working with Gallo, announced that PHA stimulation of certain T-lymphocytes caused them to release a growth factor, which they initially called T-cell growth factor (TCGF), since renamed interleukin-2 (IL-2).[32] Bernard Poiesz, also of Gallo's lab, found that certain leukemic cells would grow and multiply indefinitely on exposure to interleukin-2, even without prior stimulation by PHA. These findings were published in 1980.[33]

The dates are important. Only then, between 1976 and 1980, did the intellectual and technological means needed to recognize and isolate the AIDS pathogen become available. This is the same period American public health officials identify as onset of the AIDS epidemic.

Using the technique of stimulated lymphocyte culture, Gallo finally found the first human retrovirus. In his words:

> It was from such malignant cells [found by B. Poiesz], grown with IL-2, that we isolated the first examples of HTLV-I in 1978–79 from the cells of two leukemia patients. My colleagues and I isolated the virus, characterized it and showed it was specifically a human virus; our results were published in 1980 and early 1981. Later we isolated many other examples. My colleague Marvin Reitz then showed that these viruses were not closely related to previously described animal viruses.[34]

This narrative omits any mention of previous investigations of the Dutch virologists and minimizes the capital role of the young physician Bernard

Poiesz, then a trainee at NCI. Suffice it to say that Gallo was traveling and absent from his laboratory during the decisive period of this discovery.

The virus was first isolated from the lymphocytes of Charles Robinson, a black patient from Alabama, who suffered from an aggressive lymphoma, which was diagnosed as mycosis fungoides. It was next found in cells of patient M. B., also black, who presented with a clinical picture interpreted as Sezary syndrome, a disorder related to mycosis fungoides.[35]

Gallo named his virus Human T-cell Leukemia Virus (HTLV). The acronym stuck, but the "L" was later altered to indicate "lymphoma," still later, "lymphotropic," which means "gravitating toward lymphocytes." Ordinal numbers in Roman numerals were added after 1982, when Gallo's Bethesda team isolated another virus in the same retrovirus family: HTLV-II.[36] This virus was first detected in 1978, in a permanent cell line of lymphocytes (line MO), derived from a young white male from Seattle, and cultured by David Golde in Los Angeles. Irvin Chen's analysis of the RNA of this virus showed that it was quite different from HTLV-I.[37] The patient, M. Moore, who suffered from an extremely rare form of T-cell leukemia, known as "hairy cell leukemia," launched an unsuccessful suit against the University of California opposing the scientific use of his cells without remuneration.

Doctors recognize several different types of leukemia. HTLV-I is not the cause of the more common varieties. During the two years following its discovery, Japanese and American scientists demonstrated that HTLV-I was the cause of adult T-cell leukemia (ATL). This disease is uncommon in Europeans and North American whites, but it is endemic to the southern islands of Japan, and fairly common in Caribbean blacks and Africans. Similar to Sezary syndrome, ATL was first described in 1977, in a masterful article by Kyoto physician Kiyoshi Takatsuki. From the blood of a Japanese patient with ATL, Isao Miyoshi, Yorio Hinuma, and collaborators isolated a retrovirus, which they called ATLV. After Mitsuaki Yoshida analyzed its RNA sequences, it became apparent that ATLV and the American HTLVs were simply different strains of the same pathogen.[38] HTLV can be passed from mother to child through the placenta and through breast milk, and it can also be transmitted between adults through sexual contact and blood. It may lie dormant for a very long time, possibly even forty years after the initial infection.[39]

After the Wrong Culprit

The new disease of New York and San Francisco homosexuals began to interest the NCI in the fall of 1981. Kaposi's sarcoma had long been known as a malignant disease, but the possibility of a viral cause was a captivating notion that had an immediate impact on research. A conference on Kaposi's sarcoma and opportunistic infections was held in Bethesda on September 15, 1981. As the clinicians presented their observations, it became apparent that the virologists were far more interested in malignancy than they were in opportunistic infections. Already tension was mounting between the researchers from the Centers for Disease Control (CDC) in Atlanta and those of the NIH in Bethesda. Members of the National Institute of Allergy and Infectious Diseases, a component of the NIH, felt that the new disease was at least as relevant to them as it was to the NCI. The competition was driven by more than a conceptual debate: money played a role. Substantial grants would be awarded to those working on the new disease. Two Boston centers, the Dana-Farber Cancer Institute and the Department of Cancer Biology of the Harvard School of Public Health also announced their readiness to chase the oncogenic virus.

Beginning in spring 1982, Paul Feorino and his virology colleagues at the CDC labored to find the AIDS virus, but unlike the previous rapid successes with Legionnaire's disease and African hemorrhagic fevers, these efforts were frustrated. In early 1983 Feorino noticed the presence of a cytolytic virus (i.e., one capable of killing cells) in a lymphocyte culture derived from an AIDS patient, but he abandoned this direction, discouraged by Gallo, who claimed that the AIDS virus had to be oncogenic, not cytolytic.[40]

In his Harvard lab, Myron Essex was working on the feline leukemia retrovirus. He was struck by the similarities between this disease of cats and AIDS: both were characterized by immunodeficiency and malignancy. Serological studies had shown that the immunodeficient patients frequently carried antibodies against cytomegalovirus, hepatitis-B, and Epstein-Barr virus. In 1982–83 Essex was convinced that approximately a quarter of all AIDS patients carried antibodies to HTLV.[41] His tests were flawed, but they pointed in the right direction.

Essex and Gallo agreed, with their colleagues, that AIDS was caused by a retrovirus, most likely HTLV-I. Exactly how the virus produced the symptoms was still not known, although its predilection for T4-cells was obvious. They believed it had only recently been introduced into America. Its presence in Haiti reinforced their hypothesis of a causal link with AIDS.

Gallo was convinced they had found the culprit. He announced his discovery in a press release, a note published in the CDC's *MMWR*,[42] and in a series of articles that appeared in *Science* beginning May 20, 1983. He later reconstructed the crucial events of 1983 as follows:

> These suggestive results [of Essex on FeLV] made it seem even more plausible that a variant of HTLV-I (or its near relative HTLV-II, isolated in 1982) might be the AIDS agent. Essex's group and my own quickly began searching for such a virus. Soon we were joined by a third group, led by Luc Montagnier of the Pasteur Institute, who had been stimulated by the retrovirus hypothesis. All three groups employed the methods that I and my colleagues had developed for isolating HTLV-I: the virus was cultured in

T-cells stimulated by the growth factor called IL-2 and its presence was detected by sensitive assays for viral reverse transcriptase. Those methods quickly produced results. Beginning in 1982 and continuing throughout 1983 my coworkers and I found preliminary evidence of retrovirus different from HTLV-I or II in tissues from people with AIDS or pre-AIDS conditions.[43]

Despite these later statements, it is clear from the May 1983 publications that Gallo and Essex did not believe the AIDS virus to be "a retrovirus different from HTLV-I or II," that is, a special and till then unknown member of the HTLV group; they thought it was identical with HTLV-I or at least very close to it. From the blood of an American AIDS patient, they claimed to have found a virus that was "indistinguishable from earlier HTLV isolates" and "closely related to the HTLV-I subgroup." They also claimed to have found antigens of the HTLV virus in the lymphocytes of two French AIDS patients, whose blood had been brought in February 1983 from Paris to Bethesda by Jacques Leibowitch. They were not sure "whether these isolates from France belong to subgroup I or II of HTLV or to a new subgroup."[44] Using molecular hybridization of DNA, Gallo and his coworkers also found HTLV provirus sequences in DNA from two of thirty-three AIDS patients tested.[45]

These were highly suggestive indicators, but they did not prove that HTLV was the cause of AIDS, and they failed to answer many serious questions. Why had this fairly widespread virus not caused such an epidemic before? Why was AIDS not ravaging Japan, the country with the highest frequency of HTLV? How could a virus, known to stimulate the growth and division of lymphocytes, result in their depletion? How reliable were those tests for anti-HTLV antibodies? On this last point, for example, Essex's positive results, which had made such an impact on the direction of research, were later shown to be a lab error.[46]

The American teams had rushed down the wrong path and, encouraged by their earlier successes with the retroviruses of feline leukemia and T-cell leukemia, they lost a year in trying to justify their initial intuition.[47] In 1984 they were still trying to prove that HTLV genes were identical to those of the AIDS virus,[48] while the French immunologist, Jacques Leibowitch, flew to the rescue with an epidemiological and clinical argument as clever as it was misleading.[49]

CHAPTER 6

Discovery of the AIDS Virus

Les idées, ce n'est rien:

tout le monde en a;

ce qu'il faut, c'est

les faire passer

dans les faits.

—Luc Montagnier,

discoverer of LAV virus

IN THE UNITED STATES, where private enterprise flourishes, basic research on AIDS is done by two governmental institutions: the Centers for Disease Control (CDC) and the National Institutes of Health (NIH). Yet, paradoxically, in Western Europe, where state control over centers of higher learning and scientific research is the rule, the study of AIDS is the uncontested domain of a private foundation: the Pasteur Institute.

The Pasteurian Tradition

The Pasteur Institute, founded through public donations in 1888, was initially intended to be a vaccination center for rabies and a research laboratory for all infectious diseases.[1] The many fruitful ideas of Louis Pasteur and his successors, Emile Duclaux and Emile Roux, the Institute's first directors, gave it an auspicious beginning. Bacteriology, biochemistry, and immunology were new branches of life science just opening into major fields of endeavor. Roux once said of Duclaux that he made the Institute a "sort of scientific cooperative, where individuals could contribute to a common goal without risking their intellectual freedom." Maintaining this equilibrium was of utmost importance, but it was also a delicate balancing act between the forces of individual liberty and those of the growing needs of a working team.

André Lwoff, who won the Nobel Prize for his work done at the Pasteur Institute, claimed that in the middle of our century, medical microbiology was ahead of the disciplines on which it depended. This state of affairs could have led to a crisis in the Institute, but instead of being defeated by the "molecular revolution" in microbiology, the *pasteuriens* prepared and mastered it. Gradually the Institute grew into a multidisciplinary center for basic and applied biomedical science and teaching, microbiological reference, epidemiological surveillance, and large-scale biomedical manufacture.

Virology was always of special importance to the Pasteur Institute. After all, its original raison d'être was the combat of rabies, one of the most horrible of viral diseases. Even before the recent rise of this discipline, Constantin Levaditi worked there on polio virus, Amédée Borrel studied animal on-coviruses, and Félix d'Hérelle discovered the bacteriophage. The studies of phage and lysogenic bacteria, begun there by Elisabeth and Eugène Wollman and André Lwoff, and brilliantly continued by Elie Wollman and François Jacob, had a major impact on the developing field of molecular biology. These Pasteur scientists forged concepts that are essential to our understanding of the biological strategy of the AIDS virus and its ability to insert itself into the chromosomes of its host.[2]

Financial difficulties and a long period of agitation by dissatisfied researchers who had been striving for changes in management systems for several years resulted in the 1971 appointment of Jacques Monod as director of the Pasteur Institute, or, more properly, as the master-builder of a major reconstruction. Monod and Wollman promoted the expansion and diversification of the virology department. This expansion was accomplished in 1972 and the changes included a new unit for the study of oncogenic viruses. Its director was Luc Montagnier, a specialist in cancer-causing viruses, who came from the Institut Curie at Orsay, south of Paris.

Montagnier had welcomed two colleagues to his new unit, both from the Pasteur laboratory at Garches: Jean-Claude Chermann and Françoise Barré-Sinoussi. The latter had developed her expertise in mouse retrovirus techniques, involving the quantitative determination of reverse transcriptase, during a stay at the NIH lab of Robert Bassin in Bethesda. Chermann was working on the retroviruses suspected of causing cancer in mice and was exploring the inhibition of their reverse transcriptase by various chemical compounds. Montagnier worked on interferon, its physiological role and the possiblities for its production through genetic engineering. He was very comfortable with lymphocyte culture techniques, and for this work he used interleukin-2, produced by Gallo's lab.

All three of these scientists were working in the difficult field of retroviruses. They discovered that anti-interferon greatly enhanced the production of retrovirus in mouse cells. Searching for a virus in human breast cancer, they found a retrovirus, similar to one responsible for breast cancer in mice, in tissue taken from a young Tunisian woman with a rare type of tumor. In short, as Montagnier observed, from 1977 on, the Pasteur team was in possession of all the concepts and methods that would be needed for the isolation the AIDS virus.[3]

The Pasteur virologists first encountered AIDS during a controversy about the Institute's production of hepatitis-B vaccine. Production of this vaccine, developed in 1975 by Philippe Maupas of the Tours Virology Institute, was very lucrative. In 1982 it accounted for no less than 10 percent of the revenue of the Pasteur Institute Production (IPP), and this increased in the following year to 20 percent. The technique required massive amounts of human plasma. In 1981 the IPP had purchased 2,500 liters of plasma from American blood banks to meet their needs, a third of which (856 liters) was mixed with European plasma to prepare vaccine. The product was tested on chimpanzees: one developed a nonspecific hepatitis; another died of an arbovirus infection. The press became very excited about these events, associating them with news of the possible existence of an infectious agent in blood from the United States. For several years, this blood had already been tested for infective agents with, among other tests, an analysis for the presence of reverse transcriptase. Nevertheless, in the fall of 1982 the scientific director of the IPP, Paul Prunet, asked Luc Montagnier to examine the imported plasma for traces of HTLV-I.

Discovery of LAV

By September 1982 Jacques Leibowitch, a physician who at the time was working at the Raymond Poincaré Hospital in Garches near Paris, had been convinced that the cause of AIDS was an exotic virus of African origin that infected T4-cells and was transmitted by blood. This description pointed toward an HTLV retrovirus. In the same month, he analyzed lymphocytes taken from M. Elomata, a patient from Zaire, who presented with leukemic lymphoma, thereby testifying to the presence of HTLV in Africa.[4] On October 5 Leibowitch gave a seminar at the Cochin Hospital on "the retroviral hypothesis in AIDS." He asked, with rhetorical emphasis, "Is there a French retrovirologist present?" No one replied. Soon after, Leibowitch telephoned Robert Gallo, who told him of his research on the AIDS virus.

Leibowitch informed the French task force of Gallo's preliminary studies and promoted the idea of an AIDS virus, closely related or even identical to HTLV-I. The members of the task force accepted the notion of a retrovirus as the most probable cause of AIDS, but were not persuaded that it would be found in blood. They reasoned that since the virus destroyed and reduced the numbers of circulating T-cells, it would be difficult to find in the peripheral blood. However, enlargement of lymph nodes was a common feature in early AIDS. The researchers suspected that the virus could be more easily detected in these swollen nodes. Moreover, isolation of the virus from a patient in the initial stages of illness before the onset of immunodepression and multiple opportunistic infections would be of greater etiological significance.[5] These ideas may have been built on shaky ground, but they led to excellent results.

Françoise Brun-Vézinet, director of the virology laboratory at the Paris infectious disease center, Claude Bernard Hospital, joined Luc Montagnier in the search for retrovirus in AIDS patients and, above all, in those who presented with early signs in the lymphatic system. Clinical aspects of the work were handled by Willy Rozenbaum, an infectious disease expert who had just transferred from the Claude Bernard Hospital to the Pitié-Salpêtrière.[6]

Thus it was at the Pitié, on January 3, 1983, that a lymph node was removed from the neck of a thirty-three-year-old male identified in the laboratory notes by the first letters of his name, BRU, and in the published papers by the anagram RUB. He was later identified by newspaper reporters as Frédéric Brugière. A homosexual who had relations with fifty partners a year and who had visited New York City in 1979, Brugière had been bothered for one month by minor symptoms, sufficient to suggest but not confirm a diagnosis of early AIDS-Related Complex (ARC) with enlarged nodes.[7] Montagnier recalled:

> That afternoon, I carried the biopsied lymph node to my fumehood for the usual procedures (grinding, washing, centrifugation, and exposure to protein A to active T- and B-lymphocytes). The initial culture ought to last for weeks, thanks to the use of the T-cell growth factor, interleukin-2, which I obtained from Dr. Didier Fradelizi, of Jean Dausset's service at the Hôpital St. Louis. I added serum containing anti-interferon antibodies in order to neutralize any interferon which the cells might have been producing to combat infection and which would make it difficult to find the virus.
>
> On the fifteenth day, Françoise Barré-Sinoussi was able to demonstrate a weak but unmistakable trace of reverse transcriptase. The test was repeated to rule out lab error. Françoise Barré Sinoussi, Jean-Claude Chermann, and I deliberated on these findings. We decided to begin a more ambitious program designed to find out if this really was a retrovirus, and, if so, to see if it differed from the other known human retroviruses, HTLV-I and HTLV-II.
>
> I phoned Willy Rozenbaum to let him know the results. We held a meeting with Françoise Brun-Vézinet, Françoise Barré-Sinoussi, and Jean-Claude Chermann, on Saturday morning, February 12. The clinician [Rozenbaum] gave a brief but beautifully clear update on the knowledge of AIDS. We showed him our preliminary results: the enzyme was definitely a reverse transcriptase, not a cellular enzyme. It was associated with the viral particles and these particles had the same density as retroviruses, that is, 1.17 in a sucrose gradient.
>
> But a genuine claim to having isolated a virus requires being able to produce it at will in noninfected cell cultures. By that time, the first culture from the patient was beginning to show signs of fatigue: virus production disappeared, followed by disppearance of the cells. It was necessary to start growing the virus in noninfected T-lymphocyte culture. The only source of these was blood donors. Urgently, I phoned professor André Eyquem, the immuno-hematologist in charge of the Pasteur Institute blood transfusion service. That same day, I had the blood of a donor and half of the lymphocytes were added to those cultured from Dr. Rozenbaum's patient. We were delighted to see the production of reverse transcriptase, hence virus, re-

appear in this mixed culture. The virus in the patient's lymphocytes had infected those of the healthy donor, and they in turn began elaborating virus.[8]

In writing up this experience for his laboratory journal, Montagnier mistook the date. He cited the first day as January 4 instead of January 3, but the latter date did appear in his retrospective account and has been definitely confirmed by other sources. Later on in the journal, Montagnier recovered the right date because he entered the events of two consecutive days under the heading "January 5."

Another chronological error should be mentioned: increase in reverse transcriptase was noticed not on the "fifteenth day" (i.e., January 17 or 18), but in a small amount on January 15, and then unmistakably on January 26. Inscription of the decisive analysis in Montagnier's journal bears the date "15.1" [sic], but it is situated between entries for January 23 and 26.

The original handwritten title of this experiment in the laboratory journal clearly reveals that the point of departure for the Pasteur Institute team was the hypothesis of Gallo and Essex: the word "HTLV-1" appears, with the figure "1" less slanting and in a slightly different color and thus probably added at a later moment; this word "HTLV-1" is crossed out and replaced at an even later moment by the word "Bru 1," accompanied in the same hand and pen by the exclamation "+ + *(enfin)*" ("finally").

A page from the laboratory notebook of Luc Montagnier, indicating the first steps in the isolation of the AIDS virus. (Reprinted with permission of Luc Montagnier)

According to her laboratory notes, Françoise Barré-Sinoussi first observed the production of reverse transcriptase by the cultured lymphocytes on January 25, 1982. The activity of this enzyme was initially very weak. It increased slowly to a peak on February 7 and then declined. This was surprising and even disturbing, because HTLV, the only known human retrovirus group, did not behave in this way. HTLV caused lymphocytes to divide, and this multiplication increased the amount of reverse transcriptase. This new virus seemed to act differently: it killed the cells. From this moment on, according to Barré-Sinoussi, the suspicion was born that the new virus might be something other than Gallo's HTLV.[9]

But what exactly was the relationship between the new virus and HTLV? This was an important question. Charles Dauguet's electron microscope photos of the virus, taken on February 4, 1983, showed that there were significant morphological differences between it and HTLV, making it unlikely that they were one and the same.

Names Are Never Innocent

Montagnier quickly told Gallo about the discovery, in a letter carried to Bethesda by Leibowitch on February 2, 1983. With a great deal of circumspection, he said they had "perhaps" found something new in a case of "immunoproliferative syndrome." Gallo sent antibodies capable of recognizing two proteins of the HTLV-I virus, but they did not react with the French virus. When informed by telephone, Gallo refused to believe the result, so convinced was he that Montagnier's virus had to be a variant of HTLV.[10]

Montagnier wanted to call his new virus "RUB," an acronym formed by scrambling the letters in the name of his prototypical patient, but he gave up this idea in favor of a solid technical term that seemed harmless: T-cell Lymphotropic Retrovirus. This name, however, would eventually be used as a pretext for regrouping it with the first human retrovirus found by Gallo.[11]

The French paper appeared in the May 20, 1983, issue of *Science*, with a note indicating that the manuscript had been received on April 19, 1983. This was the same issue in which Gallo and Essex announced their findings implicating HTLV-I as the cause of AIDS. Although Montagnier's paper acknowledged only a possible relationship between the new virus and the HTLV family, the abstract left no doubt. It began with these words, announcing the discovery of "A retrovirus belonging to the family of recently discovered human T-cell leukemia viruses (HTLV), but clearly distinct from each previous isolate." The first part of this sentence did not figure in the original manuscript. The abstract was written by Gallo, at the request of the editors, and hastily approved by Montagnier over the phone.

In the main text of the article, the French authors claimed that the new isolate contained proteins normally not belonging to HTLV-I, notably p19 and p25. Some evidence in favor of HTLV was presented: antibodies that strongly reacted with HTLV-infected cells were found in the blood of Brugière, here called "patient 1," and another patient, called "patient 2," with an early AIDS-like syndrome. Later, however, it was shown that the serum of Brugière had reacted with one or more surface antigens of infected cells, not HTLV itself; the second result turned out to be a lab error. They reported on how the retrovirus had been grown in the lymphocytes taken from (umbilical) cord blood or from healthy donors. Electron microscope images revealed round particles budding through the surface of infected lymphocytes. Despite all this, the writers avoided shouting "Eureka" and ended their article with a tempered paragraph, beginning, "The role of this virus in the etiology of AIDS remains to be determined." They knew they might have found nothing more exciting than another opportunistic pathogen. Since the proliferative capabilities of the lymphocytes were not enhanced, they suggested that the lymphatic hyperplasia could have been merely an inflammatory reaction. Factors other than a specific infection by this one virus could contribute to the cause of AIDS, including the overload of the immune system by repeated viral and bacterial infections.[12]

This issue of *Science*, which contained several articles on human retrovirus infections, and the way in which the popular and medical press reacted to it, left the Pasteur Institute team with a bitter aftertaste. The specificity of "their" virus was only secondarily apparent, hidden behind the idea that the cause of AIDS was a type of HTLV.

American virologist Matthew Gonda noticed the similarities between the French virus and the lentiviruses, which are nononcogenic retroviruses of animals, and already in the summer of 1983 he made Gallo's team aware of his observations.

The first French retrovirus came from a patient who did not have full-blown AIDS. To deal with this methodological awkwardness, it would be necessary to find the same virus in patients with different and well-recognized forms of AIDS. From the end of May 1983, an informal group, known as "Les Dix" (The Ten), got together once a week at Montagnier's lab to focus and coordinate their work. A second strain of the same virus was isolated in a node biopsy from a homosexual male with multiple lesions of Kaposi's sarcoma; a third, in the blood of a young hemophiliac with neuromeningeal toxoplasmosis; a fourth, in a young woman from Zaire, who died ten days after the biopsy. In all these cases of widely differing ethnic, social, and biological settings, the virus was the same. David Klatzmann, Jean-Claude Gluckman, Luc Montagnier, and their colleagues proved that the virus invaded T4-lymphocytes exclusively, but instead of conveying a sort of "potential immortality" and causing cell division, as occurred in HTLV-I and HTLV-II infection, the virus destroyed the cells it had invaded.

Montagnier and his associates were increasingly convinced that the virus was not a member of the HTLV family and was related to the lentiviruses.

They referred to the first isolate of their virus as "Lymphadenopathy Associated Virus (LAV)" and the later isolates as "Immune Deficiency Associated Virus (IDAV)."[13] These names were not a felicitous choice, because the action of the first isolate thereby seemed restricted to lymphadenopathy alone and because the subtle differentiation in nomenclature between the various other isolates suggested more important, specific differences in structure and function. In fact, the second term, IDAV, was rapidly abandoned.

Frédéric Brugière, the patient in whom LAV was first isolated, enjoyed fairly good health for several years, but eventually the disease manifested itself with all its cruelty and, in the autumn of 1988, he died of AIDS.

Virus in Limbo

In the historic reconstruction of the discovery of the AIDS virus, Robert Gallo said:

> Beginning in late 1982 and continuing throughout 1983 my co-workers and I found preliminary evidence of retroviruses different from HTLV-I or II in tissues from people with AIDS or pre-AIDS conditions. Then in May of 1983 Montagnier and his colleagues Françoise Barré-Sinoussi and Jean-Claude Chermann published the first report of a new retrovirus from a patient with the lymphadenopathy ("swollen glands") typical of some pre-AIDS cases. The French investigators gave their find the name lymphaden-opathy-associated-virus (LAV). The initial report of LAV was intriguing, but it was hardly a conclusive identification of the cause of AIDS. The reason is that the methods available (reverse transcriptase assays accompanied by electron microscopy) can show that a virus is present but cannot specify the precise type of virus.[14]

The chronological order suggested by Gallo's presentation merits comment. His publications show clearly that until May 1983, he and his co-workers were looking for and finding isolates identical or very close to HTLV-I and HTLV-II, and up until that date they did not mention in any way "retroviruses *different* from HTLV-I or -II in tissues from people with AIDS or pre-AIDS conditions." Gallo relegated Montagnier's discovery to May 1983, yet he had known about it since February.

All this aside, by the summer of 1983, the etiological role of the Pasteur Institute virus in AIDS was indeed still unproven. In August, John Maurice published two articles in *Journal of the American Medical Association*, giving an accurate portrayal of the French discovery and popularizing the term LAV; however, he seemed to consider that HTLV-I was more likely to have a role in the cause of AIDS.[15] Distrust concerning the role of the "Pasteur virus," poor cousin of rich Uncle Sam, was shared by many European specialists. In March 1984 Leibowitch still wrote, "It's too early to assign it a place, either opportunistic or causative, in the story of AIDS."[16]

In September 1983 a Cold Spring Harbor meeting was organized by an NCI task force to present the state-of-the-art in human leukemia retrovirus studies. In spite of its eventual impact, Montagnier's paper was given a cool reception. He announced several new findings: isolation of LAV in three very different AIDS patients (one homosexual, one hemophiliac, and one Haitian); proof of selective affinity for T4-lymphocytes; demonstration by ELISA assay of anti-LAV antibodies in 63 percent of patients with pre-AIDS and 20 percent of those with full-blown AIDS; and finally, evidence of the similarities between LAV and the lentivirus responsible for equine infectious anemia (EIAV) as well as evidence for essential differences between LAV on the one hand and HTLV-I and -II on the other. Gallo intervened in a scornful and aggressive manner. He doubted that LAV was a retrovirus, and he rejected its etiological relationship with AIDS. He claimed that his team had found anti-HTLV-I antibodies in 10 percent of AIDS patients, and from some patients they had isolated parts of the virus itself. From the French point of view, the meeting was dominated by Gallo's group, which tried to minimize the French contribution.[17]

In early 1984 the Pasteur team began clarifying the morphological differences between HTLV-I and LAV. They confirmed the latter's similarities to the equine anemia virus by demonstrating that the immunological properties of the LAV protein p25 resembled those of an analog in EIAV.[18] They characterized another specific protein, p18, and isolated an LAV virus in a hemophiliac with AIDS and in his apparently healthy hemophiliac brother.[19]

In December 1983 Abraham Karpas, a hematologist in Cambridge, England, had published an electron micrograph of a virus found in the blood of a young homosexual male with AIDS. As it turned out, Karpas had found the right bug, several months after the Parisian team, but long before the Americans. He succeeded in growing his virus in a permanent cell line and began work on a serological test for its identification. From the outset, he insisted on the differences between his virus and HTLV.[20]

The proceedings of the Cold Spring Harbor meeting, published in June 1984, contained an introduction by Gallo in which appeared the virus, HTLV-III, not mentioned during the meeting of September 1983. Here also appeared a subtle but clever change in meaning of the acronym, HTLV; where "L" had meant "Leukemia," it now stood for "Lymphotropic."[21]

Isolation of HTLV-III

HTLV-III made its official debut on April 24, 1984, when Margaret Heckler, Secretary of the U.S. Department of Health and Human Services, announced at a press conference in Washington that Robert Gallo and his colleagues (Mikulas Popovic, Zaki Salahuddin, Elizabeth Read, and others) had isolated a new virus, proved that it was the cause of AIDS, and were putting the finishing touches on a test that would be made available in November. Within two years, she promised, federal laboratories would find and produce a vaccine.[22]

Gallo described his new virus first to the popular press and then in a series of articles published in the May 4, 1984, issue of *Science*. The American scientists had indeed made a significant contribution to knowledge about the AIDS virus.

According to Gallo,

The new virus (or viruses), however, resisted the early attempts at laboratory culture: when they were put in T-cells, the cells died. . . . In the fall of 1983, my colleague Mika Popovic identified several cell lines that could be infected with the virus but resisted being killed. To obtain them the blood cells of a person with leukemia were separated and allowed to proliferate into clones of genetically identical cells. . . . the most productive of them was the clone designated H9. All the resistant lines are made up of leukemic T4-cells that are immortal in culture and therefore an endless source of virus.[23]

Thus, mass production of HTLV-III was accomplished. Mikulas Popovic, an experienced virologist, had chosen a very unusual method: he infected lines of leukemic lymphocytes with a pool of virus derived from ten different individuals. The alleged heuristic hypothesis was to retrieve the most viable strains, by a sort of natural selection.[24] This procedure presented significant disadvantages from a methodological point of view: it became impossible to recognize the precise origin of the virus thus isolated. Viruses with similar immunological characteristics were isolated in forty-eight persons with AIDS or AIDS-related complex (ARC), but despite the affirmations of Gallo and his collaborators, it now seems highly unlikely that these isolates were successfully cultivated in permanent lines. None were found in 115 heterosexuals in good health.[25] Laboratory notes disprove many published results.

The advent of the Western blot technique greatly improved the sensitivity of clinical tests. In a blind study, M. G. Sarngadharan and his colleagues identified HTLV-III antibodies in 88 percent of forty-eight AIDS patients, 79 percent of fourteen gay males with ARC, and in less than one percent of several hundred healthy people. This technique also allowed for better analysis of the proteins involved in the immunological reactions.[26]

These were considerable advances, but HTLV-III could be considered a new virus only if it differed from LAV. Reporters were primed to ask about its possible identity with LAV at Gallo's press conference on April 24, 1984, but he avoided comment. They had been alerted three days earlier by a *New York Times* interview with James Mason, director of the CDC in Atlanta. In fact, CDC researchers, notably Donald Francis and V. S. Kalyanaraman, a former collaborator of Gallo, were convinced that Montagnier's hypothesis was correct. They had analyzed the antigens of the French virus and declared they were satisfied with the results. They too had isolated a virus that corresponded to that of the Pasteur team. The virus controversy revealed the tensions and conflicts existing between the government-supported institutions of the United States engaged in the fight against AIDS.[27]

The Priority Dispute

Before he isolated his own HTLV-III, Gallo had twice obtained samples of LAV: the first, carried to Bethesda by Montagnier on July 17, 1983; the second, sent from Paris at the request of Mikulas Popovic on September 22. Popovic signed a certificate to the effect that he recognized French priority and planned to use the virus for biological, immunological, or molecular research only, avoiding any commercial use of the substance without prior consent of the Pasteur Institute.[28]

The sequence of events suggests that Gallo's team effectively ignored or failed to look closely at the July samples, being more confident of their own isolates at the time. Only when confronted with repeated failure and the growing opposition of other American virologists did they decide to take another look at the Pasteur virus.

Were LAV and HTLV-III two different viruses, or were they simply one virus with two names? Once serological tests, cloning, and gene sequencing were complete, there was no doubt: the viruses were identical. But this verdict was not necessary for one to be astonished by the behavior of Robert Gallo. Before claiming he had isolated a new virus, he could have compared it with the LAV specimens he possessed, published the result of the comparison, and, if unable to prove a difference, respected the priority of the discoverers in the attribution of the name. When the term "HTLV-III" became synonymous with LAV, Gallo and certain American governmental institutions made an all-out effort to save it. For a brief period, a ridiculously cumbersome solution was reached by the use of the double acronym: LAV/HTLV-III (recommended by the World Health Organization) or rather HTLV-III/LAV (used by the American government and most of the English-language scientific literature). In May 1986 an international commission on virological nomenclature put an end to the absurd situation and baptized the bug with yet another acronym: HIV, for Human Immunodeficiency Virus. In order to strike a compromise, the Commission revoked the French team's right to name their discovery, but found fault with the American team, refusing terminological affiliation with the HTLV family.[29]

CHAPTER 7

Solution to a Controversy

Ce que nous savons est le grand obstacle à l'acquisition de ce que nous ne savons pas.

—Claude Bernard, master of experimental biology

THE AMERICAN scientists, especially Robert Gallo and his NCI team at Bethesda together with Myron Essex at Harvard, opened the way that would lead to the elucidation of the true cause of AIDS. They had forged the tools that were indispensable to attaining this goal. But these same scientists missed the discovery of HIV. No one had better intellectual preparation in the field of research; no virology team had superior technical facilities. And yet they failed to accomplish a relatively simple task, or at least a task that from today's point of view gives the impression of simplicity.

In the history of science, this situation is not an uncommon occurrence. An epistemological obstacle bars the way of would-be discoverers, a barrier to understanding that derives from the legacy of prior successes, especially their own, and from the preconvictions that accumulate along a given path of exploration. The French team's advantage was some sort of greater "ingenuity," greater intellectual freedom, and a shorter list of major triumphs. Montagnier said, "If the Americans had believed in the LAV from the very beginning, they would have rapidly left us far behind, thanks to their financial strike force."[1]

But to "believe" in another's ideas, researchers must often "forget" a few of their own, sometimes even those that have led to, or constituted, their major achievements. If Gallo had not discovered HTLV-I, he might well have been the discoverer of HIV. One can imagine and sympathize with the sense of frustration and annoyance Gallo must have felt at some moment in the summer or fall of 1983, when he realized he had spent a long time running down a blind alley. He must have felt deprived of a prize to which he was somehow entitled in view of his previous discoveries, and I believe that this sense of loss led him to construct a face-saving scenario and to fight with all available means.

Major financial considerations, often camouflaged by the demands of national prestige, intervened to play a sinister role in these events.

The Interests at Stake

Isolation of the causative agent of an infectious disease has a threefold payoff of practical importance: it opens possibilities for accurate diagnosis by serology, prevention by vaccination, and treatment by chemotherapy. Discovery of the AIDS virus raised hopes, which so far have been disappointed in the realms of vaccination and therapeutics. But it led to rapid success in the claboration of highly effective diagnostic tests. Montagnier's Pasteur team, including, among others, Françoise Brun-Vézinet, Françoise Barré-Sinoussi, Christine Rouzioux, and Jean-Claude Chermann, used standard procedures to produce reagents from the LAV retrovirus that would recognize the presence of specific antibodies in the serum of an infected person. As early as June 1983, encouraging results were obtained from a radio-immunoprecipitation technique (Radio-Immuno-Precipitation Assay, or RIPA) and the now commonly used Enzyme-Linked Immuno-Sorbent Assay (ELISA).

During an international meeting in Paris in October 1983, Montagnier announced that the IPP (Institut Pasteur Production) would make the ELISA test commercially available. This brought a strong reaction from Gallo, who questioned the specificity of the test and cautioned the Pasteur Institute about the risks of promoting an unreliable method. True, at the time, the test appeared to yield positive results in only 40 percent of confirmed AIDS patients and approximately 72 to 75 percent of ARC patients; moreover, at the time no one was certain of its exact specificity, or in other words, what percentage of the positive results were wrong (false positives).[2]

The Pasteur Institute applied for a U.S. patent for a diagnostic kit based on the ELISA test for LAV antibodies in December 1983. The originality they sought to protect was the use of the viral products to enhance the test's specificity, not the ELISA method itself. The application was duly registered and sent for study. The Pasteur Institute made an agreement with Genetic Systems Corporation of Seattle for production of their AIDS blood test.

In April 1984 the NIH applied for a patent for Gallo's AIDS diagnostic kit. A year later, while the French were still kept waiting in suspense, the NIH was awarded a patent (U.S. Patent 4,520,113), thereby obtaining the rights to an income deriving from the sale of AIDS diagnostic kits in the American market, then an estimated five million dollars annually. The annual royalties rapidly reached a total of eight million dollars, and continue to grow. The delay over the French application was not unusual; the relatively rapid processing of the NIH request was.[3] The Food and Drug Administration (FDA) also created a holdup at their level and did not approve the French kit until 1986.

Trials on the French ELISA test, published by the Pasteur team in June 1984, yielded the following results: 37.5 percent positive in AIDS patients, 74.5 percent in patients with lymphadenopathy suspected of having early AIDS, 18 percent in apparently healthy homosexuals, and one percent of all blood donors. CDC virologists repeated this trial in the United States with similar results: 41 percent positive in AIDS patients, 72 percent in lymphadenopathy patients, and zero percent in a control group of seventy individuals.[4]

At the same time, Gallo's team published the better results of their own Western blot technique: 100 percent positive in AIDS patients, 84 percent in those with lymphadenopathy, and zero percent in the control group.[5] It was not known whether the heightened accuracy came from the strain of virus used or from the technique itself.

During 1984 both teams improved the sensitivity of their test. Mikulas Popovic's lymphocyte cell line H9 allowed the production of significant quantities of viral antigens by several bioengineering firms.

The paternity of the permanent H9 line is today controversial, for it seems likely that it is a simple clone of the HUT78 line, developed a dozen years earlier by Adi Gazdar.

Soon after their isolation of LAV, the French group tried, without success, to grow it in transformed permanent T-lymphocyte culture. It was Robin Weiss and Rachanee Cheingsong-Popov of the Chester Beatty Laboratories in London who managed to grow descendants of the same viral strain in a particular permanent lymphocyte line (called CEM). If the first HTLV-III isolated was in fact a cloned strain of LAV, then the Pasteur team had been victims of a very instructive circumstance. As it turns out, the first isolate of LAV will not grow easily in permanent lymphocytic cell lines; the viral strain changed then and became more "adapted" to lymphocytic cultures. Quite paradoxically, Montagnier and his coworkers were unlucky, precisely because they moved too quickly in their attempt to establish viral cultures in immortalized lymphocytic lines. In giving their American and English colleagues a virus changed in vitro, they had unknowingly enhanced their colleagues' chances of success. Before he had heard about the American and English results, Montagnier discovered that LAV adapted to culture in B-lymphoblasts transformed by Epstein-Barr virus.[6]

Scientific rivalry intensifies when industrial competition joins the Nobel race. One year after its application for a patent, the Pasteur Institute launched a suit against the American government. French scientists pointed out that they had filed an application first and they accused Gallo of having used their isolate of LAV in defiance of the condition that he not exploit it for commercial purposes. The Americans claimed that at the time of French application, the Pasteur test was still only of doubtful value and that there was no proof that Gallo had used their isolate instead of his own. The French countered by saying that during their year-long wait, their test had been dramatically improved without alteration of the basic principles exposed in their application.

By the time of the patent award, the quality of the kit prepared with Montagnier's LAV antigens was not inferior to the quality of those containing Gallo's antigens; English and Australian trials even leaned clearly in favor of the former. According to the French, there was more similarity between the Pasteurian virus and the NIH virus than would be expected between independent isolates. The notebooks of Gallo's lab referred to "LAV" and not "HTLV-III." Gallo reportedly explained that he had used this label because, at the time, there was no other name. But, he maintained, he had worked only with his own isolates. During the inquest it was established that the French virus had been cultured in white cells in Gallo's lab, and electron micrographs of it had been taken.[7]

Two Viruses Are in Fact Just One

After the announcement of the HTLV-III discovery, Gallo was pressed to clarify the relationship of this virus to LAV. He tried to discourage other virologists, notably those at the CDC, from working on genetic comparisons, promising to get on with this himself right away.[8] Instead of this investigation, he and his colleagues undertook first the molecular hybridization of the three types of HTLV and published a series of experiments that suggested a relationship between HTLV-III and HTLV-I and HTLV-II. The published findings confirmed the expectations of the Bethesda team,[9] but it is now evident that they were inaccurate. According to Montagnier, Gallo's conclusions were founded on laboratory artefacts.[10]

In September 1984 Robin Weiss and his London colleagues, using in vitro cultures, established that antigens of HTLV-III and LAV were serologically identical.[11] To do better it was necessary to "clone" the two viruses by inserting their genes in bacteria (as phage inserts itself in lysogenic bacteria) in order to obtain sufficient quantities of pure virus for biochemical analysis. The next necessary step was sequencing, that is, the determination of all the nucleotides of the viral genome. These techniques, though extremely delicate, were already routine in any well-equipped molecular biology lab.

At that time, there were not two but many isolates considered possibly responsible for AIDS, and no one was sure of their exact relationship. Apart from the strains isolated by the teams of Montagnier and Gallo, there was, in the first place, the English virus of Karpas. Donald Francis of Atlanta and Jay Levy of San Francisco had found viruses in American homosexuals that they thought were similar to LAV. Levy named his virus, AIDS-Related Virus (ARV). In September 1984 the AIDS virus was also isolated in Italy by Giovanni Battista Rossi and his colleagues.[12]

Emulation, said Taine, leads to excess and marvels. The rapidity with which the cloning and sequencing of virus was accomplished at the same moment in North America and in Europe certainly leans toward the marvelous. Beatrice Hahn, Robert Gallo, Flossie Wong-Staal, and coworkers announced the molecular cloning of HTLV-III in November 1984,[13] and a few weeks later Marc Alizon, Pierre Sonigo, Françoise Barré-Sinoussi, Simon Wain-Hobson, and Luc Montagnier did the same for LAV.[14]

The exact nucleotide sequence of LAV was established by Simon Wain-Hobson, Pierre Sonigo, Olivier Danos, Stewart Cole, and Marc Alizon and published in the journal *Cell* (manuscript received December 26, 1984, after having been refused by *Nature*).[15] At the beginning of January 1985 this was also accomplished by Lee Ratner, Robert Gallo, Flossie Wong-Staal, and William Haseltine for two isolates of HTLV-III;[16] then by Paul Luciw, Jay Levy, Ray Sanchez-Pescador, and others for ARV on February 1, 1985;[17] and by Dan Capon, M. A. Muesing, and colleagues at the American firm Genentech for another ARV six days later.[18] This enormous task, altogether comprising the sequencing of some ten thousand nucleotides per virus, was completed in an incredible hurry.

Some of the structural data had been anticipated; some were surprising. As expected by many who began to disagree with Gallo and his circle, the AIDS virus was very different from HTLV-I and HTLV-II. Surprising, however, was the fact that the virus contained two genes that had never been described before. It had also been expected that the various isolates would have fundamental similarities, but it was astonishing to discover that Montagnier's LAV and Gallo's HTLV-III were identical to within 1.8 percent of nucleotides. While the other independent retroviral strains differed within usual limits (for retroviruses about 10 to 20 percent), LAV and HTLV-III varied no more than identical twins.[19]

Gallo himself had described the considerable heterogeneity of the AIDS virus and the remarkable variability of the "hot spots" along its genetic material. Isolates from two different patients are never identical. How then to explain the fact that the structure of HTLV-III was practically superposable on LAV? This gave birth to a rumor, a serious suspicion: had Popovic and Gallo really isolated HTLV-III from American patients, or did they obtain it by culturing the sample sent from Paris? In using the pool of agents taken from ten different individuals, did they not, accidentally or deliberately, introduce the French strain?

A press conference was held in New York in February 1985, followed by several sorry scientific debates and the judicial process over the diagnostic kit patents.[20]

At first, Gallo claimed that the Parisian isolate he had received in September 1983 had not been used at all because he had never succeeded in achieving more than a transient growth of it. In April 1986, however, he retracted this statement and acknowledged that they had used the virus for research purposes prior to their discovery of HTLV-III. He even admitted that the electron microscope images that appeared in the May 4, 1984, issue of *Science*, illustrating an article joined with his own announcing the discovery, was actually a picture of LAV and not, as the legend said, the new virus isolated by the American team. According to Gallo, a mix-up could have occurred during selection of the photos. The picture published was not that of HTLV-III.[21] In fact, this image appeared not in the main article but in an annexed article, and the principal author of the latter, Jorg Schüpbach, claimed that it was solely Gallo's decision to publish this photo.[22]

Gallo's confession was provoked by a curious discovery made by the lawyers for the French side. Following an anonymous telephone call in December 1985, they began to have doubts about the origin of Gallo's published photo and set about examining with the greatest attention the copies of the documents from Gallo's laboratory. On December 14, 1983, Matthew Gonda, a specialist in viral morphology at the NCI Laboratory of Cell and Molecular Structure in Frederick, Maryland, wrote to Mikulas Popovic that out of the electron microscopic photographs of thirty-three serum samples considered infected with AIDS virus, the virus was seen only in samples no. 6 and 7. A copy of this letter had been included in the inquest, but two passages were suppressed. In the original text, Gonda indicated that samples 6 and 7, the only two containing electron microscopic images of retrovirus, were labeled ''HUT78/LAV'' and ''T17.4 LAV.'' Thus, manifestly these were Popovic's cell lines infected with Montagnier's virus.[23]

Whatever lay behind this imbroglio, today it can be accepted as established that Gallo, Popovic, and collaborators had cultured LAV before or at the same time as their own isolates, and that when they announced their discovery of HTLV-III they knew that it was at least similar enough to confuse their photographic images. Gallo's laboratory notebooks make quite likely the conclusion that, at the time of the supposed discovery of the HTLV-III virus, his team had not yet succeeded in cultivating any permanent lines of the American isolate of this virus.

A Political Compromise

The dispute was settled in March 1987 with an amiable agreement between the U.S. Department of Health and Human Services and the Pasteur Institute. Removing all doubt about the political expediency of such a move, the agreement was announced in Washington as a common declaration by U.S. president Ronald Reagan and French prime minister Jacques Chirac, a conservative who was beginning to emerge as the Right's candidate for president against socialist leader François Mitterand. The French would abandon the judicial process and renounce rights to damages for income already acquired by the opposite party; the Americans would add the name of Montagnier to that of Gallo to their patent for the diagnostic kit, henceforth to be recognized as a common invention to which both parties held equal rights. In the future, each party could make liberal use of the technological achievements and discoveries of the other, and 80 percent of all profits were to be donated to a joint foundation to finance research in AIDS and other retrovirus diseases.[24]

As an integral part of the agreement, Gallo and Montagnier published a ''by no means exhaustive'' chronological history of AIDS research, promising not to "make nor publish any statement which would or could be construed as contradicting or compromising the integrity of said scientific history." A confidential protocol was signed at the same time by the two sides. Lawyers of both parties declared that all those not expressly bound by the agreement were able to examine the terms freely and carefully. In fact, the published document is scarcely more than a bibliographical list, by date of publication, including summaries but not interpretations of the published texts. All that a historian finds litigious or somber in this affair was carefully glossed over in silence.[25]

The Structure and Life Cycle of HIV

Many theoretical and practical questions were resolved with cloning and sequencing of the AIDS virus. Its structural organization is decidedly different from that of the HTLV family. It is indeed a lentivirus, related to the visna virus of sheep. These features were demonstrated by comparative morphology, particularly by the work of Matthew Gonda using electron microscopy, and by comparison of sequencing of the visna virus done in 1985 by Pierre Sonigo at the Pasteur Institute, together with Ashley Haase of the University of Minnesota.[26]

The structure of HIV and its mechanism of action came to be understood between 1984 and 1986.[27] It is an RNA virus, a typical retrovirus, with a roughly globular shape and fairly high molecular weight. Its string of genetic information, its payload, is encased in a protein capsule, called the "core" or "nucleoid," which in turn is packaged in an envelope made up of lipid and two glycoproteins. Each virion (single virus) contains two copies of RNA, reminiscent of chromosome pairs.

The genome of HIV is more complicated than that of most other known retroviruses. As in other retroviruses, three genes code for the structure (*gag* for internal proteins, *pol* for transcriptase, and *env* for the envelope), but HIV has a particular genomic organization with several other genes that code for regulation of the viral processes. William Haseltine in Boston and Flossie Wong-Staal in Bethesda began to understand the extremely refined machinery of this virus, especially the role of the gene *tat*, which "turns on" the structural genes. This is a system of feedback loops which apparently allows the virus to adapt to different circumstances and modify its life cycle according to the state of the infected cell. In other intracellular parasites, nothing like it had ever been seen before.[28]

HIV has a particular affinity for T4-lymphocytes. The glycoprotein, gp120, of the external envelope recognizes and reacts with a molecule, known as CD4, on the surface of the lymphocyte and certain other cells, thereby fixing the virus to the cell. This glycoprotein was identified independently by both Myron Essex's team at Harvard and Luc Montagnier's team in Paris.[29] The receptor role of the CD4 molecule was also demonstrated by two independent groups: David Klatzmann with a group of scientists at the Pasteur Institute, and Angus Dalgleish and Robin Weiss of London. The virus is attracted to this molecule, and its binding with it results in cellular damage. After lymphocytes have been incubated with antibodies directed to the CD4 molecule, they cannot be infected by the AIDS virus.[30]

When the viral RNA enters the cytoplasm of the infected cell, it is transcribed into DNA by the action of reverse transcriptase, a biochemical apparatus made up of two specific enzyme activities contained in the virus itself. The viral DNA then enters the nucleus of the cell to become part of the chromosomal material. Integrated like this into the cell genome, the virus temporarily loses its individuality and can remain latent for a number of years. During this period, the cell appears to be normal and the virus seems to disappear. Its essential part is hidden in the form of a so-called provirus, a piece of viral DNA attached to the host DNA. In this state, the virus is invulnerable to drugs; it can be destroyed only by killing the cell.

The proviral DNA may be silent, but it is still "alive" because it is transmitted to every daughter cell after each cellular division. This elegant parasitism penetrates the very heart of the host's control center and thereby differs from the classic model of infection, which places the invading microbe in frank opposition to the cell. Fortunately, research conducted in the middle of our century on the mechanism of integration of the bacteriophage into bacteria and on the genetic determinism of lysogeny permitted a rapid comprehension of the life cycle of human retroviruses.

The provirus can be activated to take over the enzymes and ribosomes of the host cell, inducing them to make viruses. Activation of viral replication depends on the functional state of the lymphocyte. It can be provoked in vitro by certain chemical compounds and bacterial toxins and is very likely unleashed in vivo by antigenic stimulation. The virus comes out of hiding during another infection, which activates the lymphocyte infected with HIV.

During viral replication, cell division is turned off and the cell dies. Unlike the oncoviruses, including HTLV, the AIDS virus does not kill the host organism by causing its cells to reproduce uncontrollably; it kills by destroying a particular set of host cells. Presently, the mechanism of cellular destruction provoked by the burgeoning of viral particles is still only poorly understood, because cells not directly infected also die. Dani Bolognesi and his colleagues have demonstrated that the gp120 envelope glycoprotein by itself can also bind with CD4 on healthy cells; thus gp120 molecules spread by the virus could kill cells, either directly by damaging them (cytotoxicity), or indirectly by causing the host's immune system to attack its own "marked" cell.[31]

The capacity of HIV to damage cells (its cytopathogenicity) varies greatly from strain to strain. This corresponds with the remarkable genetic heterogeneity of strains isolated in Africa, Europe, and America.

Haunts of HIV

Contrary to early medical ideas, HIV does not attack lymphocytes only; it infects all cells having the CD4 molecule on their membranes. Targets include certain white cells called monocytes, especially the macrophage, which is derived from monocytes. They probably constitute the most important reservoir of the virus. Macrophages can provide virus to sustain the infection of lymphocytes for a long time after the virus enters the organism.[32] Actual numbers of infected lymphocytes circulating in an HIV positive individual, or even in a person with full-blown AIDS, are relatively small. The virus can be found in monocytes of the lung and brain; its action in these organs is not due solely to immunodepression.[33]

The AIDS virus was first isolated from lymph nodes and blood taken from both sick and healthy persons. In October 1984 Daniel Zagury, Jerome Groopman, Robert Gallo, and colleagues reported its isolation from the semen of two AIDS patients. At the same time, David Ho, Martin Hirsch, and their colleagues found it in the semen of an apparently healthy homosexual,[34] while Groopman and Gallo et al. located the virus in the saliva of one AIDS patient and in several other people either healthy or sick with AIDS-related conditions.[35] In blood and semen, HIV is found inside lymphocytes (more in semen than in blood), but it can also be free ouside of cells.[36] Epidemiological studies suggested that the virus was present in cervico-vaginal secretions, although proof of this took some time.[37] It has also been identified in tears, breast milk, and cerebro-spinal fluid.[38] In March 1985 George Shaw and others in Gallo's lab demonstrated the presence of the virus in the brain tissue. This was confirmed by several groups: Simone Gartner and colleagues, who managed to isolate a neurotropic form of HIV from a brain sample taken from a patient; Rozemay Vazeux, Luc Montagnier, and others in Paris; Marc Stoler and collaborators, who detected the virus inside brain macrophages and microglial cells using in situ hybridization.[39] The teams of E. Tschachler and of Daniel Schmitt found that HIV infiltrated certain cells of skin and mucosa (epidermal Langerhans cells).[40]

The virus may come to the body surface, but it cannot be transmitted by touch. It is highly susceptible to heat and disinfectants. Virologists confirmed the conclusions of epidemiologists: the principal vehicles of spread are semen and blood. The virus is found in the vagina, but only in relatively small numbers. This explains the possibility of infection from female to male through vaginal intercourse, and the even greater ease with which this can occur in the opposite direction.

DNA sequences identical to those of HIV were found in the genomes of African insects by Jean-Claude Chermann and his team in 1986. This, however, is insufficient to implicate insects as vectors of the human disease,[41] especially since, at the time of writing, epidemiological evidence argues strongly against this hypothesis. Nevertheless, it is not impossible that insects could play some role in the natural history of the retrovirus.

Other Viruses Associated with AIDS

In October 1985 the Portuguese biologist, Maria-Odette Santos-Ferreira, came to Paris to learn virus isolation techniques at the Pasteur Institute. She brought blood samples from a patient from Guinea-Bissau, who had been treated at the Egas Moniz Hospital in Lisbon since early 1985. Clinically, the patient suffered from unmistakable AIDS, yet his blood was negative in ELISA and RIPA tests. Luc Montagnier and his team used the same techniques on this patient's blood that they had employed when they first isolated the previously unknown LAV from a lymph node. The virus displayed preference for T4-lymphocytes and cytopathic effects, similar to those of HIV, but hybridization experiments, done by François Clavel, revealed that only a small amount of the genetic material bore any relationship to the genome of the old LAV. There were similarities in genomic structure, but the details were quite different.[42]

In spite of the considerable genetic variability of HIV, previously isolated strains from all over the world contained the same antigenic sites on their three main proteins (p24/25 inside, and gp120 and gp41–43 outside). The prototypical strains, LAV and HTLV-III, had been used as a source of antigens to identify antibodies of all known strains. Here was a new virus with antigenic proteins so different from the others that none of the commonly used diagnostic reagents could detect its presence. If this new virus could also cause AIDS, a negative test for HIV antibodies would lose its reassuring significance.

Research was focused on AIDS patients who were seronegative. In early 1986 such a patient was identified at the Claude Bernard Hospital. He came from Cap-Vert off Senegal and had been hospitalized in Paris since 1983. A second representative of the new virus was found in his blood. It was named LAV-2, and later changed to HIV-2. Diagnostic tests to recognize this virus were soon made available, and their application revealed that HIV-2 was responsible for a large epidemic focus in West Africa. It is transmitted mainly through heterosexual relations.[43] The cloning and sequencing of the genome of the new virus was accomplished between the fall of 1986 and the spring of 1987, in a united effort by several French research workers, including the Centre National de Recherche Scientifique (CNRS), the Institut National de Services et Recherches Médicales (INSERM), and the Pasteur Institute.[44]

In September 1984 Ronald Desrosiers, M. D. Daniel, and Myron Essex isolated a new type of retrovirus in the blood of macaques raised in captivity and suffering from a syndrome analogous to human AIDS.[45] To reflect its relationship to HTLV-III, it was named STLV-III$_{mac}$, later altered by the international virus nomenclature commission to SIV. In the blood of wild

African green monkeys from Ethiopia and Kenya, Essex's team found antibodies that reacted better with the antigens of the macaque retrovirus than they did with those of HIV.[46] From these monkeys, they isolated a retroviral strain, which they named STLV-III$_{agm}$.[47] The first isolate turned out to be a laboratory contaminant, but eventually several strains of SIV were found in the blood of apparently healthy green monkeys. Another species of African monkey, the sooty mangabey (*Cercocebus atys*), frequently carries a strain of this virus (STLV-III$_{smm}$) inside lymphocytes with no obvious problem.[48]

The Tours virologist Francis Barin examined blood samples collected by Souleyman M'Boup, a doctor at a public health clinic for prostitutes in Dakar, Senegal. These women were not sick, but their blood revealed a relatively high level of seropositivity. Barin had spent a study period at Essex's lab in Boston and thus had the opportunity to compare these results with the analyses made on the blood of green monkeys. He discovered that the Dakar people had been infected with a virus that was serologically closer to SIV than to HIV.[49]

Myron Essex and Phyllis Kanki isolated a retrovirus in blood taken from apparently healthy citizens of Dakar and found it to be antigenically similar to the AIDS virus.[50] They named it HTLV-IV, but its existence was short-lived. It is still discussed in scientific publications as an isolate of HIV-2, the American counterpart of the French LAV-2, but the sad truth is already known. James Mullins and other Harvard researchers soon cloned this virus to reveal that it was none other than STLV-III (SIV), Desrosier's macaque virus, which had contaminated their cultures in the lab.[51]

At the time of writing, there are still a few well-respected scientists who refuse to recognize HIV as the ''cause'' of AIDS. One of the rebels against current opinion is Peter Duesberg, professor of molecular biology at Berkeley, who, contrary to generally accepted thinking, sees HIV as an innocuous, or only slightly harmful, opportunistic retrovirus. According to this scientist, HIV, which is frequent in conditions that favor the true and still unknown cause, would be only a reliable indicator of exposure to risk. He is ready, he claims, to be injected with HIV as long as he can be assured that the isolate is purified beyond suspicion. Obviously, he only theorizes and has not carried out the experiment. Duesberg's criticisms of the official thesis are not without value inasmuch as they indicate zones of uncertainty and show that satisfactory solutions to certain significant problems are yet to be found. But perhaps he has been too quick to jump from methodological difficulties to negative conclusions.[52]

Strong criticisms of the etiological role of HIV in AIDS may have been dealt with, but a few weak criticisms remain. Today it is said that HIV is the cause of AIDS, just as Koch's bacillus is the cause of tuberculosis and Schaudinn's pale spirochete is the cause of syphilis. Their presence in an organism is necessary but not sufficient to produce the disease. The pathological action of this virus occurs only under certain conditions that depend on the constitution of the host organism and on its milieu. This may seem obvious, but is the analogy between HIV and the agents of tuberculosis and syphilis really perfect? Does the AIDS virus act alone like the other two, or does it require an accomplice? The answer is still not known.

CHAPTER 8

The Stages of AIDS

Περὶ δὲ τῶν ἀφανεστάτων

καὶ χαλεπωτάτων

νοσημάτων δόξῃ μᾶλλον

ἢ τέχνῃ κρίνεται.

As for the most hidden

and most difficult diseases,

conjectures are more

decisive than (established

medical) art.

—Hippocrates,

personification of the

ideal doctor

IN 1985 THE AIDS epidemic entered a new phase. Recognition of HIV seropositivity altered the social dimensions of the disease and introduced serious medical, ethical, and legal problems of surprising complexity. In addition, the African focus began to reveal other epidemiological facets of AIDS that were even more disturbing than those of the American focus. All over the world, the most dismal prognoses were being confirmed; the exponential rise in numbers of seropositives and the geographic expansion of the infection took on the proportions of an international catastrophe. From this time on, AIDS was a true pandemic.

AIDS therapy is improving progressively, but in the absence of a miracle drug against the virus, it remains only palliative. The search for a protective vaccine has been even more disappointing. Nevertheless, enormous scientific effort, unprecedented in medical history, has elucidated the pathogenetic mechanisms and characterized the different stages of AIDS.[1]

Every disease has its own natural history, its own spectrum of abnormal conditions ranging from the moment of infection, in the strict sense of the word (penetration in the host organism), to recovery of health, chronic illness (permanent equilibrium between the pathogen and the host defenses), or death. At the outset, physicians were fascinated by the original and unexpected aspects of this disease, manifested not through specific lesions, but through the intermediary of other diseases. After 1985 it became increasingly clear that, in spite of these undeniably original features, HIV infection did correspond, at least in part, to a "classic" pathogenetic pattern: not all virus particles that had entered the host organism and multiplied there disappeared in the nuclei of lymphocytes to become the latent proviral constituent of the genome. Some viruses continued to propagate and cause particular symptoms. The effect of the infection is concurrently immunopathogenic and cytopathogenic.

Seropositivity: A New Epidemiological Dimension

How can it be known if someone has been infected with the AIDS virus? The procedure used to isolate a specific retrovirus is too long, too complicated, and too expensive to be applied as a routine diagnostic test to all suspected individuals. Indirect proof of the presence of the virus in the host organism is necessary. After the identification and isolation of HIV retrovirus (back in the time of LAV and HTLV-III), the teams of Montagnier and Gallo both designed specific tests using standard technical methods. These tests detect the presence in the examined serum of specific antibodies, which are produced whenever the immune system comes into contact with a foreign organic substance, such as bacterial, or, as in this case, viral proteins. Antibodies are biochemical correspondents of viral antigens, that is, a sort of "complementary" molecule that "fits" the proteins of the viral envelope and internal core.

The ELISA (Enzyme-Linked Immuno-Sorbent Assay) is the easiest and quickest of these tests. The presence of molecules that combine specifically with purified viral antigen is detected by a color reaction. The ELISA method is adapted from the immuno-diagnostic technique invented by Swedish scientists E. Engwall and P. Perlman in 1971. The Western blot and RIPA (Radio-Immuno-Precipitation Assay) are sophisticated tests that make use of electrophoretic analysis of immunoglobulins, which are fixed by incubation of the test serum with viral proteins. Proviral DNA can be detected by hybridization through molecular probes, but this procedure often fails.

The name "Western blot" has an amusing origin. In 1974 the Scottish biochemist E. M. Southern invented an electrophoretic procedure for identifying DNA by the position of spots made by the substance on gel or on blotting paper after exposure to an electric current. Hence the name "Southern blot." When this same method was applied to the analysis of RNA, it was nicknamed "Northern blot." When Southern's technique was applied to proteins, the play on words was extended to "Western blot."

As a result of the elaboration of these serological tests, a new concept came to alter the dimensions of AIDS: seropositivity. This concept overturned the epidemiological data concerning the frequency and distribution of HIV infection, introduced semantic difficulties and, on the practical side, created tremendous ethical and psychological problems.

A clearly defined and unambiguous notion began to replace the ill-defined and frequently humiliating term "high-risk group" (used for the lack of anything better by epidemiologists to indicate a segment of the population statistically more exposed to infection). A person is "seropositive" if the result of tests done on his or her serum is positive. The precise meaning of this result became an important scientific and social problem. Beginning in 1984, studies of seroprevalence (the frequency of seropositivity in a determined population) were begun first on limited groups in France[2] and the United States,[3] and then on a representative sample in England.[4]

At first, the diagnostic tests were not sensitive enough, because the viral components used had not been sufficiently concentrated and purified. Improvements were steadily made and, by the summer of 1985, AIDS kits using ELISA became commercially available as a routine diagnostic procedure. From this moment on, governments of several industrialized countries ordered the mandatory testing of all blood donors for HIV.

Thus a previously hidden portion of the viral invasion suddenly became visible. After testing several thousand samples in 1985, the French transfusion centers announced a rate of 0.5 to 1 seropositives in every thousand healthy donors. These figures matched those among blood donors in the French army. Since October 1985 all civilian applicants for the United States military service have been routinely tested for evidence of HIV infection. The overall prevalence of seropositivity in this population was over one per thousand. Results of several surveys and of testing in blood collection centers suggested that the number of seropositives in France and the United States was between fifty and one hundred times that of the number of patients who suffered from overt AIDS. In 1985 the CDC anounced their estimate of five hundred thousand to one million Americans presumed to be seropositive, a staggering figure at the time. The WHO placed the estimate for the whole of France at fifty thousand (out of a population roughly one quarter that of the United States). In equatorial Africa, studies of seroprevalence among blood donors, prostitutes, and patients hospitalized for other conditions revealed that the situation went far beyond the worst expectations.

Since 1984 a fact of major significance has been recognized: seropositives were known to be infectious. In classical epidemiology, seropositives might be called "healthy carriers." This term was part of the explanatory baggage of past disorders, but its use with respect to HIV introduced difficulties. Healthy carriers in other epidemics, like typhoid, could endanger other people without themselves succumbing to the infection they harbored and spread. This was certainly not the case with HIV seropositivity.

Here was a curious paradox. Seropositivity did indeed indicate the presence of antibodies to the AIDS virus, but it was not a good prognostic sign. In other diseases, this type of seropositivity is to some extent a measure of the degree of immune protection. Even after the virus is completely eliminated, antibodies can remain as a form of chemical memory to provide future protection against another infection by the same virus. Nothing of the sort occurs in AIDS. The paradox comes from the fact that, on one hand, the antibody level reflects the extent of infection in AIDS while, on the other, immune mechanisms are generally ineffective. Anti-HIV antibodies can neutralize the virus in a test tube, but they are not efficient enough in life. It is for this same reason that it has not yet been possible to create a vaccine against AIDS, at least by the so-called classic methods aimed at raising antibody levels. It seems that, through some perverse effect, a high level of anti-HIV antibody may even favor the entry of the virus into macrophages and its propagation in these cells.

Extremely serious psychological and ethical problems relate to the fact that seropositivity is not only a precarious state for affected individuals but also a source of danger for their sexual partners and for others who come in direct contact with their blood. Should all persons tested be told the truth? The whole truth? And how to tell them? Should the sexual partners of seropositives be informed? What should be done to help the newly aware seropositive person cope with life under the threat of terminal illness, both to prevent social ostracism and to protect others? In Bavaria an AIDS patient was found criminally responsible for having consciously taken the risk of transmitting the disease to another. In Sweden, in the case of a seropositive prostitute addicted to heroin, a court decided on forced incarceration—for life, it appears, since there is no hope of reversing her condition. Similar cases involving charges of criminal behavior have preoccupied the media in the United States, Canada, Belgium, and Italy. Such judicial decisions have outraged those who, in the name of human rights, seek to defend the freedoms of individuals. The profusion of publications on these issues since 1986 illustrates only too well both the novelty of the situations and the exquisite pain of the moral conflicts provoked by the AIDS pandemic.[5]

Reliability of the Tests

The consequences of a positive test are so great for the future of the person tested and, especially in the case of blood donations, for the health of others, that it is imperative to know exactly to what extent the test can be trusted. Reliability means sensitivity and specificity. The more sensitive a test, the less often it will miss a truly positive serum; the more specific a test, the fewer cases that are truly negative will be reported as positive. The ELISA test is quite sensitive, usually with less than one percent false negatives, but it is not very specific, leading sometimes to 2 to 3 percent false positives even under ideal conditions. The Western blot and RIPA assays are highly specific, with only rare false positives, but they are more costly and require qualified technologists.[6] As a result, broad screening is done with ELISA, but no serum is considered to be a true positive until the reaction has been confirmed by at least one of the other two tests available. The great drawback to all these modalities aimed at detecting the presence of antibodies is the fact that seroconversion does not occur until some weeks or even months after infection.

Obviously, things became more complicated when the second AIDS virus (HIV-2) was found. Immunological cross reaction between the two viruses is weak for the envelope proteins, although it is strong for internal proteins. This means that serum from a person with antibodies to HIV-2 might appear negative in tests for HIV-1. An ELISA test for HIV-2 was made commercially available at the end of 1986.

So-called second-generation AIDS testing is now in the works. New tests based on enzymatic gene amplification can directly detect either viral RNA or proviral DNA or specific viral proteins. The amplification method PCR (Polymerase Chain Reaction) allows confirmation of the presence of minute quantities of viral nucleic acid.[7] These tests are positive soon after infection, overcoming the problem of delay before seroconversion. Direct detection of proviral DNA has permitted the identification of infection in some high-risk persons who had been seronegative by earlier tests (e.g., homosexuals who have had frequent relations with seropositive partners).

Paths of Transmission

In the last five years, clinical observations, epidemiological statistics, and laboratory experiments have all confirmed that HIV is not very contagious and that its routes of transmission are quite limited. It is transmitted only by three routes: sexual contact, direct inoculation or injection of blood in tissues or blood vessels, or mother-child transmission through the placenta or breast milk.

Sexual contact is without doubt the most common means of infection. In semen and vaginal secretions of infected persons, the virus is present in small quantities in a free state and in much greater quantities in close association with the infected cells. It seems that infection is realized mostly by contaminated living cells, although free viral particles can also spread disease.[8] Historically, transmission between homosexual partners was the first recognized path of infection. The pernicious role of infected sperm inside the rectal mucosa was easy to demonstrate and to comprehend, but epidemiological inquiry revealed that infection could operate in the opposite direction too, from the passive to the active partner during anal coitus.[9]

Since the epidemic began, with an outbreak in the American homosexual community, there was a fairly long delay before doctors recognized the possibility of spread by heterosexual relations. This was established when the illness was observed in the female partners of a few males who had been infected via contact with blood.[10] Biologists demonstrated infection of female chimpanzees by vaginal introduction of the virus.[11] Clinicians described cases that could have occurred by no route other than infected sperm in the vagina. But this path is still the exception, at least in the United States and Europe. Statistics suggest that no more than 2 percent of all occidental adult AIDS patients are women who have contracted the disease through heterosexual relations, including anal coitus. The latter may be a more risky practice than vaginal intercourse because the intact epithelial lining of the vagina offers a significant barrier to the passage of HIV, whereas the cells of the rectal mucosa are particularly receptive.[12]

The sexual transmission of HIV, never perfectly controllable in the usual circumstances of life, was fully demonstrated by a sort of involuntary experiment in Australia. An Australian woman developed lymphadenopathy and became seropositive after artificial insemination by a previously frozen mixture of semen. A search for the eight sperm donors revealed that one was seropositive and that his semen had been used in eight different inseminations. Among the eight recipients, one developed clinical disease, three became seropositive, and the four remaining escaped harm. At the time of writing, three children born of these inseminations are well.[13]

For several years, female to male transmission was considered to be an unlikely event, but epidemiological surveys in Africa have dispelled all doubt that this does occur.[14] In Europe and the United States, however, it is not common. It increases from year to year, but still remains secondary: as of January 1988, only 0.5 percent of all AIDS cases known to the CDC were males infected by heterosexual contact.[15] It is entirely possible that this situation could change and that the epidemiological patterns of American AIDS may come to resemble those of Africa.

No serious study provides an accurate estimate of the chance of contracting AIDS from a single sexual contact. In heterosexual couples who have had regular, unprotected intercourse for months or even several years, seropositivity in one partner does not automatically mean seroconversion for the other. In this setting, diverse surveys have shown that the infection rate varies widely from 10 to 60 percent with a mean of 25 percent. The situation in North America and Europe differs from that observed in Africa, where it appears there is a much higher risk of spread through heterosexual contact. Cofactors must therefore facilitate or hinder infection. It appears that some infected subjects transmit the infection more efficiently than others. If this is true, then relations with multiple infected partners would usually carry a greater danger than the same number of encounters with a single infected partner.

According to recent epidemiological surveys, an individual's risk of becoming infected as a result of homosexual or heterosexual relations can be positively correlated with the number of partners, the frequency of other sexually transmitted diseases they have had, and with the practice of traumatizing sexual activity.

HIV virus can be found in the saliva of AIDS patients and seropositive individuals, but only in minute quantities. According to in vitro studies, saliva contains substances that seem to inactivate HIV.[16] An impassioned debate, of great practical import, rages over the significance of saliva in AIDS infection. A few cases have implicated transmission from the mouth during homosexual fellatio[17] and lesbian orogenital practices,[18] but at the time of writing, there is no well-documented case of AIDS having been transmitted by deep kissing or even by biting.

The most efficient mode of spread is transfusion of infected whole blood or concentrated blood products. Nevertheless, even when given this direct introduction of the virus into a healthy person, HIV does not always take hold—or at least, does not always provoke an immune response. About 10 percent of those who have received HIV positive blood did not undergo sero-conversion.[19]

Transfusion is not the only therapeutic intervention that can offer exposure to HIV infection. People on hemodialysis and those who have had organ transplants are not beyond the reach of this new danger. In Germany, a patient contracted AIDS following an initially successful renal transplant. The kidney had been taken from the dead body of an infected man. It was then learned that two other cadaver donors in that country had been seropositive and that the infection had been "transplanted" to five kidney recipients.[20] In recent years, several other cases of HIV infection have been documented via kidney, cornea, and especially bone marrow transplants. It became urgently necessary to perform systematic tests on all brain-dead individuals who might serve as potential organ donors.[21]

In drug addicts who inject themselves with heroin, cocaine, or other substances, infection is spread by the sharing of nonsterilized needles and syringes. An accidental needlestick can also transmit the disease, but so far this has been quite rare.[22] Until 1987 seroconversion has occurred in only five of several hundred health-care workers who have had such accidental contact (two American cases, three French). Four other persons—three nurses and a medical technician—have been infected by accidental external contact with infected blood. The first of these, an English nurse, had a chronic skin condition of the hands. The second, an American, had a chapped finger that was touched by blood oozing through a dressing. The third was splashed in the face with blood from the explosion of a vacuum test tube. She had facial acne and some blood probably came in contact with her mouth as well. The last, an American laboratory technician, was splattered on her hands and forearms by blood from a cell separator. She had a rash on her ear, which she may have touched with her soiled hand.[23] At least two other cases are known in which the infection was transmitted in the laboratory as an occupational accident during virological manipulations.[24] In France, there is one case of infection by the AIDS virus in a person who had been treated by the Chinese method of acupuncture.

An infected mother can transmit the disease to her child during intrauterine life. HIV has been positively identified in fetal tissue. A seropositive mother can also infect her child through breast milk. This explains how AIDS passed to three newborns whose mothers had received transfusions of infected blood after delivery. It is difficult to give an accurate estimate of the risk of vertical transmission from the infected mother. About a 40 percent chance of contracting the disease is given for a baby born of a seropositive mother (figures range from 25 to 50 percent). If the first child was infected, the risk for the second may be as high as 65 percent.[25]

From an epidemiological point of view, all these routes are relatively sheltered: the infection is not spread by air, ingestion, dirty objects, nor by simple contact with the carrier. Nevertheless, a "crisis" was announced in the summer of 1988 by the famous American sexologists William Masters, Virginia Johnson, and Robert Kolodny, who claimed to publicize their fears in the name of humanity and concluded, "categorically, that infection with the AIDS virus does *not* require intimate sexual contact or sharing of intravenous needles: transmission can, and does, occur as a result of person-to-person contact in which blood or other body fluids from a person who is harboring the virus are splashed onto or rubbed against someone else, even if this is a single, isolated occurrence."[26]

The arguments advanced for this opinion are epidemiological. According to their survey, the epidemic has spilled over, from the original U.S. male homosexual population, to flood other sectors to a previously unimagined extent. Concerning modes of transmission, these writers present suppositions and fears as if they were documented facts. Masters and his coauthors are unable to give any proof of the actual danger of a simple external contact with the blood and secretions of an AIDS patient. American epidemiological services have investigated over two thousand such cases without finding a single consequent seroconversion.[27]

It still seems that the virus is unable to penetrate normal skin. This cannot be said often enough: there is absolutely no evidence that AIDS has ever been spread under normal living conditions—not in schools, not in crowded buses or trains, not in restaurants, not at the hairdressers', not in business meetings, not even between members of the same family who live in abject poverty and share the most dismal of sanitary conditions. AIDS cannot be contracted from a handshake, a swimming pool, or a toilet seat. It breaks through the barrier separating individuals only by sexual activity, the biology of maternity, the injection of drugs, or medical intervention.[28]

The Silent Stages

Is it justified to use the term "healthy carrier" to describe anti-HIV seropositive individuals when it evokes a fundamentally false analogy with other infectious diseases? The risk conveyed by seropositivity requires that the notion of health be replaced by that of a state of latency. After the initial invasion, the AIDS virus does seem to vanish, yet it persists in the organism, mostly integrated in the genome of certain somatic cells. This type of latency, not to be confused with the incubation period, was an unforeseen phenomenon, an un-expected complication in the host-parasite relationship.

Most people put lesions, symptoms, syndromes, disease states, illnesses, and diseases into one fairly vague general concept. Even medical discourse suffers from this type of confusion, and this is the source of certain difficulties that arise in the analysis of clinical cases of possible AIDS from the period before 1980. It is necessary to know that a lung abscess is a lesion; cough, a symptom; chronic pneumonia, a syndrome; consumption, a state of disease; a patient's suffering from a cluster of ills, an illness; or, tuberculosis, a disease. These terms do not share the same degree of logical abstraction, and it is annoying to find that, in many clinical descriptions, these different pathological realities are mixed together and considered on an equal level.

The incomplete, even erroneous conceptualization of AIDS, at the beginning of clinical investigations, has left an unfortunate confusion that persists in present terminology: AIDS simultaneously means a "state of disease," that is, a cluster of particular clinical manifestations of an acquired immunodeficiency; and a "disease," in the strict sense, that is, the pathological condition resulting from HIV infection.

It has been confirmed that HIV has a special affinity for cells with the CD4 molecule on their surface membrane. When it enters the host by a route providing direct access to the circulating blood, the virus penetrates T4-lympho-cytes, macrophages, and other monocytes, and certain cells in the central nervous system. It remains quiescent in resting T4-cells and does not immediately reproduce itself. Activation of these T4-cells causes the virus to enter the cell's genome. In the first few days after infection, the virus multiplies rapidly and the number of infected cells increases, but there is still no measurable alteration in the host's body functions or immune reactions. This is the *incubation period*. It can last from six to eight weeks, and occasionally much longer. Sometimes antibodies do not appear until several months after the infection.

After the incubation period, the patient suffers from the *primary infection syndrome*: fatigue, mild fever, sweats, swollen lymph nodes, joint and muscle aches, occasional sore throat, fleeting diarrhea, and a maculo-papular cutaneous rash on the trunk. These disturbances may last up to two weeks and disappear spontaneously. Neurological signs have also been reported during this period, but they are slight and irregular.[29] This flulike syndrome seems so ordinary that its association with AIDS was not appreciated for a long time. Most often, it is subclinical and passes unnoticed, but an outstanding event, *seroconversion,* takes place, which marks the beginning of the next stage.

This first plateau of equilibrium between the virus and the host defenses is generally called *latency*. In fact, latency, when the virus is completely silent or "sleeping" in the infected cells, must be distinguished from the state of *chronic infection*, which is also clinically mute but can be detected by biological signs (such as seropositivity, determined by testing for the presence of antibodies, increased neopterine in urine,[30] etc.). Most doctors do not clearly differentiate between these two states, and the word "latent" has been applied both to the absolute silence of the virus and to conditions in which its activity is reduced to infraclinical manifestations, without obvious symptoms. The discovery of the virus inside macrophages and nervous-system cells suggested that these sites were the main source of ongoing infection and thus the period following seroconversion, originally thought to be quiescent, came to be seen as one of low-grade chronic infection in the vast majority of cases.[31]

The state of latency or low-grade infection can last for a long time, perhaps an entire normal lifespan. Time is still lacking for a precise determination of its average duration or its possible upper limit. Posttransfusional AIDS has been the model for this determination, since the exact moment of infection is known. A mathematical model was used to analyze the data of 297 patients who were transfused with infected blood between April 1978 and February 1986 and in whom lymph node enlargement or overt AIDS was diagnosed between January 1982 and June 1986. The results suggest that the time lag between infection and first clinical manifestations varies with age: approximately two years in children aged four or under years; eight years in persons five to fifty-nine years; and five and a half years in people over sixty. The average duration is longer in females (8.6 years) than males (5.6 years). These results underestimate the actual mean duration. The longer such observations are made, the more the mean duration is corrected upwards. It is possible that the duration of this subclinical state is dependent on the route of transmission, and that it is longer when the virus enters the host across mucous membranes rather than through direct inoculation of blood.[32]

Advanced Clinical Forms

Viral antigens are present in blood before the appearance of antibodies, then they decrease sharply only to rise again with the onset of clinical symptoms. This is when the latent or chronic form of AIDS changes into the active form. The patient's immune system maintains a sort of balance between its normal function and the alterations induced by HIV. It might be tempting to say that the immune system held control over viral reproduction. In fact, this system has itself already been invaded by the enemy. When a certain biochemical signal turns it on, the viral agents kill T4-lymphocytes, creating a chink in the cellular defenses of the immune armor and opening the way for opportunistic infection.

HIV infection is responsible for numerous disease states of severities ranging from mild asymptomatic immunodepression and relatively benign infections to aggressive malignancies, severe neurological damage, and life-threatening opportunistic infection. In 1986 the Walter Reed Army Institute of Research (WR) and the CDC proposed a classification of HIV infection and its associated conditions.[33] The WR system grades the evolution of disease in six hierarchical stages reflecting the chronological and biological status of infection: WR1 is silent, asymptomatic; WR2–WR5 encompasses prolonged lymphadenopathy and related symptoms, which have also been called ARC (AIDS-Related Complex); WR6 represents full-blown AIDS defined by systemic immune deficiency and heavy opportunistic infections.[34]

Swelling of lymph nodes and the most varied but minor clinical manifestations begin quietly and increase slowly. They can persist for several years, progressing gradually toward proven AIDS, or they can abruptly convert into terminal immunodeficiency. The final stage, or AIDS in the strict sense, appears in diverse clinical forms, where serious opportunistic infections, Kaposi's sarcoma, and non-Hodgkin's lymphoma predominate.[35]

The duration of each stage is not fixed. It can be altered by the exposure of the organism to "cofactors." This offers the hope that, in some fortunate individuals, the silent stage might persist for a very long time or even indefinitely. Laboratory exposure of infected cell cultures to various carcinogens and antigens (other viruses, pathogenic bacteria, etc.) can arouse the dormant virus, hidden in the cell genome. In the human body the destructive process is unleashed by immunostimulation, which is the activation of the cells that "police" the organism. The immune response, the very process that should defeat a virus, has, in the case of HIV infection, the perverse effect of increasing viral reproduction. It is possible that other factors leading to immunodepression, such as intestinal absorption of sperm, drugs, malnutrition, and some diseases, can have the same effect via a different pathogenic mechanism. Whatever the case may be, it seems that superinfections do play an essential role in AIDS, not only as the opportunistic diseases resulting from the breakdown of the immune system, but also as a sort of detonator for the viral explosion.

Prognosis of Seropositivity and Cerebral AIDS

In the five years following infection, 10 to 20 percent of people will progress to proven AIDS and another 20 to 40 percent will have minor symptoms. In San Francisco, between 1978 and 1980, a cohort of 6,700 homosexual and bisexual males voluntarily donated blood for an epidemiological survey on hepatitis-B. By September 1987, this group was found to have 75 percent seropositivity for HIV. Sixty-three of those infected prior to 1982 were randomly selected for careful monitoring. Five years after the most likely moment of infection, 15 percent had proven AIDS; in one more year, this had risen to 24 percent; another year after that, to 31 percent; and during the next year, the figure approached 40 percent. In 1987, seven years and four months after the most likely date of infection, 40 percent had persistent lymphadeno-pathy or a related condition, but approximately 20 percent of these seropositive individuals still had no clinical symptoms whatsoever.[36]

It is impossible to predict the overall risk of progressing from seropositivity to the final stage of AIDS. The observations to date indicate that the risk does not decline with time, suggesting a pessimistic outlook for all seropositives, but these estimates are based on limited periods of study, not long enough to permit pertinent conclusions. In a few rare cases, spontaneous disappearance of seropositivity has been observed, perhaps because the virus has been effectively eliminated. This inversion has occurred only when the seroconversion resulted from a single contact with a minimal quantity of virus, such as an accidental needlestick.[37]

Given the present state of our knowledge and therapeutic possibilities, the onset of immunodeficiency is irreversible. The prognosis is gloomy: approximately half the patients die during the first year following a diagnosis of AIDS; at three years, 85 percent are dead. In a few rare cases, survival is prolonged.

The severity of the disease in children and the effects of cerebral AIDS further darken the already somber picture. Pediatric AIDS progresses rapidly and relentlessly to a terminal phase. As for newborns infected in utero, approximately 20 percent will become sick during the course of the first year of life, and the rest fall ill at the fairly constant rate of about 8 percent per year over several years.[38] Half of all pediatric patients have disturbances in psychomotor development, due to the direct cytotoxic effects of the virus on brain tissue.[39]

Neurological and psychiatric symptoms were recognized in adults as early as 1982, but they were attributed to opportunistic infections and reactive depression. By 1985 treatment of opportunistic infections of the nervous system had improved, revealing that many of the residual neurological problems obviously linked to the cytopathogenic effects of HIV. The virus was found inside brain macrophages and other cerebral cells[40] and Jay Levy isolated it from the cerebrospinal fluid of a patient with neurological problems.[41]

Pathologists have found evidence for an AIDS encephalitis, and psychiatrists have described an AIDS dementia, all without any identifiable cause other than direct retrovirus effects. Psychological testing of asymptomatic seropositives sometimes reveals loss of motor control and higher intellectual functions such as memory, concentration, and rapid recall. Psychiatric symptoms are a common finding in advanced AIDS.[42]

A 1983 medical thesis included the clinical history of one of the earliest AIDS patients in France, in which mention was made of a series of psychiatric problems. Rereading this text today, one would be prompted to think of cerebral AIDS. The typewritten description dwelled on how the patient's reaction to his illness became tiresome for his physicians and created serious problems.

And yet, when the same case came to be published in a medical journal, this psychiatric aspect of the case was practically eliminated, probably to avoid burdening the crisp scientific account with seemingly unrelated baggage.[43] What we think we know often obscures what we see.

Discovery of the presence of the AIDS virus in the central nervous system came as a surprise, a real shock. The parallel action of HIV on two different fronts, as one might say, diminished the chances that some seropositives might remain symptom-free and called for more complex therapeutic strategy.

PART THREE

A LOOK BACK

CHAPTER 9

The Historical Lesson of New Diseases

La nouveauté se fait par arrangements inédits de choses anciennes.

—Jacques Monod, biologist

IS AIDS A NEW DISEASE? A difficult question, or perhaps even badly put, too vague. What exactly does the syntagma "new disease" mean? "New" because the disease went unrecognized by physicians before a certain date or because it "really" did not exist? "New" to a certain place or to the whole world, "new" in the recent past, or in all human history?[1]

Recent Anglophone authors distinguish between two aspects of conceptualizing disease: "illness," meaning the experience of being sick as lived by the patient and perceived by his or her entourage; and "disease," meaning the pathological condition as a concept constructed within the framework of a nosological system. Distinction between these two aspects of sickness is essential. The newness of a disorder (in the broad sense) appears both in the suffering, on an individual or a collective level, and in its scientific recognition ("medical model of the disease").

In order to grasp the significance and extent of the problem, we will briefly examine several diseases that have been perceived, rightly or wrongly, by patients and doctors to be "new."[2] The review will be confined to those diseases now considered to be infectious.

Origin of the First Great Scourges

Some infectious diseases are as old as humankind. They are caused either by agents, such as common pyogenic bacteria, that affect all mammals and even some other metazoa, or by pathogens transmitted to humans "vertically" from their primate ancestors. The latter case applies to malaria and almost all intestinal parasites.[3]

During the Neolithic age, several "new" diseases appeared as the result of "horizontal" transmission of pathogens from domesticated animals. Examples are tuberculosis and acute eruptive fevers provoked by the pox viruses. The agents that cause these human diseases are similar to those that provoke epizootics in cattle and poultry.

Smallpox probably goes back to this prehistoric period, as does measles, the virus of which is closely related to those that cause rinderpest and canine distemper. These viruses did not originate in Europe, but were imported to the Mediterranean region from Africa, or more likely from Asia.[4]

Viruses are not primitive biological systems; they do not have their origin at the origin of other life forms. They are the product of degenerative evolution of cellular genes. Viruses cannot propagate in a free state; in other words, they reproduce only when they parasitize cells with protein-synthesizing apparati.[5]

Continuity of the existence of a pathogenic virus requires conditions propitious for intraspecific transmission (within a species) and the possibility of interspecific passages (between different species). Exclusively human viruses can persist only if certain demographic conditions are realized.[6] This requirement is absolutely imperative for the pathogens of acute diseases, which terminate quickly either in the death or in the complete cure of the patient. Viruses that cohabit with humans, either without provoking major difficulties or by persisting in a latent form after the disappearance of clinical symptoms, can be transmitted vertically and thus come from phylogenetic ancestors of humans and not from animals that live in their immediate surroundings. This is most likely the situation with the herpes simplex virus and possibly also that of chicken pox and shingles.

As for sexually transmitted diseases, the fifth century B.C. Hippocratic treatises refer directly to genital herpes and indirectly to lymphogranuloma venereum.[7]

The Outbreak of Pestilences in Greece

The Homeric epic mentions *loimos*, a pestilence suffered by the Achaian army during its siege of Troy. The ravages of this disease are presented as an extraordinary event, a manifestation of divine wrath.

In the archaic period, deadly epidemics were fairly rare and well circumscribed in time and place. The populations of European regions were below the critical threshold of numbers and density needed to guarantee permanence of the afflictions.

The first major epidemic of a collective disease with high mortality for which a historical description survives is the pestilence that broke out in Attica in 430 B.C. It was thought to be a new phenomenon. According to Thucydides' magistral account, "No pestilence of such extent nor any scourge so destructive of human lives is on record anywhere." Thucydides, an erudite historian who was familiar with medical texts, said doctors were unable to cope with the disease, "since they at first had to treat it without knowing its nature" (see *History of the Peloponnesian War*, II, 47-54, translated by C. Forster Smith, 1919).

I deliberately refer to this disease as a "pestilence" and not by its usual label, "plague of Athens," because it had nothing to do with "plague" in the modern sense of the term. Historians of disease have been unable to agree on what the retrospective diagnosis might have been. Each new generation of scholars proposes new hypotheses. The CDC specialists in Atlanta have participated in this too. Alexander Langmuir, former CDC director, claims that "the Thucydides' syndrome" was influenza complicated by Toxic Shock Syndrome (TSS). TSS is a dangerous disease that the very old and ubiquitous bacteria, *Staphylococcus aureus*, can provoke under certain particular situations.[8] A small epidemic of TSS affecting American women appeared in 1978. Medical opinion regarded this syndrome as a "new" disease. This outbreak was related to the use of vaginal tampons. Now it is associated with other factors. The American epidemic was only a local outbreak of a very old syndrome. TSS stands as a remarkable example of a "new" clinical entity due to changes in the habits of human life, and not to the transformation of a pathogenic agent.[9]

In spite of many opinions to the contrary, I continue to think of the pestilence of Athens as an outbreak of exanthematous typhus in immunologically virgin territory, complicated by nutritional deficiency and secondary infection. Whatever its identity, this disease may indeed have been new to Greece, as the Athenians thought, but it was probably not new to all humanity. Thucydides mentioned that the disease was said to have begun "in Ethiopia beyond Egypt." Since the most ancient past, Africa was saddled with the ignominious reputation of being the cradle of diseases that passed as being new.[10]

The Microbial Unification of the Roman Empire

Several previously unknown diseases appeared in the first century A.D., at the height of the Roman Empire. "The face of man has also been afflicted with new diseases, unknown in past years not only to Italy but also to almost the whole of Europe" (Pliny, *Natural History*, XXVI, 1, trans. W.H.S. Jones).

Thus Pliny described as new diseases "lichen" or "mentagra," "carbunculus," "gemursa," "elephantiasis," and "colum."[11] Today and with only one exception, it is impossible to tell what the true nature of these ills might have been. "Lichen" began on the chin, called *mentum* in Latin and hence the name "mentagra." It was a sycosis-like ailment, but it extended downward from the face to involve the neck, chest, and hands. Considered to be an Asian import, this "lichen" was contagious and limited to only one social group: "Women were not liable to the disease, or slaves and the lower and middle classes, but the nobles were very much infected through the momentary contact of a kiss" (Pliny, *Natural History*, XXVI, 3, trans. W.H.S. Jones). This is the first historical reference to a "kissing disease."

The ''carbunculus'' of Pliny may actually have been today's anthrax, a zoonosis, with a frequency that depends on cattle-raising conditions. Roman ''elephantiasis'' was certainly leprosy. With a long history in the Far East and known to the Hippocratic authors only in a few rare imported cases, leprosy did not begin its expansion into the eastern Mediterranean region until the Hellenistic age. It did not exist in endemic form in Europe before the dawn of the Roman empire.[12]

Seneca also spoke of new diseases in the middle of the first century (*Letters to Lucilius* XV, 95, 15–30). As Plato had done before, he blamed the intemperate habits of the new age.

In the second century, Plutarch constructed a theoretical debate around the idea of new diseases by opposing two opinions that seemed to him to be equally surprising: either the diseases were completely new and a change had taken place in Nature itself; or all diseases had always existed, but had simply not been noticed by physicians (*Quaestiones convivales* VIII, 9, in *Moralia*, translated by Edwin L. Minar). During this fictive debate, the guests at Plutarch's banquet offered three explanatory hypotheses: (1) all diseases have existed always and everywhere, but they are recognized only with time; (2) some diseases are new, because it is clear they come from another country; (3) some diseases are new, because they come from the outside world, the cosmos.[13]

According to Plutarch, Democritus had taught that some diseases have a cosmic but nevertheless nondivine origin. He meant that they were provoked by the extraterrestrial descent of harmful particles. Curiously enough, a similar opinion was invoked in a recent discussion on the origin of microbes, by Francis Crick, who cut the Gordian knot of virology with a radical cosmic solution.[14] Of all the diseases that spread in pandemic fashion in the Roman world, the most deadly was smallpox. The famous physician Galen suffered from it. Measles was likely introduced to the Mediterranean on several occasions, but the earliest certain historical description dates only from the end of the ninth century A.D. Rhazes succeeded in distinguishing measles from smallpox, yet he still confused it with scarlatina and rubella. The modern reader learns with surprise that this Persian physician considered measles to be more dangerous than smallpox.

Plague and the English Sweate

True plague, which is the dreadful disease caused by the bacillus *Yersinia pestis*, did not appear in Europe until the early Middle Ages. As an epidemic disease of humans, it may not have existed anywhere in the world until the historical era. The first probable but not ascertained record of plague goes back to Africa of the third century B.C.

There were three devastating pandemics of true plague, each thought not to have immediate precursors: the sixth-century plague of Justinian (supposed to have begun in Egypt); the grimly famous Black Death of fourteenth-century Europe, the most deadly pandemic in all human history thought to have come from China; and the nineteenth-century plague of Manchuria.[15]

The exceptionally high lethality of the plague agent and its devastating effects would not be biologically justified if its survival were to depend only on its parasitism of human hosts. In fact, plague is a disease of rodents, and attacks humans only secondarily.

Why did the plague bacillus ever make incursions into human populations? Why is there no interspecific transmission now in those regions of the world, like the western United States, where at this very moment plague thrives among sylvatic rodents? There are continuous reports of isolated cases, but none of these ignite epidemic outbreaks. Hygienic measures are thought to control plague, but this may not be the entire story, or even the most important factor. Recent work has shown that a single mutation at one genetic site on *Yersinia pestis*, or at two sites on its close cousin *Yersinia pseudotuberculosis*, can radically alter the virulence of a strain. Long-lasting plague enzootics of rats and other rodents are probably due to less virulent strains favored by natural selection. From time to time, a mutation at a critical locus could result in a hypervirulent strain, which, when passed to humans under specific conditions, would bring a disastrous epidemic.[16]

Mystery surrounds the origin and nature of the disease called the English Sweate, or sweating sickness. This serious epidemic disease was characterized by such special clinical symptoms that it can be easily distinguished from all other pestilences. Victims died quickly, usually only twenty-four hours after the onset of a brutal fever and a drenching, stinking sweat. This latter symptom became the pathognomonic sign and gave its name to the disease.

When the Sweate first appeared in England around 1480, and when, especially by autumn of 1485, it had decimated a population already severely drained by war, doctors were convinced it was a new disease. None of the ancient or medieval medical authors had ever described a pestilence that could be compared to it. Some physicians, for example the illustrious John Caius, thought it was somehow limited to the British temperament: he observed that foreign visitors to England escaped illness, and when the epidemic appeared on the Continent in 1529, it seemed to afflict British travelers exclusively. This may have been a false impression or, like AIDS in homosexuals, it may have had an approximate reliability only during the first phase of the epidemic. In his article for Diderot's *Encylopédie*, the French physician Jean-Jacques Ménuret de Chambaud swept away the explanations of those who wished to see it as divine retribution for the crimes of the English and asked if their blood did not contain a hereditary predisposition that could render harmful some foreign substances, which are innocuous for others.

Until 1551 the Sweate smoldered principally in England, then flared in continental Europe, where it vanished quite rapidly, only to reappear abruptly in France and northern Italy a century and a half later. There is every reason to believe that the Sweate was a viral disease, but it has not been possible to identify its pathogen nor to find any satisfying correspondence between its pathological manifestations and various other acute syndromes observed at other times and places in the world. It has been related to some influenza-like epidemics and more recently to the African hemorrhagic fevers.[17]

In human infectious diseases, a sort of equilibrium settles down between host and pathogen, the result of which, as a general rule, is a decline in the mortality rate. Natural selection operates in this direction, since it is not in the biological interest of a parasite to rapidly kill its host. This equilibrium between humans and living pathogenic agents is usually achieved by a gradual change of an acute disease into a chronic disease: thus mortality wanes but morbidity increases. This process takes place within a larger network of relations with other diseases. The transformation of syphilis in sixteenth-century Europe offers one of the most striking historical illustrations of this phenomenon.

The Microbe Exchange between the Old and the New World: Syphilis, Smallpox, and Flu Syndrome

Syphilis made a startling appearance in the French army of Charles VIII during a 1494 campaign in Italy. It was called the "disease of Naples" by the French and "French disease" by the Italians, so banal was it to see strangers as the carriers of unusual diseases. The venereal contagion of the late fifteenth century seems rather to have been an "American disease." In fact, its true history is quite complex: on the one hand, it is likely that varieties of the causative organism, *Treponema*, had already been in Europe before this epidemic; on the other, a particularly virulent mutant, which did not previously exist in the Old World, was brought from the New World by the crew of Christopher Columbus.[18]

There are some curious parallels between the expansion of syphilis at the beginning of the modern era and the present epidemic of AIDS: the sexual and maternal-child transmission, the moral and ethical implications, the impact on mores, the closing of public baths and so-called places of debauchery, the reactions of social alienation, and, to a certain extent, even the extreme danger of the disease. When syphilis first appeared in Europe, it was an acute disease. Pustules erupted all over the body. Many patients died during the phase of secondary dissemination, only a few months or years after the initial infection. Syphilis was dreaded even more than smallpox itself, which was relegated to the ranks of "small" cousin next to this major killer, the "Great Pox."[19]

The principal relay-focus of the Renaissance pandemic seems to have been the island of Hispaniola, now the site of Haiti. This pathway of intercontinental diffusion of syphilis also offers a striking analogy with AIDS. The similarities go even further: an inapparent or mild treponematosis is indigenous to the baboons and gorillas of Africa. Antitreponema antibodies were found in the serum of dog-faced baboons of West Africa in 1963 by Andre Fribourg-Blanc and Henri H. Mollaret. Three years later these same researchers detected the presence of treponema in the popliteal lymph nodes of several apparently healthy primates.[20] The hypothesis of a distant African origin for syphilis is, therefore, quite seductive. It is in Africa that the disease could have passed from apes to humans, or more likely, that their common ancestor might have been already parasitized by a "paleo-treponema." After thousands of years, the bacteria could have returned from America to the Dark Continent in a much more virulent form.[21]

After the discovery of the New World, the trans-Atlantic microbe exchange operated in both directions. Sailors and conquistadors were at the origin of a sort of biological warfare, bringing powerful allies with them in the viruses imported from Europe inside their own bodies or in those of their animals. Smallpox and measles ravaged the indigenous population of America. These diseases, new for the Indians, struck with a violence that was unknown in European countries.[22] Other viruses also came into play: their selective impact on indigenous populations had serious military and demographic consequences. Swine flu virus seems to have been responsible for devastating epidemics.[23]

According to the Spanish chronicles, the breath of the white man was death to the Indian. The truth of these old accounts has been confirmed by modern epidemiological experience. Thus for example, Robert Gessain, the physician-anthropologist director of the Paris Musée de l'Homme, tells how, in 1935, he wintered on the east coast of Greenland with a sheltered population of eight hundred Inuit, who had been living there for centuries. In spring, an extremely rare event took place: a Norwegian ship arrived and the sailors came to shore. One of them had an ordinary cold. He sneezed, and within a few months, a tenth of the Inuit population died of the pulmonary complications of a viral disease, against which they had no natural defense.[24]

New Diseases in Modern Times

In the seventeenth century, European doctors described several diseases for which they found no corresponding account in the ancient literature. To explain what was to them the unexpected apparition of new nosological entities, they invoked the intrinsic variability of diseases, conjunctions of the stars, increase in population, contact with foreigners, and degeneracy of the human species in general and of the white race in particular.

This harvest of "new" diseases, for the most part mild and endemic, had two main causes: on the one hand, a change in living conditions that had altered the structure of morbidity in Western Europe; and, on the other hand, a rise in clinical medicine that fostered a subtle distinction between clinical conditions. Thanks to the neo-Hippocratic movement, epitomized in the work of Thomas Sydenham, a powerful intellectual tool was forged, permitting the description and definition of "new" diseases. Of course, these diseases were not really new; they had been around for a long time but were not "visible" to the medical eye. New nosological identities were granted, and names were given to poorly defined, ancient humoral dyscrasias.[25]

This situation recurred with increased intensity in the early nineteenth century with the advent of the new anatomo-clinical method. At that time, cholera began its advance into Europe from endemic strongholds in India, as the slow movement of ancient caravans was supplanted by the relatively rapid, long-distance travel of merchants, colonial armies, and pilgrims bound for Mecca. Since 1817 seven pandemics of cholera had swept the world. All were thought to have originated from the Ganges delta, where, according to most historians of medicine, it has been endemic since the mists of time. Nevertheless, recent investigations endorse the hypothesis that cholera may actually have been relatively new even for Asia: it may have arisen as serious illness, sometime in the eighteenth or nineteenth century, through a genetic transformation of a saprophytic *Vibrio*.[26]

Among the many diseases that, at the beginning of our century, passed for new, encephalitis lethargica is the most remarkable. Described in 1917 by Constantin von Economo, this viral disease first appeared in epidemic form in China, whence, by 1928, it had spread over the entire world, killing approximately half a million people before vanishing completely. The pathogen, most likely a virus, was never identified, but there are good reasons for believing it was a mutation of the influenza virus.[27]

Legionnaire's Disease and the African Hemorrhagic Fevers

In the recent past, several highly lethal infectious diseases were described as new, among them Legionnaire's disease, Lassa fever, Ebola fever, Marburg fever, and Toxic Shock Syndrome. In a few cases, these could be the result of genetic mutation of a relatively harmless pathogen, but in others, likely the majority, it is thought today that the causative agent existed before the obvious epidemic, and that visible outbreaks were precipitated by socioecological factors.[28]

In July 1976 an unusual acute febrile illness overcame several delegates to an American Legion conference at a luxury hotel in Philadelphia. The respectability of the victims and the high mortality—16 percent of those affected died—resulted in a public outcry and attracted media attention on a global scale. An exemplary epidemiological investigation, led by Joseph McDade for the CDC in Atlanta, discovered the causative organism, a previously unknown species of bacteria. It was named *Legionella pneumophila*.

From any point of view, "Legionnaire's disease" seemed to be a new phenomenon; yet microbiologists were able to show that various Legionella species had been around for a long time in our environment and were even quite widespread. They were pathogenic, but fairly benign. The agent of the Philadelphia epidemic was not a mutant. The real culprit was the hotel's air conditioning system. Benign microbes had become dangerous through multiplication in the stagnant water of the cooling towers and through aerosol distribution.[29]

Other small *Legionella* epidemics followed, always in places with highly updated sanitary installations. This experience taught an unexpected lesson: contemporary technology could cause "new" diseases, not only through degradation of the natural environment by all sorts of pollutants but also through methods designed to make living conditions more "hygienic." The undesirable effects of civilization never cease to amaze.

The viral agents of the African fevers, designated by the toponyms, Lassa, Ebola, and Marburg, are not really new either; they simply became "visible" to occidental physicians when they were displaced from their usual small ecological niches.

In 1967 a previously unknown virus infected some thirty people who were working in two laboratories in Marburg, West Germany, on organ tissue taken from Ugandan green monkeys. They suffered from acute fever complicated by bleeding. Seven patients died. The same illness appeared in Belgrade, Yugoslavia, at another lab working on African monkeys. The causative virus was isolated from the blood of those infected and, because it was also found in sperm, sexual transmission was considered a possibility. There was at least one case where a husband had passed the disease to his wife, probably through intimate contact. All efforts to locate the virus in African monkeys have failed, and it is not certain that they are the true natural reservoir. Brought from Uganda in 1967, the monkeys may well have been infected via an arthropod vector from a different African animal group, which was an endemic carrier of the virus. Once the virus was accidentally transmitted to humans, it spread by interhuman contact. Strict isolation of those affected led to rapid extinction of the virus in Europe, but a few other isolated cases were later recognized in Africa (Rhodesia, 1975; Kenya, 1980),[30] and Ebola, an apparently closely related virus, was recently identified in several imported monkeys in a laboratory in northern Virginia.

The fever named for the Nigerian village of Lassa is a zoonosis, accidentally transmitted to humans by direct or indirect contact with west African rodents. In 1969, two North American nuns died of the fever in Nigeria. The disease spread to the United States in the same year via a missionary who had tended the nuns. Strict isolation eradicated the American outbreak, but small, well-circumscribed epidemics still occur in Africa, and human carriers with subclinical symptoms have been identified.[31]

In 1976 an acute fever mysteriously appeared at two sites on the Sudan-Zaire border, separated by a distance of roughly five hundred miles but connected by a truck route. Several hundered persons died, including four Belgian missionaries. WHO experts intervened. Fortunately, the outbreak did not traverse the tropical forest. The pathogen was isolated from the blood of its first victim, who came from the village of Yambuku near the Ebola River. It was a virus, morphologically similar to the Marburg virus but with different antigenic properties. Its presence in blood, sperm, and all solid or liquid excretions accounts for its routes of transmission from one human being to another. Conditions in African hospitals and the multiple use of syringes favored the outbreak of epidemics. Like Marburg and Lassa fevers, Ebola fever is a very serious, acute condition, frequently aggravated by hemorrhagic complications. It is highly lethal.[32]

Retrospective serological investigation has shown that these viral diseases had existed before the epidemics that made them apparent to the Western doctors. They testify to the existence, in Africa, of silent endemic viruses with potential pathogenic properties and a capacity for interhuman transmission. A conjunction of unusual circumstances is necessary to bring them into view.[33] The coincidence of such circumstances, extremely rare until the middle of our century, has become a more likely possiblity since the Second World War. Alteration in the natural environment, social upheaval, as well as certain new habits and the advent of Western medical practices have created an absolutely unprecedented epidemiological setting in Africa.

The viral agents of hemorrhagic fevers are not related to the AIDS virus, but there are analogies in their transmission by blood and sperm. Margrethe Rask, one of the first European AIDS patients, contracted her disease at roughly the same time and place.

AIDS: A New Disease?

A disease can appear to be new in at least five different historical settings: (1) it already existed, but escaped medical attention because it was not recognized as a nosological entity; (2) it already existed, but did not appear until there was a qualitative or quantitative change in its manifestations; (3) it did not exist in one region of the world and was introduced there from another; (4) it did not exist in human populations, but did affect an animal population; (5) it is absolutely new, the causative agent had never existed as such until the first clinical manifestations. Even the last situation has some continuity with the past: then, disease results from an adaptive transformation of a previously saprophytic microbe, or a benign commensal for humans or animals. The theoretical possibility of another subgroup of the last category of absolutely new diseases cannot be excluded, but it is very improbable: diseases artificially produced either by intention (as in preparation for biological warfare), or by accident in a biotechnology laboratory.

AIDS is necessarily new with respect to the first category. Its pathological manifestations could not even have been understood as a disease before the advent of new concepts resulting from recent developments in the life sciences. In the past, a disease was defined either by clinical symptoms or by pathological lesions, which are morphological changes in organs, tissues, or cells. Nothing of the sort, neither clinical symptoms nor lesions observable by the old means, characterizes AIDS. It is not a disease in the sense given to the term before the mid-twentieth century. Persons affected by HIV virus suffer and die with the signs and lesions that are typical of other diseases. As recently as twenty years ago, these opportunistic disorders were the only reality that physicians could observe and conceptualize.

To use outdated medical terminology, AIDS appears as an "acquired diathesis" or a strange sort of "genius epidemicus" (local particularity of an epidemic). It is not a disease in the old sense of the word, inasmuch as the virus is immunopathogenic, that is, it affects the immune system and produces symptoms only through the expedient of opportunistic infection or malignancy. However, AIDS can be partially conceived as a disease in the classical sense inasmuch as the virus can also exert a direct cytopathogenic action, that is, it can directly affect, impede, or destroy certain cells. Any pernicious result of such direct action can be considered a lesion. The interest of this distinction is purely theoretical, because the lesion in question is situated at a level that was inaccessible prior to recent developments in biological investigation.

AIDS is definitely new in its present epidemiological dimension. In the past, biological and social conditions prevented a major outbreak of a retroviral infection transmitted in such a special manner, and especially one that so ruthlessly attacks the immune system. A disastrous epidemic of this type could not have occurred before the mingling of peoples, the liberalization of sexual and social mores, and, above all, before progress in modern medicine had accomplished the control of the majority of serious infectious diseases and introduced intravenous injections and blood transfusion. All this does not necessarily imply that the virus in question is a newborn in the absolute sense, a mutant whose ancestors were never pathogenic. Nor does it exclude the possibility that, even in the distant past, similar retroviruses may have provoked small epidemics of immunodepression, visible only by fluctuations in the morbidity and mortality attributed to other diseases.

CHAPTER 10

Is AIDS an Ancient Disease?

History is a hard core

of interpretation

surrounded by a

pulp of disputable

facts.

—Sir George Clark,

historian

HIV-1 AND HIV-2 have certainly not afflicted most human populations in the recent past: no serological traces have been found either in people, geographically or socially segregated from the current epidemic, or in tests done on blood collected before the middle of our century. This virtually eliminates the possibility of an AIDS pandemic earlier in our century, but not the possibility of surreptitious activity of another retrovirus with similar pathogenic properties, nor even, in a more remote past, the activity of a virus very close to the HIVs isolated today.

The pathological "archeology" of AIDS remains unexplored and preliminary results are disappointing.

Fantastic Hypotheses

A biologist and two American physicians thought they recognized AIDS in the ancient Egyptian disease *âaâ*, described in medical papyri of the pharaonic era.[1] This idea does not stand up to criticism. Egyptologists have recently expressed doubts about the grounds for identifying this "divine mortification" with parasitic hematuria (in other words, with schistosomiasis), as was suggested sixty years ago by Bendix Ebbell and supported by the excellent medico-philological analysis of Frans Jonckheere. However, this attempt to identify it with AIDS is even more daring, since it rests solely on the serious nature of the disease and on the fact that it had an effect on semen and/or the male generative organs.[2]

John Gwilt, vice president of an American pharmaceutical company, has found an even more arbitrary precursor: according to him, AIDS was already brewing in the time of Moses, as witnessed by a description in the Book of Numbers.[3] The Bible does indeed mention a terrible pestilence that caused the death of several thousand Jews, supposedly as a result of the sexual relations they had had with Moabite women. The biblical name of this disease, *mag-*

gepha, designated an affliction that killed many people. No symptoms were described. The identification of this biblical disease with AIDS is completely arbitrary, based only on the delusion that AIDS is divine punishment for sexual transgressions.[4]

A Marseille tropical disease expert wondered if the disease that ravaged Europe following the voyages of Columbus and that medical historians regard as an acute form of treponematosis may actually have been an outbreak of AIDS, coming, even at that time, from the island of Hispaniola.[5] Some aspects of fourteenth-century syphilis are indeed reminiscent of present-day AIDS, but it is impossible to confuse the two diseases, which differ greatly, both clinically and epidemiologically. Paleopathological evidence, especially signs found in ancient skeletal material, supports this distinction and suggests that the Renaissance syphilis was caused by a virulent strain of the treponema.[6]

In 1984 three Belgian physicians, Thierry Appelboom, Daniel Désir, and Jean-Louis Herweghem, considered the hypothesis that Erasmus, Rotterdam's celebrated humanist, was the first known casualty of AIDS. He died in 1556 at the age of sixty-nine. Toward the end of his life, he had suffered from relapsing fevers, diarrhea, painful arthritis, skin swellings, and generalized lymph-node enlargement. Certain aspects of his biography suggest that he may have been a homosexual. He traveled widely and is said to have had many amorous friendships. The clinical picture of his last illness does in fact correspond fairly well with the syndrome of immunodepression, but this is not the only possible retrospective diagnosis, and there is nothing to support its having been caused by a specific viral infection. Paleopathological analysis of the skeletal material thought to be the remains of Erasmus, exhumed at Basel in 1930, revealed signs of syphilis. Appelboom himself has abandoned his initial hypothesis and now considers syphilis to be the most likely retrospective diagnosis of the ills of Erasmus.[7]

We should not be surprised if the only concrete historical case cited as having presented possible symptoms of immunodeficiency is not an anonymous patient. The rich details of Erasmus's complaint are known only because of the survival of his correspondence. No physician of his era left an account.[8]

Before the nineteenth century, doctors did not make a practice of describing atypical cases. For the purposes of retrospective epidemiology, medical records do not become a reliable and sufficiently exhaustive source until the nineteenth century.

The First Description of Kaposi's Sarcoma

Since AIDS itself does not present characteristic clinical manifestations that lend themselves to retrospective diagnoses, we must trace the abnormalities in the appearance of "opportunistic" diseases. Kaposi's sarcoma occurs often, but not always, within the context of AIDS.

It is a malignant tumor of skin, first described in 1872 by the Viennese physician, Moriz Kaposi. He had in fact been born "Kohn," at Kaposvar, whence his second name. The clinical instruction of the famous Ferdinand Hebra awakened his interest in skin diseases and led him to orient his research to their morphologic description. Eventually, he too became one of the great professors of the Viennese school and a founder of modern dermatology.[9]

Kaposi described five cases of a previously unknown and rapidly fatal skin condition, which he named "multiple idiopathic pigmented sarcoma of skin" (*idiopathisches multiples Pigmentsarkom der Haut*). All his patients died within two years of diagnosis and no treatment was effective. No doubt, Kaposi had observed just the tip of a small iceberg. At the time, he was not yet a professor and attended only a limited clientele. Nevertheless, he saw three cases of this dermatosis between July 1868 and October 1869, one case in 1870, and another in 1871. All were male and over forty, but Theodor Billroth had supplied details on another case in a younger male in Zurich who had died within a year.[10]

Nothing is known about the sexual practices of Kaposi's five patients, and nothing in the description indicates the presence of other concomitant opportunistic disease or immune depression. A dedicated dermatologist like Kaposi would not have missed the additional complication of herpes or thrush.

Kaposi's autopsy of the cadaver of one patient, who died while in hospital, allowed him to discover the dissemination of sarcomatous lesions in the internal organs. There were also lesions in the lungs that, in retrospect, are suggestive of atypical pneumonia.[11]

Kaposi viewed the condition as a generalized disorder from its outset, not as a local malignancy with metastases. If the microscopic appearance of the tumors with angiosarcomatous disorganization and epithelial and fibroblastic infiltration was compatible with the definition of cancer, other characteristics failed to conform to this nosological designation. In short, one thing was clear from the very first description: this was a cancer unlike any other.

According to Lars Breimer, the clinical descriptions of Kaposi and Billroth are compatible with what we know of AIDS today and "consequently, it is possible that this syndrome had already been described in the Austro-Hungarian Monarchy and in Switzerland during the last century."[12]

This is an exaggeration. The acquired immunodeficiency syndrome was certainly not "described" by Moriz Kaposi. It is possible, however, that two of the cases Kaposi published were in reality the only manifestation observable at the time of immunodeficiency induced by infection. Nothing in the description permits a refutation of the hypothesis that they had AIDS, but neither is there anything to prove it.

Other Early Reports of Kaposi's Sarcoma

A few years later another quasi-epidemic cluster of Kaposi's sarcoma was observed in Italy. In 1882 twelve cases, collected since 1874, were reported by Tommaso De Amicis, professor of dermatology in Naples. All were male of Italian origin, living in the Naples area. With the exception of a five-year-old child, they were between the ages of thirty-nine and forty-four. The course of the disease was fairly slow with long periods of remission, except in the case of the child and the youngest adult, both of whom died rapidly with disseminated lesions and fever.[13]

The sexual orientation of these patients was not mentioned. Is it a coincidence that this cluster of Kaposi's sarcoma was identified in Naples, which, like Vienna, was a well-known destination for homosexual encounters at that time?

In the early twentieth century a third series of Kaposi's sarcoma was recorded in the medical literature. At least seven of these cases meet the criteria for a diagnosis of AIDS, using current CDC standards. These were all males between the ages of twenty-four and fifty-eight, who suffered weight loss, diarrhea, and generalized weakness. They died rapidly, within four months to two years from the onset of their cutaneous symptoms. In one case, autopsy revealed widespread tuberculosis. Although these cases had been diagnosed at many different sites in Europe, they were all of Italian origin or had contacts with Italy. What appeared, at the time, to be an ethnic link gives, in retrospect, the impression of a geographic connection. Once again, it seemed improper to publish particularities of the sexual behavior of such patients.[14]

Most of the cases of Kaposi's sarcoma described in Europe and America during the first half of the twentieth century were relatively benign. The disease turned up here and there in a sporadic fashion, affecting older males of Mediterranean or Jewish (particularly Ashkenazi) origin. Based on these observations, the features of Kaposi's sarcoma, also known as hemorrhagic sarcomatosis, wandered from the initial descriptions. It had become a milder local malignancy, with a median survival of ten or more years, most often restricted to the lower limbs and characterized by spontaneous remissions.[15]

This relatively benign Kaposi's sarcoma established in the pre-1960 medical literature has nothing to do with AIDS and cannot be used as an indicator for epidemic acquired immunodeficiency.

Early Presence of Kaposi's Sarcoma in Africa

The first reported case of this disease in Africa was observed by the German colonial doctor, K. Hallenberg, in a Cameroon native who suffered the typical skin lesions without any major illness.[16] In 1934 a more severe form was recognized in Nigeria.[17] Following this, English, Belgian, and French doctors reported isolated cases in Uganda and the Congo, without seeing them as indicators of an important endemic. The epidemic dimensions were not apparent until 1948.[18]

Paul L. Gigase, a Belgian pathologist, has shown that the small number of cases observed before 1945 were only a pale reflection of the actual situation. Underestimates were inevitable due to the undermedicalization of the "Dark Continent" and the tropical health-care worker's general lack of familiarity with the clinical and histological appearance of this skin condition. The Shi natives of South Kivu in Zaire called the disease *lubambo* and were able to distinguish it from endemic elephantiasis, called *bikimbo*. According to the inhabitants of the Belgian Congo, the incidence of this disease had not altered within human memory.[19]

Several surveys done throughout the 1950s—by J. F. Murray in South Africa, by A. Thijs along the Congo River, by Jack Davies in Uganda, by Alfred Quenum in French Equatorial Africa, and by several other dedicated doctors—revealed, on the one hand, that there was an elevated incidence of Kaposi's sarcoma in the sub-Sahara and, on the other, that children and young men were frequently afflicted with a severe form having a grave prognosis. It seemed that there was an apparent predilection for this condition in people of the "Bantu ethnic type." But one thing was clear: the Kaposi's sarcoma then seen in Africa was quite different from that described in the earlier European medical manuals.[20]

Did a new disease really appear in Africa during the 1930s and 1940s? Was an old disease somehow exacerbated, or had the scales simply fallen from medical eyes?

Reflections on Unexplored Vestiges

To prove or refute the presence of AIDS or an analogous disease in the past, research can be directed along two different paths: one, for the biologist, the investigation of indications of retrovirus infection in human remains; the other, for the historian, the study of temporal and geographic variations in records of opportunistic infections.

Properly stored samples of blood taken before 1950 are scarce. But no inventory has been made of these few, and even fewer have been subjected to systematic study from the point of view of retroviral serology. Scientific institutions, hospitals, and museums of anatomical pathology around the world maintain a great collection of organs and human tissue, often going back to the last century, and, in some cases, as far as the seventeenth century. Is it not possible that today's sophisticated techniques, perhaps PCR (Polymerase Chain Reaction), could detect the presence or absence of specific antibodies or, even more surely, fragments of a retrovirus similar to that of AIDS?

A documented history of opportunistic infections has not been written. These are numerous and include fungi and protozoa, as well as bacteria and viruses. They may be numerous, but they are fairly well delimited. AIDS patients do not pick up just anything. Apart from Kaposi's sarcoma and non-Hodgkin's lymphoma, the most common opportunistic conditions are *Pneumocystis carinii* pneumonia; lymphoid pneumonia; cytomegalovirus disease of lymph nodes, retina, and blood; oral or esophageal candidiasis; herpetic manifestations of skin and mucous membrane; cerebral toxoplasmosis; progressive multifocal leukoencephalopathy; *Cryptococcus neoformans* meningitis; chronic enteritis due to either the protozoal agent *Cryptosporidium* or forms of *Salmonella* bacteria; generalized histoplasmosis; and, last but not least, disseminated tuberculosis due to the classical Koch's bacillus (*M. tuberculosis*) or atypical mycobacteria, notably *M. avium-intracellulare*. Aside from tuberculosis, these agents are relatively nonpathogenic for healthy individuals. They are widely distributed, but were thought to be "rare" until only recently, because their presence normally caused no disturbance.

It might be surprising that the infections that attack AIDS patients are not due to the more "banal" type of pathogens, such as the common pyogenic bacteria. This results from the selectivity of the damage to immune defenses during HIV infection: humoral immunity and neutrophils, little altered by the AIDS virus, are sufficient to protect the host from staphylococci, streptococci, and many other pathogens. Collapse of the cellular arm of the immune system, due to the alteration of T4-lymphocytes and monocytic cells, leaves the patient vulnerable, immunologically "naked," to certain microbes (especially those that reproduce intracellularly), but not defenseless to all forms of invasion.

Nothing is known of the possible relationship between AIDS and some endemic diseases, such as leprosy, malaria, typhoid, or schistosomiasis, that have forged the destiny of civilizations.

Opportunistic infections are not mutually exclusive. Quite the contrary. Their accumulation is a valuable sign pointing to the retrospective diagnosis of acquired immunodeficiency. These infections vary with the environment of the affected subject: generally, according to observations made during the first years of the present pandemic, American and European patients suffer most often from *Pneumocystis*; those in Zaire, from toxoplasmosis and cryptococcosis; those in Haiti, from disseminated tuberculosis.[21] The historico-geographic setting influences the situation not only by the various routes of infection but also by the agents present.

An Outline History of Opportunistic Infections

Herpes and thrush have been known since antiquity, but except in the case of young children, medical literature rarely recognized serious outcomes. To my knowledge, there are no ancient records of any simultaneous occurrences of these infections.

As was noted with respect to the illness of Erasmus, until the triumph of the anatomo-clinical method in the early nineteenth century, physicians rarely saw an interest in the study or publication of cases where the disease ran an atypical course. As a result, our sources are often silent on certain points that now seem to be particularly important.

In 1905 the German pathologist, David Paul von Hansemann, described a case of meningitis, which at the time seemed very curious because the condition manifestly resulted from the presence of a microscopic fungus in the cerebral tissue. The organism was named *Torula hystolytica*. During the First World War, the disease it provoked in humans and animals was conceptualized under the name of "torulosis." It was only later, after the Second World War, that this seemingly rare fungus was found to be identical to the cosmopolitan fungus, *Cryptococcus neoformans*, exceedingly common in nature. *Cryptococcus* had been known by its present name since the end of the nineteenth century, but only as a saprophyte.[22]

Toxoplasmosis is a common and probably very old zoonosis. It was often confused with other parasitic disorders in the past. The protozoal pathogen, *Toxoplasma gondii*, was first identified in animals in 1908 by Charles Nicolle and Louis Manceaux. In 1914 Aldo Castellani claimed it could also be harmful for humans. However, it was not until 1937, when Abner Wolf and David Cowen described toxoplasmic granulomatous encephalomyelitis, that toxoplasmosis was brought into the realm of pathology as a "new human disease caused by protozoa." And it was only toward the 1960s that the extremely high frequency of subclinical toxoplasmosis was appreciated.[23]

After official recognition of a nosological entity, an extraordinary medical blindness to past instances of the disease is often uncovered. Favism represents a good example of a disease that had been invisible for ages despite the fact that patients suffered the highly noticeable symptom of red or even black urine caused by hemoglobinuria.[24]

Pneumocystis pneumonia also had a long prehistory of confusion with other poorly defined lung problems before it became its own diagnostic entity. The parasite was first described by Carlos Chagas, in 1909. Subsequently, its presence was detected in the organs of various animals. In 1942 it was isolated from the lungs of a newborn baby, but its role in human pathology was not demonstrated until the 1950s. Before AIDS and before the advent of immunosuppressive drugs, *Pneumocystis* pneumonia was a disease only of newborns infected in utero, malnourished children, and a few adults with leukemia.[25]

Cytomegalovirus disease also has an origin lost in the mists of time. Without doubt it is old, but it was not recognized until 1881. Clinicians confused it with other infectious disorders and could not agree on its features, nature, and cause. This might have continued for years if its peculiar histological appearance had not been recognized by Hugo Ribbert, who described the condition as a "disease with cells resembling protozoa" (*"Krankheit mit protozoenartigen Zellen "*). In 1950 John P. Wyatt redefined the concept of "cytomegalic inclusion disease," and six years later, Margaret Smith isolated the virus from infected cells.[26]

Deadly for newborns, this disease seemed to be of only minor consequence for adults. It affected especially those who had received many blood transfusions. Nevertheless, a few exceptions were reported: the disease could brutally kill previously healthy young men. One of these, a patient of John P. Wyatt, died of cytomegalic inclusion disease complicated by *Pneumocystis* pneumonia and *Pseudomonas* septicemia.[27]

The protozoan *Cryptosporidium* has been known for a long time, but only as a commensal nonpathogenic organism.

Written sources do not given any valid impression of the incidence or clinical manifestations of opportunistic infections before the beginning of the twentieth century. In fact, reliable observations of most of these infections in humans were made only shortly before the onset of the AIDS epidemic. Perhaps a detailed reexamination of old anatomical and histological specimens may give a little more information.

Finally, there is tuberculosis, by far the most important opportunistic infection from a historical point of view. In AIDS patients, tuberculosis can be severely debilitating and atypical, with dissemination to extrapulmonary sites. At first, North American AIDS experts were reluctant to consider *Mycobacterium tuberculosis* as an opportunistic organism, but they changed their minds when they learned of observations made on Haitian patients. Instead of the Koch's bacillus, fairly controllable with antituberculous medications, atypical and resistant forms of mycobacteria were often isolated. But old phthisis is reawakening in a certain clinical setting, and the appearance of galloping tuberculosis is now considered to be a reliable sign of AIDS.[28]

Doctors in the last century sometimes noticed capricious outbreaks of tuberculosis, especially those curious and isolated outbreaks of acute and highly lethal miliary forms. Certain clinical descriptions of a "galloping consumption" that seemed to appear and disappear in front of the helpless practitioner have become medical classics. Decrease in the morbidity and mortality of tuberculosis has been attributed to general improvement in living conditions, especially nutrition. This theory may hold when applied to the alteration in overall allure of tuberculosis, but informed historians know that it cannot account for some local anomalies. A careful and detailed study of these small epidemics of severe forms within the context of the great endemic setting of chronic tuberculosis may shed new light on the history of infectious diseases.[29]

If historical events are not negligible for the correct appreciation of certain aspects of the present AIDS pandemic, the reverse is no less true. The discovery of an infectious agent that selectively erodes immune defense offers an opportunity to take another look at the scourges of the past.

CHAPTER 11

Prodromes of the Epidemic in the Americas

Ce n'est pas la faute

de l'histoire, mais la

faute des médecins,

si l'histoire ne rend

pas plus de services

à la médecine.

—Charles Daremberg,

medical historian

ACCORDING to the official investigations, the AIDS epidemic began in the United States in 1978.[1] Using epidemiological cross-checking, this date can be pushed back to the bicentennial year of 1976. Retrospective diagnosis of AIDS in Europe can be applied to cases treated in December of 1976.[2] But was this the real beginning? In 1930 Charles Nicolle, bacteriologist, novelist, and Nobel laureate for his work on the role of lice in the spread of typhus, wrote a beautiful book on the destiny of infectious diseases, in which he predicted:

> Nature's attempts to create new infectious diseases are as constant as they usually are vain. What happened in antiquity when, by exception, nature succeeded in an attempt is repeated at every moment now and will continue to be repeated always. It is inevitable. Equally inevitable is the fact that we will never be able to track their origin. When we become aware of these diseases, they are already fully formed, "adults" one might say. . . . How could we recognize these new diseases? How could we suspect their existence before they had donned their attire of characteristic symptoms? We must equally resign ourselves to perpetual ignorance of the first cases. They will always pass unnoticed, confused with other diseases, and only after a long period of trial and error, will the new type of pathology be released from the already classified disorders.[3]

With respect to AIDS or any of the other "new" diseases of our era, this rule of Nicolle's still applies. There is every indication, in fact, that the present epidemic began insidiously, with sporadic cases that passed unnoticed under the guise of opportunistic disease or a wasting disorder of obscure diagnosis and uncertain etiology.

A New Look at Old Medical Records

Once AIDS became a specific nosological entity, several physicians in North America and Europe had the feeling that they may have already encountered the syndrome in patients treated long before the official onset of the epidemic. Unfortunately, all these patients were no longer living, when new diagnostic techniques finally provided a possibility for a definite revision of the former diagnosis.

In this domain, memory without written proof does not count. However, the health-care activity of our era is heavily bureaucratized, and medical archives in many countries contain a wealth of detailed documentation concerning its most diverse aspects. The protohistory of AIDS is hidden there, a filigree thread embedded in a matrix of outdated knowledge. Someday these documents of hospitals, medical offices, and public health and medical research institutions should be searched with a fine-toothed comb.

In the meantime, scrutiny of the published literature does offer a precious glimpse. Medical literature, already abundant at the beginning of this century, has become voluminous since the Second World War. It contains a great many reports or clinico-pathological observations of cases presenting what were thought to have been curious and unusual pathological situations. In rereading these reports, in the light of our present understanding, one discovers, not without surprise, some descriptions that resemble the clinical pictures of acquired immunodeficiency syndrome.

A clinical definition of the acquired immunodeficiency syndrome was set down in March 1983 by the CDC in Atlanta as part of an attempt to standardize epidemiological surveillance in the United States.[4] The consecutive use of serological tests confirmed the great diagnostic value of these clinical criteria, at least in the present situation. Whenever the CDC have revised their definition (for instance in 1985 and 1987), it has been to broaden rather than restrict the significant clinical manifestations.[5]

The CDC criteria can be applied to retrospective diagnosis. A major difficulty, however, is that information concerning lymphocyte typing and immune response is often lacking, or at least incomplete in older descriptions. I use two supplementary restrictions to heighten the reliabilty of these criteria in the retrospective situation: age under fifty-five (instead of sixty); and death shortly after onset of the illness. In the literature prior to about 1950, there are very few cases amenable to a diagnosis of AIDS. Not only are they extremely rare, these few cases are mostly surrounded by circumstances that make room for several conjectures. After that date, cases become more and more frequent, details more abundant, and symptoms more and more in conformity with the clinical definition of AIDS.

Therefore, an HIV-type virus seems to have been present in human populations since at least the middle of the twentieth century. These suggestive case reports were sporadic and scattered over several continents. They were published because they seemed rare and atypical. The documentation supporting the existence of this condition long before its official recognition proves, at the same time, that no epidemic wave preceded the present pandemic. Before 1978, in North America and Western Europe at least, AIDS does not seem to have been a collective disease.

At least sixteen cases, published in American medical journals between early 1940 and June 5, 1981 (when the CDC announced their observations of *Pneumocystis* pneumonia in homosexuals), have been found to fit the present clinical definition of AIDS. Data concerning lymphocyte function may not always be satisfactory, but physical, histological, and parasitological findings leave no doubt about the presence of opportunistic diseases in the setting of otherwise unexplained immunodeficiency. Several other cases described during the same period were rejected, because clinical data were thought to be insufficient, or because other immunodepressive states and malignancies could not be excluded. In about a dozen of these incomplete or questionable cases, a retrospective diagnosis of AIDS is quite possible, but less probable than in the sixteen accepted cases.[6]

It goes without saying that this kind of historical survey is necessarily far from exhaustive. Conducted with the help of bibliographic compilations (*Index Medicus, Current Contents, Excerpta Medica, Index Catalogue of the Library of the Surgeon General's Office*), selection was dependent on the more or less felicitous choice of a descriptive title.

AIDS in 1952?

The oldest case in our series is a medical "classic" because John P. Wyatt of St. Louis, one of the leading experts on cytomegalic inclusion disease, used it to show that "on exceedingly rare occasions" serious forms of this disease are not necessarily confined to newborns and can strike adults.

In February 1952, a twenty-eight-year-old male, called R.G., was admitted to the Baptist Memorial Hospital in Memphis, Tennessee, with a diagnosis of "viral pneumonia." He had always been well until two weeks earlier, when he developed general malaise, fever, cough, and respiratory difficulties. Chest X-ray revealed diffuse nodular opacities. Biopsy of a macular skin lesion showed a nonspecific, chronic inflammatory reaction. Unlike most pneumonia cases, there was no elevation in the white cell count; in fact, his lymphocytes had dropped from forty-seven to fifteen. Syphilis and lymphogranuloma serology, as well as blood cultures for diverse organisms, were negative. Antibiotics had only a transient effect. He was placed on cortisone, but only in the late stages of his illness. Three months after admission to hospital, an exploratory operation was done on his left lung. Attempts to isolate a virus failed; however, microscopic inspection of the lung biopsies revealed giant inclusion bodies in some of the pulmonary cells—the first time in the history of medicine that this finding had been made in tissue taken from a living adult. The patient apparently made some improvement and left the hospital three weeks after his biopsy. Two and a half months later he was readmitted with an infection in the scar of his thoracotomy incision caused by pyocyanin-producing bacteria (*Pseudomonas aeruginosa*), a gram-negative organism refractory to most antibiotics until the 1970s. He died of overwhelming sepsis.[7]

Autopsy confirmed the diagnosis of cytomegalic inclusion disease made by the biopsy. Wyatt and colleagues also noted in histologic sections of the lungs a curious necrotizing arteritis of pulmonary vessels and a mononuclear inflammatory response so intense that it resembled lymphomatous infiltration. A few years later, the German pathologist, Herwig Hamperl, took another look at these slides and made a retrospective diagnosis of *Pneumocystis carinii* pneumonia superimposed on the cytomegalovirus infection.[8] The material was reexamined, in 1982, by Peter Nichols of Los Angeles, who confirmed Hamperl's diagnosis and drew parallels between this case and acquired immunodeficiency syndrome. He emphasized the absence of any mention of the patient's sexual orientation in the original publication.[9] Wyatt said that appropriate portions of the lower lobe of R. G.'s lung had been frozen.[10] Are these samples somewhere to be found?

Features of the American Cases

From a geographic point of view, the sixteen cases had the following distribution: continental United States, 12; Hawaii, 1; Canada, 2; Central America, 1. The only peculiarity of the distribution within the United States was the fact that it corresponded fairly well to regional densities of medicalization. The patients either lived or were attended in cities with major medical centers. This probably has more to do with regional medical practice than it does with the actual incidence of the disease.

The South American medical literature has not yet been systematically subjected to the same scrutiny, but even if the absence of such cases is eventually confirmed, it cannot be taken as a faithful reflection of historical reality. As noted above, publication of this kind uncovers more about medical interests than it does about epidemiological realities.

The most southerly of the sixteen early cases was published in Mexico in 1957. It was that of a forty-three-year-old male, who died rapidly with shortness of breath, spitting of blood, weakness, vomiting, and anemia. Autopsy revealed the presence of visceral Kaposi's sarcoma with a primary lesion in the heart.[11] In 1958 and 1959, aggressive Kaposi's sarcoma leading to death within one year was reported in three North American males twenty-four to thirty-two years old.[12]

The oldest known case in Canada was a thirty-six-year-old man who died of an enigmatically severe *Pneumocystis* pneumonia.[13] Following this, a few other instances of equally severe *Pneumocystis* pneumonia were noticed in the United States. One of these was a forty-eight-year-old male agent of the merchant marine in New York City, who died rapidly of an atypical pulmonary condition in 1959. Autopsy revealed *Pneumocystis* pneumonia. George Hennigar, the pathologist who did this post-mortem inspection and immediately recognized that the case was unprecedented, later said that, a posteriori, he considered a diagnosis of AIDS in this case was a "strong possibility." The fact that the patient was a Haitian black is not negligible in the eyes of certain American epidemiologists.[14]

A 1964 case of *Pneumocystis* pneumonia was of special interest because it involved a couple. The female partner was included in our series, but her spouse was not, because he also suffered from lymphocytic leukemia.[15]

In those cases reported before 1979, there is a definite predominance of males: eleven males, five females. But the chronological distribution is strange: all seven cases prior to 1960 were male, but in the nine cases after that date there were five females and four males.

Between 1964 and 1981, there were three reports (two in the United States, one in Canada) of progressive multifocal leukoencephalopathy, suggestive of a retrospective diagnosis of AIDS. In addition, there were three case reports of aggressive Kaposi's sarcoma and two of intestinal cryptosporidiosis (all in the United States). One of the patients with Kaposi's sarcoma also suffered from *Chlamydia*. The organs of this patient were removed and frozen. Both patients with intestinal cryptosporidiosis had other opportunistic infections: the first, a female from Hawaii, had generalized toxoplasmosis; the other, an East Coast male homosexual, had disseminated cytomegalic disease. A defect in lymphocyte function was described in the latter two patients.[16]

Intelligence from the Cold

The clinical descriptions cited above are strongly suggestive but not definitively diagnostic of AIDS. Nevertheless, the record is impressive, since it is the residue of a double filtration. The selection is made not only by time, which inexorably destroys essential elements of the evidence, but also by physicians who are inevitably blind to what has not been scientifically codified.

In one of the sixteen probable cases, serological testing has confirmed the retrospective clinical diagnosis. Robert R., a fifteen-year-old American black male, was admitted in 1968 to St. Louis City Hospital for edema of his external genitalia and legs. The pathogenic mechanism of this nontropical elephantiasis was a blockage of the lymphatic vessels, but the underlying condition was unknown. *Chlamydia trachomatis*, a microbe that can be sexually transmitted, was isolated from his lymph, serum, prostatic secretion, and various biopsy samples. It was thought that he had lymphogranuloma venereum, a disorder caused by a *Chlamydia*, which is usually benign and clears up rapidly with antibiotics.

In the case of Robert R., however, all attempts at treatment met with failure. To the great surprise of his doctors, the boy seemed to have no immune defenses. His flesh literally melted away and he died on May 15, 1969. Autopsy revealed the typical lesions of Kaposi's sarcoma. One detail was ascertained, the significance of which did not appear until much later. When pressed to identify a possible source of his *Chlamydia* infection, the boy had admitted to only one furtive sexual encounter with a girl. Something else became clear from the anatomical examination: he carried signs of anal trauma resulting from intense homosexual activity. His partners were unknown. Robert R. had never left the United States and no link with foreigners could be established.[17]

Memory Elvin-Lewis, a biologist, and Marlys Witte, a surgeon, were puzzled by this case because *Chlamydia* was not supposed to be so aggressive and Kaposi's sarcoma did not normally occur in adolescents. Thus they took steps to freeze blood and lymph from Robert R. in order to preserve it for some future studies. The boy's case was published in 1973 as a medical mystery, but in 1984, Witte and her colleagues updated their conclusions and suggested that Robert R. represented an early case of AIDS. This announcement was greeted with skepticism. In 1987 the blood and lymph samples were taken out of the freezer and sent to Robert Garry, a microbiologist at Tulane, who confirmed the presence of specific antibodies: using the Western blot technique, all protein markers for antibodies to HIV-1 were positive. Moreover, in all samples significant levels of antigens related to a present strain of HIV-1 were found.[18]

In spite of this evidence, some specialists still have difficulties believing this story, because it challenges the neat scenario whereby AIDS is presented as having been imported into the United States, at the end of the 1970s, where it was rapidly recognized, if not intercepted, by the public-health network.

Screening tests for anti-HIV antibody have been entirely negative when applied to a vast series of serum samples collected, frozen, and stored in 1976 by the CDC of Atlanta. This was the blood of volunteers participating in a medical survey on a completely different subject. Some of these donors did develop AIDS after 1981, offering thereby the proof of a relatively recent date of their initial infection.[19] In another study, David Madden and coworkers tested 310 serum samples collected between 1959 and 1964: no examples of seropositivity were found. This result is noteworthy, since the blood had been drawn for a study of high-risk pregnancy: fifty-three of the patients were drug addicts and several others were suffering from cancer or other debilitating conditions.[20] In a series of tests done by Bruce Evatt and his colleagues on blood taken from American hemophiliacs, the first appearance of seropositivity coincided with the official onset of the AIDS epidemic.[21]

But we must clearly understand what all this means. Negative results cannot rule out the possibility of HIV being present in the population. Even if the results were completely reliable, they offer no more than an indicator of how rare the virus may have been in the study group. The logical consequences of a single positive result are much stronger. Many negative tests may fail to prove the absence of a virus, but one positive result indubitably proves its presence. This conclusion is justified in purely logical terms, but it presumes the absolute specificity of the tests utilized. The ELISA test is not sufficiently specific; false positive results do occur, fortunately many fewer when the Western blot method is used. Nevertheless, virtually all our confidence levels for the reliability of the tests have been based on fresh specimens; it is not known if they apply when it comes to very old serum. Some trials suggest that the usual tests are less reliable when applied to older samples, especially when the ELISA method is used alone.

James Moore and coworkers identified anti-HIV antibodies in some of the 1,129 samples collected from drug abusers in forty-three states between 1971 and 1972. The frequency of positivity varied with the tests used. With the ELISA test, forty-five (about 4 percent) were positive, but only fourteen (1.2 percent) could be confirmed by the Western blot method. One serum that was strongly positive by Western blot testing was negative by ELISA. None of the eighty-nine samples from non-drug-user controls, collected during the same period, were positive. The authors of this investigation think that serum derived from drug users could yield false positive results.[22]

Virus Endemic to Amazonia?

Surprises can come out of South America. Results obtained on testing the blood of aboriginal Amazonian people greatly perplexed researchers because they were so different from the epidemiological schemes presently in vogue. Out of 224 samples collected, prior to the present epidemic, from apparently healthy Indians living in the Orinoco River valley of Venezuela, nine (4 percent), five females and four males, contained antibodies to HIV-1. Three of these seropositive samples had been taken in 1968. The tests were done with the utmost care, using RIPA and Western blot assays.[23] In another study, a contemporary group of Venezuelans suffering from a particularly severe form of falciparum malaria were found to have anti-HIV antibodies.[24] Were these false positives, or did they open the way for a new explanation? Was this virus, if indeed it was a virus, really HIV-1, or perhaps a close relative? Was it endemic to the isolated Amerindian populations living on the margins of modern civilization?

A Yale University expedition, led by Francis Blake, to the banks of the Tocantins River of Brazil identified anti-HIV antibodies in the blood of monkeys and of a few human females who prepared the flesh of these animals for food. This evidence seems to suggest that a particular nonpathogenic retrovirus, closely related to HIV, may be endemic to this region.[25] However, other serological studies of several aboriginal tribes have been entirely negative.[26]

CHAPTER 12

The Old World before AIDS

Porta itineri longissima est.

—Varro,

encyclopedic writer

HOW DID the situation before AIDS in Europe, Africa, and Asia resemble or differ from that, just described, in the New World? The answer to this question has a bearing on the many speculations about the origins and peregrinations of AIDS.

For Asia, the problem is quickly solved. On the one hand, the sporadic appearance of the disease sometime and somewhere in the vast territories of the Far East seems entirely possible, if not probable, but nothing on this subject has been published; on the other, epidemic AIDS is definitely new to Asia and was introduced only recently.

Europe: A Clinical Case in 1959

Application of the same criteria mentioned in the previous chapter to the search for patients in the European medical literature since the Second World War until the first announcement by the CDC, has permitted the identification of fifteen patients in whom a retrospective diagnosis of AIDS seems possible.[1] In fact, these medical descriptions fall into two well-separated chronological groups: the first group contains six cases observed between 1959 and 1969; the second contains nine cases seen since 1976. The hiatus between the two groups is doubtless of considerable epidemiological significance, since a few cases in the second group represent the not immediately recognized beginnings of the present epidemic.

Rigid application of the adopted criteria requires the exclusion of several cases at the extreme ends of the series. At the more recent end, a few of those patients observed since 1974 are omitted, because they were still alive several years later; and at the most distant end, one case of a man who died in 1948 of fairly typical symptoms (disseminated Kaposi's sarcoma, lymphoid hyperplasia, intestinal hemorrhages, etc.), because he was more than fifty-five years old.[2]

Leaving aside the last-mentioned patient, the earliest possible AIDS case in this series is that of an English sailor who died in Manchester in 1959. He had been a previously healthy twenty-five-year-old male who presented in November 1958 with chronic inflammation of the gums (gingivitis) and nonpruritic skin lesions on his back. By December, he was bothered by a litany of problems: breathlessness, persistent fatigue, weight loss, nocturnal fever and sweats, productive cough, and hemorrhoids. In February 1959, when he developed a large painful anal fistula and a small papule in one nostril, he was admitted to the Manchester Royal Infirmary. Chest X-ray showed scattered nodular opacities in both lungs. A diagnosis of miliary tuberculosis was made despite the fact that his TB skin test was negative and his sputum was free of tubercle bacilli. A mild elevation of his white count was noted, apparently without any decrease in lymphocytes. Both the anal fistula and the nasal lesion progressed to ulceration, the latter eroding nasal cartilage and spreading to the upper lip. Antibiotics, steroids, and eventually radiotherapy were used to no avail. He died in September 1959.

It was only at the autopsy that pathologist George Williams found the presence of an interstitial pneumonia with cytomegalic inclusion bodies and evidence of *Pneumocystis carinii*. A peculiar brownish nodule was observed embedded in the gray matter of the left parietal lobe of the brain. The case was published in the October 29, 1959, issue of *Lancet* as an extraordinary coincidence of cytomegalovirus and *Pneumocystis*. Williams and his colleagues remembered this patient in 1983 and wondered if he might have had AIDS. He had been single, they recalled, but absolutely nothing was known of his sexual orientation. He had been a sailor and had traveled widely between 1955 and 1957. Homosexuality is common in the navy, and anal fissures can be a diagnostic indicator of such practices.[3]

This history could be included in a present-day medical textbook as an illustration of the typical unfolding of AIDS. Although the retrospective diagnosis is based solely on clinical and pathological evidence, it is difficult to envisage any other coherent explanation for this death in the bloom of youth. The possibility of confusing such a picture of wasting with galloping consumption is also instructive.

To my knowledge, at least two other convincing European cases of AIDS have been identified in the literature prior to 1976: one from England in 1961; the other from Sweden in 1967. These cases may have been separated in time and space, but they did have some common features: both had opportunistic infections of atypical mycobacteria (*M. avium intracellulare* in one case; *M. kansasii* in the other) and both occurred in girls.[4]

Is the European Virus an Import?

As soon as AIDS was recognized in the United States, undisputed cases were found in Europe. As discussed in Part One of this book, European doctors grasped the significance of their observations only after they had been alerted by their American colleagues. Some early European cases played an important role in the eventual formulation of ideas concerning the origin of the epidemic. Exemplary, from this point of view, were the Danish, Belgian, and French cases that pointed to equatorial Africa as the source of the disease. In particular the case of Margrethe Rask, a surgeon from Denmark, who died in Copenhagen of a mysterious infection that she had contracted in Zaire; a French woman and a Portuguese male chauffeur, both treated in Paris after journeys to Africa; and a female secretary from Zaire who worked for a Belgian airline. The medical care of these patients went back to 1976, but it was only in 1983 that their histories were published.[5]

These sparks from Africa did not ignite a blaze, but when the virus was brought from America the epidemic broke out. One of the French patients, in whom symptoms of opportunistic disease began prior to 1981, was a thirty-two-year-old male, hospitalized in 1980 following travels in Haiti and the United States. Contact with the Caribbean and North America was common in the past history of Parisian homosexuals, through whom the AIDS epidemic would emerge in late 1981 and early 1982. Copenhagen's second AIDS patient was infected by homosexual relations in which he had engaged during a 1979 stay in New York. Similarly, the first English case of AIDS was due to infection resulting from a homosexual escapade in Miami.[6]

In Germany a male homosexual had been followed for Kaposi's sarcoma and anemia since December 1976. In January 1978 he was hospitalized at the University Clinic in Cologne where he was found to have aplastic pancytopenia, lymphadenopathy, and seropositivity to cytomegalovirus. He recovered from a nonbacterial meningitis, but succumbed in January 1979 to thrombocytopenic hemorrhage. No autopsy was performed, but his history was published within the year as a rare example of Kaposi's sarcoma coinciding with aplastic anemia. In 1983 Wolfram Sterry and Arno Konrad, the doctors who had cared for this patient, realized that in all probability he had had AIDS.[7] This patient had made no secret of his numerous homosexual affairs. In the first report, the attending physicians did not mention these activities, convinced that they had nothing to do with his medical condition. He had been a violinist and had traveled widely, but never, it seems, to the United States, Haiti, or Africa; however, in no way does this exclude direct contacts with American homosexuals, much less those with intermediaries.

Another German case, of a twenty-one-year-old male whose symptoms of disseminated mycobacterial histiocytosis began in 1978, is worth mentioning because it was the first in Europe to report a T4-lymphocyte count. While it is now certain that this patient suffered from AIDS, the source of his infection is not known.[8]

One other highly probable case from a relatively early date was that of a fifty-nine-year-old Israeli male whose symptoms of Kaposi's sarcoma began in 1969. In spite of his age, he was included in our series because examination of his blood revealed a decreased cellular immunity that could not be attributed to medication.[9]

Devastation of a Norwegian Family (1966–1976)

In 1966 a twenty-year-old Norwegian sailor developed persistent lymphadenopathy, musculo-skeletal pain, recurrent colds, and dark spots on his skin. He had traveled extensively in Europe and Africa and had twice been treated for venereal disease. Doctors in Oslo's Rikshospitalet diagnosed an autoimmune connective tissue disorder and placed him on corticosteroids and a powerful immunosuppressive drug. Immunological tests, done in 1971, revealed a decrease in lymphocyte reaction and a considerable increase in serum gamma globulins. The disease smoldered until 1975, when he suddenly developed a severe pulmonary disorder and progressive neurological disturbances, including partial paralysis of the legs, urinary incontinence, and dementia. He died in April 1976. Autopsy revealed giant cell encephalitis and lymphocyte depletion in spleen and lymph nodes.

By the time of his death, the patient was married and the father of three children. There was no history of homosexual activity. From 1967 his wife, aged twenty-four at the time, suffered from repeated attacks of cystitis and pulmonary problems, candidiasis, and unexplained fever. In 1973 her condition progressed to weight loss and signs of encephalitis. Acute leukemia was diagnosed in 1976, and her neurological status declined further to partial paralysis of the legs and dementia. She died in December 1976, eight months after her husband. Autopsy revealed approximately the same findings. A daughter born to this couple in 1967 developed normally until age two. Then she suffered a series of major infections, including bronchial candidiasis resistant to all forms of therapy. She died of disseminated chicken pox four months before her father, in January 1976.[10]

These clinical descriptions are in themselves sufficient to suggest the retrospective diagnosis of AIDS. The probability became certainty in 1988, when several serum samples, taken and frozen between 1971 and 1973, were tested by ELISA and Western blot: anti-HIV antibodies were present in all three members of this unfortunate family.[11]

The father was infected prior to 1966, most likely on one of his voyages. He had transmitted the infection to his wife sexually and she in turn may have passed it to their child through the placenta. This is the earliest known case of proven AIDS in a child. Two older sisters are still well and seronegative, with no sign of immunodeficiency. With the death of these three persons, this small outbreak of AIDS in Norway came to an end. It did not reappear in that country until after the introduction of the American viral strain.

Other Serological Testimony: How Old Is HIV-2?

Anti-HIV-1 antibodies have been measured in plasma samples collected from Scottish hemophiliacs between 1974 and 1984: results confirm the relatively late introduction of the virus through contaminated blood products.[12]

A forty-three-year-old Portuguese male was admitted to London's Hospital for Tropical Diseases in 1978 for a four-year history of a bewildering ensemble of exotic complaints, including intermittent fever, cryptosporidiosis and enterovirus enteritis, candidiasis, herpes, relapsing pneumonia, hepatitis, and scabies. For ten years between 1956 and 1966, he had lived in Portuguese Guinea (now Guinea-Bissau). While in hospital, he continued to lose weight and suffered a chronic diarrhea refractory to all treatment. After three months in hospital, he returned to his homeland to die. A retrospective diagnosis of AIDS in this patient seemed very probable, but tests on his serum done in 1987 were negative for anti-HIV-1 antibodies. In 1988, however, ELISA and Western blot assays were found to be strongly positive for HIV-2.[13]

In February 1989, M. Kawamura and colleagues published the results of a serological study of over three thousand serum samples collected from eleven west African countries between 1966 and 1977 and stored by the WHO Serum Bank in Japan. Anti-HIV-2 antibodies were detected even in the oldest of these specimens (two seropositives in the series of 207 samples collected in 1966 in the Ivory Coast). Seroprevalence did not increase significantly until the end of this series. The Japanese scientists considered only those cases clearly confirmed by Western blot testing.

This serological evidence supports the opinion of some Parisian virologists who believe, because of the structural properties of HIV-2 and the epidemiological profile of the disease caused by it, that HIV-2 existed long before the present AIDS pandemic due essentially to HIV-1.[14]

Africa: The Mystery of Aggressive Kaposi's Sarcoma

European physicians working in postwar equatorial Africa after the Second World War noticed that Kaposi's sarcoma occurred more frequently there (with an incidence perhaps two hundred or three hundred times greater than elsewhere) and assumed forms that were more serious than those encountered in European and American patients. Nevertheless, it was not possible to determine if this was a new or an old disease. Most tended to think of it as a relatively new disease, because Alphonse Loewenthal, a well-trained and meticulously observant dermatologist, claimed to have seen only one case, while he was working in Uganda from 1931 to 1941. Sporadic instances of Kaposi's sarcoma could be traced back a long way in some African countries, but doctors familiar with these regions were under the impression that there had been no epidemic before the mid-twentieth century.[15]

In 1961 and again in 1980, international symposia were held in Kampala, Uganda, to focus on this preoccupying outbreak of African Kaposi's sarcoma.[16] Papers were presented on its epidemiology and clinico-pathological appearances, and conclusions were drawn. No one mentioned the possibility of an infectious disorder of the immune system. AIDS was still unknown.

The AIDS epidemic began sometime in the period between these two conferences. At the second, no particular change was reported in the characteristics or distribution of the disease during the preceding ten years (1970–1980). Things were quite different by 1984, when various aspects of African Kaposi's sarcoma were reexamined by specialists at a Nairobi conference on cancers associated with the AIDS virus. They ascertained that, in some African countries, Kaposi's sarcoma had recently increased in frequency and become decidedly more aggressive, more generalized, and more lethal.

To help appreciate the incidence of Kaposi's sarcoma in Africa, one can make use of its relative proportion in some series of biopsies and in clinical cases of cancer. In the pre-AIDS era, it was most frequent in eastern Zaire, then in Rwanda and Burundi where it made up roughly 10 percent of all cancers; decreasing to 6 percent in Cameroon; 3 to 5 percent in Tanzania, Uganda, and the countries of the former French Equatorial Africa; 1-3 percent in Mozambique, Botswana, and Nigeria; and, finally, less than one percent in South Africa, Ghana, and West Africa. These figures are much higher than those observed in Europe, the United States, or even North Africa. According to the observations of P. L. Gigase, made in the Lake Kivu region of Zaire between 1953 and 1960, there was a fairly stable rate of six to eight new cases per year for every one hundred thousand males. The endemic of Kaposi's sarcoma was limited to regions south of the Sahara, and this situation has not changed significantly for a quarter of a century. The incidence of this disease is, as a general rule, highest near the equator and decreases with distance from it.[17]

In African countries, Kaposi's sarcoma seemed to depend on a genetic factor, since it was usually confined to aboriginal peoples. However, in the United States it occurred less frequently in people of African origin than it did in those of European extraction. In Africa tribal differences in incidence were observed, but they seemed less important than the geographic factors. "African Kaposi's" attacked younger adults more often than did the European form; it did not spare children. Among the adults there was still a predominance of males, but children of both sexes were affected equally. It seemed to favor rural environments as much as, if not more than, the cities.

Clinico-pathological observations in Zaire and Uganda allowed distinction of three forms of Kaposi's sarcoma:

    1. A relatively benign form of growth limited to nonulcerating cutaneous nodules and plaques, like the "classic" European form.

2. A locally aggressive or florid form with rapid ulceration, but limited visceral involvement. The prognosis is poor, but survival can be prolonged.

3. A rapidly progessive and highly lethal lymphadenopathic form (''pseudo-Hodgkin's'' type), with visceral dissemination from the outset. This form constitutes approximately 10 percent of all African Kaposi's. It affects mostly young adults and children.[18]

With good reason, a professor of surgery at Kampala, S. K. Kyalwazi, wondered, as early as 1969, if African Kaposi's sarcoma might be two quite different diseases.[19] The fact that the microscopic appearances of the lesions in the two forms were identical did not necessarily imply that the underlying pathogenetic mechanisms could not be remarkably different.

None of the many autopsies done, since 1970, in African medical centers has revealed the simultaneous existence of Kaposi's sarcoma and *Pneumocystis* or *Cryptococcus* infection. In the nodular form, cell-mediated immunity was intact, but it may be altered in the other two more aggressive forms. After 1970 several patients with the third, lymphadenopathic form of the disease were reported to have decreased cellular immunity without any impairment of humoral immunity. This deficit was an irregular and often transitory finding.[20]

In May 1984 Robert Biggar's international team conducted a systematic survey of hospitalized patients in Katana, near Lake Kivu in Zaire. None of the fourteen patients between the ages of fourteen and sixty-four with biopsy-proven Kaposi's sarcoma were found to have anti-HIV-1 antibodies, although three of the reactions were borderline (too weak to be considered positive). In a control group of twelve patients admitted for surgical problems, there were two seropositives. In another group of 250 young people attended in the outpatient department of the same hospital, 12.4 percent had HIV-1 antibodies.[21]

Other serological testing by ELISA and Western blot revealed that African patients with endemic Kaposi's sarcoma did not usually have antibodies to HIV-1. Robin Weiss and colleagues examined blood samples collected in 1984 from sarcoma patients in Uganda and Zambia: in patients with endemic nodular Kaposi's sarcoma only 17 percent (five of thirty) were seropositive, but in patients with aggressive Kaposi's sarcoma as many as 92 percent (twenty-four of twenty-six) were positive. In two large control groups of people who did not have Kaposi's sarcoma, seropositivity was 2 percent in Zambia and 20 percent in Uganda.[22] In another study, several Nigerians with Kaposi's sarcoma were seronegative.[23] According to the Lusaka physician, Anne Bayley, the most aggressive forms of Kaposi's sarcoma did not appear until after the onset of the present AIDS pandemic.[24]

These investigations confirmed the clinical impression that there were a number of common features between some forms of African Kaposi's sarcoma and the same disease in AIDS patients, but they did not support the notion of a common pathogenesis. Kaposi's sarcoma seems to be an opportunistic disease of unknown, probably viral, origin.[25] It can just as well unmask the presence of an underlying AIDS, as it can result from a completely different pathogenic constellation.[26]

Jonathan Weber and Kevin De Cock have proposed the oversimplified hypothesis whereby AIDS is viewed as an epidemic form of African Kaposi's sarcoma. This hypothesis may not be acceptable in its strong formulation, but it is not completely unjustified.[27]

Although it may not be linked to AIDS, the presence of the very aggressive form of Kaposi's sarcoma in Africa's past is of considerable historical importance, not necessarily in revealing the existence of a virus with properties like HIV, but possibly in concealing it. Suspicion persists concerning the role of the HIV in the recrudescence of the Kaposi's sarcoma, as it has been observed in equatorial Africa since the middle of this century.

True Blood May Not Lie

Except for references to Kaposi's sarcoma and lymphoma, the African medical literature, before the American communiqué of June 1981, is relatively silent on the subject of opportunistic diseases before 1977. In that year, Zaire's earliest AIDS cases were seen (a woman from Kinshasa and her little girl), as well as a Rwandan family, in which the twenty-seven-year-old mother and her children presented with symptoms that, in the light of present knowledge, make a diagnosis of acquired immunodeficiency highly probable. A retrospective diagnosis of AIDS has also been made in a Canadian who died in 1978, having received a blood transfusion in Zaire two years earlier.[28]

With respect to observations made directly in Africa, I know of only a few publications on cryptococcosis in equatorial Africa and the Ugandan report of a single fatality from disseminated *Strongyloides*. The latter was a forty-five-year-old male who died in 1973 of an infestation of these tiny worms of eel-like appearance. The infestation involved several organs including the meninges, possibly the result of immune depression.[29]

As for African cryptococcosis, an opportunistic infection that became one of the best indicators of the AIDS epidemic at its explosive beginning in Zaire, the first exact observation was made by a team of colonial physicians, led by P. Ravisse, just before 1958 when French Equatorial Africa acquired political freedom. During the 1960s, approximately one new case of cryptococcal meningitis was noticed each year in Kinshasa's hospital admission records. The rate began to increase noticeably in the early 1980s, at the very moment when the AIDS epidemic began its expansion.[30]

Hasty conclusions should not be drawn from comparison of the rudimentary medico-historical information out of Africa and the documentation of the pre-AIDS era in North America and Europe. There were vast differences in the levels of medical care and research between the continents. Well-informed experts on the working conditions of doctors in Africa before 1980 emphasize the enormous, practical difficulties that made it almost impossible to recognize *Pneumocystis* and other unusual forms of opportunistic infections. It is no accident that the first definite cases of African AIDS were recognized not in situ but in patients who were treated in Europe. In the tropics, the wealth of lethal infectious pathology is matched by the poverty of diagnostic facilities, rendering undetectable sporadic appearances of AIDS. It is entirely possible that localized or even moderately large epidemics have passed unnoticed.

The situation did not change until the advent of serological tests. Essential for the appreciation of the extent of the present-day epidemiological situation, these tests can also shed light on the past.

In 1986 Myron Essex and his team tested a total of 1,213 stored plasma samples, of which 818 were collected in 1959 from a variety of African countries (672 in central Africa, i.e., the Belgian Congo, southern Sudan, Rwanda, and Burundi; and 146 from bushmen of South Africa); 118 in 1967 from Mozambique; and 277 in 1982 from rural Bantu tribes in Zaire. These specimens had been collected and frozen as part of a systematic study on the relationship between malaria and the geographic distribution of certain human genes. ELISA was slightly positive in twenty-one of the 1959 samples from central Africa and negative in all others. Only one of the twenty-one samples with positive ELISA tests remained positive for anti-HIV-1 antibodies after confirmation by Western blot and immunofluorescent microscopy. This was the blood of a donor from Leopoldville (now Kinshasa),[31] whose identity is no longer known. It seems that he was an adult male thought to have had tuberculosis (Myron Essex, verbal communication).

This retrospective analysis is very important from a medico-historical point of view because it makes three conclusions highly probable: (1) HIV-1 or a close virus with similar antigenic properties was present in Zaire as early as 1959; (2) epidemic AIDS is relatively new to Africa, since the prevalence of HIV seropositivity seems to have been very low until 1982; (3) ELISA tests on stored frozen plasma are unreliable and yield many false positives.

A Belgian team from Louvain collected and carefully preserved large numbers of serum samples from young postpartem mothers at Kinshasa in 1970 and again in 1980, for an epidemiological study of hepatitis-B in central Africa. Luc Montagnier, Jan Desmyter, and others found that two of the eight hundred specimens collected in 1970 were seropositive. Thus, 0.25 percent of these women in a sample group representative of the capital of Zaire and its surroundings showed evidence of contact with HIV-1. In the 1980 samples, this had risen to 3 percent—a twelvefold increase—in an otherwise epidemiologically identical group of young mothers.[32] In 1985 this was probably higher than 5 percent seropositivity, and at the time of this writing it is estimated to be more than 12 percent. Montagnier says that these figures show ''that the epidemic is equally new in this African country, because there were still very few persons infected in 1970 and that diffusion of the virus had been relatively rapid between 1970 and 1985."[33]

Other retrospective studies of early seropositivity yielded similar results from frozen and stored serum taken from a group of west African children[34] and in samples preserved for a 1976 study of Ebola fever in Zaire (5 out of a total of 659 specimens were positive). One of the latter specimens, kept in the CDC lab at Atlanta and examined by J. P. Getchell and colleagues, contained an intact HIV virus, which was isolated (HIV-1$_{Z321}$) and presently is the oldest known strain of the AIDS virus.[35]

Surprising results were obtained in the laboratory of Robert Gallo. In December 1984, Carl Saxinger and others tested a series of random serum samples collected between August 1972 and July 1973 from healthy Ugandan children, with an average age of 6.4 years, for a systematic study of the epidemiology of Burkitt's lymphoma. Two thirds (fifty of seventy-five) showed evidence of exposure to the AIDS virus.[36] In the light of more recent knowledge, these results are highly improbable. The samples were first screened by ELISA assay and then subjected to a more refined technique that had just been developed by this same lab ("unlabeled antibody-peroxidase procedure"). If the samples have been preserved, they should be retested with newer reagents to rule out false positives.

It seems that AIDS may have begun its expansion into certain regions in Africa during the 1970s, but the rate of infection was still very low. Several other retrospective serological studies done on African serum samples taken before 1975 have uncovered no positive results.[37] In a 1986 Kampala survey, all of ninety-six elderly residents tested were found to be seronegative, while 15 percent of 716 young adults showed evidence of AIDS infection.[38]

An enormous series of forty-two thousand serum samples taken between 1972 and 1976 from Ugandan children of ages ranging from a few days to eight years is kept in liquid nitrogen in Lyons. According to Guy de Thé (verbal communication), a survey of these samples has revealed a fairly high frequency of HTLV-I antibodies, but no traces of HIV.

Harry Meyer, a scientist with the U.S. Food and Drug Administration, found two positives out of 144 specimens collected in 1963 from children in Upper Volta (now Burkina-Fasso).[39] Were these true results or were they false positives?

A warning is necessary. It is now clear that ELISA tests must be controlled to avoid the false positives that must be suspected in all samples coming from Africa, especially in those collected and frozen more than ten years ago. In tropical countries there is a remarkable parallel between positive serology for HIV or HTLV and the presence of antibodies associated with malaria. Since no immunological cross-reaction has been demonstrated between AIDS and malaria, explanations for this correlation must be sought elsewhere. Several possibilities can be entertained: geographical coincidence between AIDS and malaria, especially tertian fever caused by *Plasmodium falciparum*; an as yet ill-defined role of mosquitos in retrovirus transmission in Africa; humoral immune stimulation in retrovirus carriers also suffering from chronic malaria; and, last but not least, a high incidence of false positives for retrovirus in Africa.[40] False positives are more common in Africa than elsewhere, but the reasons for this have not yet been elucidated.[41] Blood may not tell lies, but we must learn to understand its language.

PART FOUR

DISASTER: ITS EXTENT AND CAUSES

CHAPTER 13

The Origin and Spread of the AIDS Agents

Je ne suis quand même

pas assez insensé

pour être tout à fait

assuré de mes

certitudes.

—Jean Rostand,

"man of truth"

RETROVIRUSES capable of causing AIDS have certainly existed for at least several decades, quite probably for several centuries, and perhaps for millennia. Knowledge of their origin clarifies certain biological conditions without which the current pandemic could not have occurred. But such knowledge does not answer the fundamental question: why now? The question goes beyond the framework of virology. To resolve this problem of the origin of the current pandemic, we must consider a complex of factors in which the biological and the social are inextricably entwined.

The pandemic raging now resulted from at least two different epidemics superimposed. They were triggered by two distinct agents, genetically related to one another only by an indirect lineage. The first epidemic, caused by HIV-1, was identified by American doctors as a specific disease previously unknown; the second epidemic, caused by HIV-2, would probably have gone unnoticed if the gravity of the first had not sharpened the attention of physicians and guided the research of virologists. This second epidemic was at first centered in one place, West Africa, whereas the worldwide spread of HIV-1 began in three places, one in central Africa and the other two on the coasts of North America. The two American centers surely had a common origin, but it is unknown whether the brushfires on the two continents were independent and somehow parallel, or whether one touched off the other. Which, therefore, was first: Africa or America?

The Infection in Monkeys

Between 1969 and 1982, four epizootics had decimated a colony of macaques (*Macaca arctoides* and *Macaca mulatta*) used in research at Davis, California. Since the first appearance of this disease, malignant lymphomas and immune depression were discovered in these animals, along with opportunistic infections. By the time of the fourth epizootic, in 1981–1982, the connection with AIDS could be made. Published at the beginning of 1983, the data on this new disease of monkeys rapidly attracted the attention of AIDS researchers.[1] This disease, soon dubbed SAIDS (Simian AIDS), was doubly interesting: it could be used to support the hypothesis on the role of monkeys in the origin of AIDS, and it provided an animal model for experimental studies of the human disease.

Tissues harvested from the macaques in California that succumbed to this disease in the winter of 1982–1983 were injected into four living animals of the same species. Within several weeks all had developed generalized lymph-node enlargement and opportunistic infections. Two died rapidly, and one had skin lesions resembling Kaposi's sarcoma.[2] By the beginning of 1984, Murray Gardner and his Davis colleagues had isolated the retrovirus responsible for the 1981–1982 monkey epizootic. This virus, called SRV-1, was quite distinct from HTLV-I.[3]

In September of the same year, M. D. Daniel, Ronald Desrosiers, Myron Essex, and their collaborators at Harvard University isolated another agent from a macaque with SAIDS, this time with serologic properties close to HTLV-III. Though no STLV-II was known, these workers designated the new virus by the acronym STLV-III (later STLV-III$_{mac}$, renamed SIV$_{mac}$), doubtless thus to underscore its hypothetical kinship with Gallo's HTLV-III.[4]

Serologic tests were performed in 1987 on samples of frozen sera from the Davis-colony macaques that succumbed to SAIDS in 1976–1978. These studies showed the cause of this first epizootic would have to be a strain of the SIV. These investigators succeeded even in infecting a monkey with tissue frozen ten years earlier and isolating the virus of the previous epizootic from the new host's lymphocytes.[5]

Since these were captive animals, it was very difficult to say if humans had infected these monkeys or vice versa. The human AIDS virus can be transmitted to chimpanzees in laboratory conditions by introducing it either into the bloodstream or the vagina.[6] These infected chimps became seropositive and carried the virus in their blood, but evidenced no clinical disturbance.

The macaques that suffered, while captive, from a disease closely resembling human AIDS, had originated in Asia. In 1985 Myron Essex therefore tested a series of blood samples obtained from wild Asiatic monkeys. He found no trace of SIV. The same negative result was obtained from examining the blood of African chimps and baboons. By contrast, more than 50 percent of green monkeys examined (principally *Cercopithecus aethiops*) had anti-SIV antibodies in their blood. This seroprevalence varied in different parts of Africa between 30 and 70 percent.[7] Some mangabey monkeys (*Cercocebus atys*) were themselves highly infected. Several strains of SIV virus were isolated from green monkeys, mangabeys, baboons, and mandrills.[8] Remarkably, though, these animals infected in natural circumstances, running wild, seemed to suffer no symptoms of disease that could be linked to the virus in question. The entry of SIV into their bodies remained without visible pathogenic effect.

From a healthy mangabey, Patricia Fultz had isolated a strain of SIV that was entirely inoffensive to this simian species. Macaques infected by this viral strain suffered from a chronic illness not dissimilar from the minor forms of human AIDS. After passage through the bodies of several macaques, the agent became progressively more virulent. A viral strain isolated after such passages, when inoculated into a healthy macaque, elicited acute, severe pathological reactions. Inoculated back into a mangabey, it sickened the animal despite its natural resistance (Colloque des Cent Gardes, 1988). This experience illustrates the possibility that the recent form of HIV-1 had its virulence potentiated by an analogous process.

Numerous Asian and African monkeys, belonging to several dozen species, carry a leukemia retrovirus called STLV, which is the simian counterpart of HTLV-I.[9]

The Genealogy of the AIDS Retroviruses

No pathogenic virus is entirely new. They do not spring up ex nihilo. They come from ancestors that must have similar genetic characteristics and must replicate somewhere, be it in an animal population or a human population, in which they have struck a sort of biological equilibrium.

It is difficult to believe that there was a very recent origin of the HIV-1 and HIV-2 viruses by means involving two sets of sudden and parallel mutations over a relatively brief period of time. New data on related animal retroviruses, and molecular analysis of their various strains, make a slower process seem probable, with successive selection pressures operating on a highly variable viral genetic pool.

Today we know the exact biochemical composition of a considerable number of retroviral strains. An enormous amount of work has been completed in the last several years, unsuspected by the layman, in the area of sequencing molecules that carry biological information. By analyzing the frequency of amino acid substitutions in specific proteins, or better yet, of nucleotide substitutions in the genomes of various strains, it has become possible to calculate evolutionary distances and hence establish pedigrees, to retrace the steps of evolution and try to guess its rhythm.[10] The American group of M. A. McClure has calculated genetic distances in the molecular phylogeny of the principal retroviruses. The group's analyses are based on the differences between the viral protein sequences.[11] Gerald Myers, and Shozo Yokoyama, Takashi Gojobori, and other Japanese investigators working in the United States have gone beyond this to compare the genomes themselves.[12] Matthew Gonda and his colleagues, concentrating their attention on the *pol* segment, a relatively stable structural gene, published in December 1988 a phylogenetic tree of retroviral relationships, with a calculation of the relative length of each of the branches.[13] These investigations now replace the more or less fortunate intuitions of earlier authors with the rigor of scientific method, but nonetheless remain speculative.

The evolutionary past of the AIDS agents can be presented as a tree with many branch points, of which the most significant are

1. The point of origin of the retrovirus;
2. The divergence of the lentivirus and the oncovirus lineages;
3. The separation of the lentivirus lineage affecting primates (SIV/HIV) from the lineage whose descendants infect certain other mammals;
4. The divergence of the HIV-1 and HIV-2 lines;
5. The diversification of the HIV-1 line.

The origin of the retroviruses is lost in the depths of time. They probably derived from movable elements in the cellular genome, shearing off from the mother cell at some point before the appearance of the mammals.[14]

The lentiviruses, including HIV, form a natural strictly monophyletic group. Although the agents of AIDS and the retroviruses of the HTLV line have certain common characteristics, in form as well as in function, they are clearly distinguishable by their nucleotide sequences. The HTLVs are closer to the bovine leukemia virus (BLV) than to SIV/HIV. Genetic analyses have confirmed Montagnier's hypothesis that the AIDS virus is linked to the lentiviruses, namely, to the visna virus and the virus of equine infectious anemia (EIAV), and not to Gallo's two HTLV species.[15] The bifurcation that gave rise to the lentivirus lineage and which, from an evolutionary point of view, thus separates Montagnier's virus from Gallo's HTLVs, probably dates back to prehistory.

Early lentiviruses diversified to infect a wide variety of mammals: primates, horses, cattle, and cats. In the cells of primates, a new retrovirus branch detached itself and exploited a T4 tropism. Doubtless there was a slow evolutionary process involving several steps. We know practically nothing about the phases of this development. The lentiviruses find their host either in primates (including humans) or in domestic animals. If this is not an artifact of the research itself, the key link seems to be man.

Whatever the case, the lentiviruses divided into several quite distinct branches: all the isolates of HIV and SIV form a homogeneous cluster, separate from the EIAV of horses, the visna in sheep, and the bovine AIDS virus (BIV) which, in turn are clearly further in genetic distance not only one from the other but also each of them from the HIV.[16] Although the isolation of the BIV and the description of a sort of AIDS in cattle dates back to 1972, the retroviral nature of this agent and its analogy with human AIDS was not recognized until 1987.[17] It is now known that domestic cats can be affected not only by Jarrett virus leukemia (feline leukemia virus), but also by another disorder resembling human AIDS, in which the causal agent is a lentivirus.[18]

The appearance of the common ancestor of the SIV/HIV line surely goes back several decades, but probably much further. The sequencing of the HIV-2 genome demonstrates that it differs significantly from that of HIV-1.[19] According to Gerald Myers and T. F. Smith, the differences between three homologous sites on the viral nucleotide sequences would require a period of some forty years as their minimal mutational distance; Paul M. Sharp and Wen-Hsung Li put at 140 to 160 years their estimate of the actual age of the branch from which HIV-1, SIV_{agm} and HIV-2 stem, while the calculations of S. Yokoyama indicate the evolutionary distance between the genomes to necessitate a longer period of at least 280 years.[20]

The AIDS agent thus existed in its ancestral form well before the recent epidemic. The ancestor of the line was not necessarily pathogenic. Minimal differences between certain decisive loci on a retrovirus can render it inoffensive, accentuate its virulence, or change the clinical picture that it causes.

The evolutionary relationships between the different strains of SIV and the HIV-1 and HIV-2 lines have not yet been clarified. SIV isolates sequenced so far have been clearly closer to HIV-2 than to HIV-1.[21] The SIV_{mac}/HIV-2 group members notably bear the gene called *vpx*, which is not found in HIV-1.[22] All signs point to the notion that the HIV-1 and HIV-2 viruses cannot be descended from each other, and that HIV-1 cannot have descended from most known strains of the simian virus. On the one hand, the SIV_{agm} (African green monkeys) virus is situated between HIV-1 and HIV-2: it appears to be the cousin of HIV-1, but at a considerable genetic distance. On the other hand, the SIV_{mac} virus is very close to the HIV-2, though the virologists were still unable to determine which of the two forms is older.[23]

The SIV_{mac} virus probably derived from the SIV_{smm} (sooty mangabey monkey) virus. Macaques, Asian monkeys, were not infected in the wild; the relationship of their viral strain to HIV-2 rather than HIV-1 strongly suggests that their infection came not from man but from African monkeys in captivity. The existence of a special simian viral strain similar to HIV-1 has just been discovered in two Gabonese chimpanzees. We do not know whether the primordial infection was vertically transmitted from a common ancestor to both humans and certain monkeys, or if one of the primates passed it horizontally to the others. And in the second hypothesis, we do not have conclusive arguments to settle the issue of whether the infection arose in the first instance from monkey or human.[24]

The heterogeneity of the HIV-1 virion populations allows the calculation of their minimum age. The variability of the African strains of this virus is greater than that of the American strains. Practically all HIV-1 strains isolated from European patients are closer to the American than to the African strains. According to Shozo Yokoyama's calculations, the degree of diversification of the American and French HIV-1 isolates require a span of at least twenty years. The evolutionary distances between the African isolates require a lapse of at least forty to fifty years. These numerical results are founded on the supposition that a stable site on the viral genome evolves at a constant rate of 10^{-3} nucleotide substitutions per year.[25] According to the calculations of Robert Gallo and Howard Temin, HIV-1 has existed as a human parasite for no less than twenty years but not more than one hundred years.[26]

These are provisional estimates. If the calculation of the minimum threshold seems reliable enough, the determination of the maximal value is quite uncertain.

Opinions on the Origin of the Agents of the Current Pandemic

Infection with viruses similar to HIV-2 is endemic among African primates, especially in green monkeys.[27] They are hunted, handled, and eaten. They sometimes bite a hunter or a child. According to Gallo, interspecies transmission of a retrovirus could have been facilitated by the consumption of raw monkey brain, of which certain Zairean tribes were fond.

It is therefore unnecessary to invoke the possibility of zoophilic sexual contact. One curious ethnographic detail warrants remembering. In his work on the sexual customs of the tribes inhabiting the Great African Lakes region, Anicet Kashamura wrote, "To stimulate a man or woman, and arouse intense sexual activity in them, one injects their thighs, pubic region, and back with male monkey blood (for a man), or she-monkey blood (for a woman)."[28]

Hence there was ample opportunity for the virus to breach the barrier between monkey and man. Why then did such interspecies transmission not take place in some distant past? Certain authors have noted that only in the 1950s was there an intensification of the trade in living African monkeys and their exportation to the United States and Europe to meet the needs of biotechnology and medical experimentation. Several new techniques, for example the use of in vitro culture of monkey kidney cells to study enteroviruses or to prepare vaccines, multiplied potential instances of blood contact, thus rendering human infection with simian retrovirus more likely.[29] According to this hypothesis, the place of passage could have been a Western breeding center or laboratory as easily as the African forest.

It is quite common for an agent to pass from its animal reservoir to a human population. This occurred at other times in Africa with the yellow fever virus and, more recently, with the viruses causing hemorrhagic fevers. These infections were generally benign for the "natural host," which was well adapted to the parasite, but brutally struck down the "occasional host." Survival of a parasitic microbial species depends only on the survival of its natural host.

According to the "simian hypothesis" of Myron Essex and Phyllis Kanki, the SIV virus, endemic among African monkeys, may have been transmitted to man somewhere in western Africa, and may have given rise, through adaptation to its new host, to the current human AIDS virus.[30] Writing in *Scientific*

American, Robert Gallo noted the possibility that "STLV-III [= SIV] somehow entered human beings, initiating a series of mutations that yielded the intermediary viruses before terminating in the fierce pathology of HTLV-III."[31]

This explanation is plausible with respect to the HIV-2 and the origins of the recent epidemic in Senegal and Guinea-Bissau. The HIV-1 epidemic, however, more widely dispersed and much more serious in its clinical and epidemiologic characteristics, cannot have had the same biological source as the HIV-2 epidemic.

The virus designated by the number 1 was first in order of discovery but not necessarily in actual order of appearance. Immediately after HIV-2 was discovered, some thought it represented an intermediate form between the SIV and the HIV-1. That would have implied an ideal evolutionary lineage: SIV would have spread to humans, there to become HIV-2, then with successive passages between humans would have acquired virulence and, as a result of clonal selection, been transformed into HIV-1. Molecular analysis gave the lie to this hypothesis. Though it might be more recent than HIV-2, the HIV-1 virus cannot be descended from it, but rather from a common ancestor. Its simian origin is thus possible but not proven.[32]

The agent of the current HIV-1 pandemic could equally stem from interhuman contamination. According to the "Afro-African hypothesis" set forth by Luc Montagnier, "The virus existed for quite a long time in certain isolated African tribes without causing the least damage: there was no AIDS because the tribe had genetically adapted to the virus, and tolerated it, all the while transmitting it to successive generations. And then, for reasons that remain to be determined, the virus would have been recently passed on to other African populations much more sensitive to the virus, because they had not been heretofore exposed to it. And there, the disease appeared."[33]

It is not even necessary to suppose that this hypothetical tribe should have acquired a strong resistance to the virus. A relatively closed population, with high birth and death rates and a relatively low life expectancy, could have survived the endemic presence of even a rather virulent AIDS virus.

It was not impossible, said Montagnier, for a primitive virus to have undergone a mutation, suddenly rendering it more virulent. So the question again: why now?

One American scientist, Ernest Stirnglass, maintained that the AIDS virus arose from a mutation stimulated by—the experimental atomic explosions! According to him, the beginning of the epidemic in central Africa and the recent prevalence of AIDS in that part of the world were due to the increase in radioactivity in the equatorial zone, from the fallout of strontium-90, the radioactive element brought by wind and rain from the Saharan sites of French nuclear tests.[34] Notwithstanding its scientific appearance, this hypothesis cannot be taken seriously. Without real foundation in known facts, it seduced the imagination by coupling disasters symbolizing today's twin peaks of horror.

According to Guy de Thé, "The probable, yet unproven, hypothesis would be that in humans, as in all animal species, there are one or more retroviruses that are perfectly adapted and hence with but rare pathological consequences. For unknown reasons, a genetic recombination may have occurred between human and simian retroviruses." A genetic recombinatory event, occurring somewhere in central Africa, between two ancient viruses, one originating in the monkey and the other in man, may thus have given rise to the new, highly pathogenic virus.[35]

We may recall in this connection that the origin of the agent of Indian cholera is now explained in terms of just such a recombination. As to the AIDS agent, the hypothesis is audacious. It is neither refuted nor supported by the most recent genetic analyses.

A Black Death or a White Plague?

In our epidemiological speculations, tropical Africa is the ideal place to situate a tribe hit by proto-AIDS. Numerous investigations along these lines have, however, provided no conclusive results. Blood samples from pygmies living in the brush of the Central African Republic were tested: in eight hundred cases, only one AIDS patient was found—a woman who had recently been infected through sexual relations with a Bantu.[36]

Among certain tribes living in rural regions of eastern Zaire and Kenya, Robert Biggar found a greatly increased number of individuals whose blood seemed to contain antibodies to a virus similar to HIV-1. Despite this marked seroprevalence, full-blown cases of AIDS and related conditions are rare in that locale. It thus seems possible that such confined and relatively isolated populations were infected before the outbreak of the present epidemic and, over time, adapted themselves to the virus.[37]

The Afro-African hypothesis need not omit the possibility of an autochthonous source in South America. In our current state of understanding, the American hypothesis is not excluded. Serologic observations on the Amazonian Indians provided certain clues that favor it.[38]

Since 1983 the early presence of malignant forms of Kaposi's sarcoma in Africa was interpreted by Jonathan Weber as a sign of the prevalence of AIDS on this continent well before the recent epidemic.[39] Kevin De Cock defended this hypothesis by adding to the identification of Kaposi's sarcoma with AIDS certain new epidemiologic considerations, notably the comparison with African hemorrhagic fevers and Burkitt's lymphoma.[40] His argument was largely demolished by a group of Belgian physicians, specialists in African medicine. According to Peter Piot and his colleagues, even if one admitted that AIDS might be an old disease, its epidemic emergence in Africa appeared to represent some radically new event. Endemic AIDS would not have escaped the notice of colonial physicians in the former Belgian Congo.[41]

It remains no less true today that strong arguments can be advanced favoring the African origin of HIV-1. The great variability of the strains isolated from natives of the continent is an indicator of the original agent's antiquity. According to this criterion, it should be older than the ancestor of the strains currently raging in America and Europe. The high seropositivity rate in certain parts of central Africa also suggests that the epicenter be situated there.

In the earliest European cases of overt AIDS, the infection had African roots, but less certainty prevails with the earliest American cases. Despite the peremptory statements of certain authors, the African origin of the recent American epidemic has not been proven.

One of the champions of the African hypothesis is Robert Gallo, whose authority and media charisma weigh heavily in the world press, shaping Western public opinion. Gallo's ideas on the origin of AIDS are the logical continuation of his conviction that the pathogenic agent belongs to the HTLV group. From the start he applied the same historico-geographical model of explanation that he had used to depict the world distribution of the HTLV-I virus.

Endemic infection by HTLV-I was first recognized on the islands of Kyushu and Shikoku in southern Japan. In the course of 1982 and 1983, it was confirmed that this virus had spread to several regions of the United States, the Caribbean, in the northern part of South America, and, especially, in Africa. In 1982 Isao Miyoshi showed by means of serologic tests that Japanese macaques were carriers of a virus quite similar to the HTLV; then, in 1983, he isolated this simian virus (STLV). Miyoshi supposed that the HTLV-I was in fact an animal virus passed from macaque to man. Subsequently the STLV was found in a number of Asian and African monkeys. It was conspicuously absent in New World primates.[42]

How to explain this curious geographical distribution of the human infection, and how to link it to the monkey data? A. F. Fleming and Gerhard Hunsmann had the idea that the slave trade could be the key to the enigma. According to them, it was in Africa that the virus had passed from monkey to man, and it was from there that it had subsequently been propagated into the other current epidemic zones.[43]

Robert Gallo developed and fleshed out this hypothesis.[44] He presented it as follows. "HTLV-I originated in Africa, where it infected many species of Old World primates, including human beings. It reached the Americas along with the slave trade. Curiously, it may well have arrived in Japan in the same way. In the 16th century, Portuguese traders traveled to Japan and stayed specifically in the islands where the HTLV-I is now endemic. Along with them they brought both African slaves and monkeys, as contemporary Japanese works of art show, and either one or the other may have carried the virus."[45]

This explanation met with lively opposition among certain Japanese scientists. HTLV-I infection could also be found among the Ainu living in the northern island of Hokkaido with no history of contact with Europeans. Moreover, if the Portuguese had brought the virus to Japan, they should have been themselves infected. But no such findings could be discerned either in Portugal or in the Portuguese colonies of Goa and Macao. Some Japanese preferred the hypothesis according to which the ancestor of HTLV-I had already infected their country's prehistoric inhabitants,[46] but others advanced new genetic arguments in favor of the African origin.[47] It seemed more and more probable that HTLV-I effectively derived from Africa, but nevertheless the role of the Portuguese in its transmission seemed more and more unlikely.

Gallo extended his original hypothesis and averred that the AIDS agent, the HTLV-III virus (the name he still used for HIV-1), was born in Africa. In the genesis of this new human virus he saw a sort of repetition of what had occurred much earlier in the appearance of HTLV-I.[48] Jacques Leibowitch had had this idea even before it had been formulated by the American scientists, and he defended it ardently. The lay press popularized it throughout the world.[49]

It became banal to consider Africa as the cradle not only of humanity but also of its most important infectious diseases. The San Francisco biologist Jay Levy set forth a widely accepted opinion when he declared: "The AIDS virus probably originally occurred in Africa, was present in Africa and existed in balanced pathogenicity in that area, and either came from indigenous animals in Central Africa or from human populations who had grown resistant to its pathologic effect and were just carrying it around without much harm. That's true for many viral diseases and I would guess that's true for the AIDS virus."[50]

In defending the African hypothesis, William Haseltine asserted that humankind evolved over a period of several million years in Africa and that, after the prehistoric migrations, the western part of it lived for tens of thousands of years separate from the milieu that initially formed both humans and their parasites. Humans in Europe and in America had lost their resistance against parasites that still flourish in the rich brew of tropical climate and primate speciation. "Recently, however, the shape of the world has altered. Dakar in West Africa is now a six-hour plane ride from New York City. We are once again knit to our African heritage, once again in touch with those parasites that evolved with us—parasites that are still present in the primates of Africa. We peoples who have separated from Africa are now in the position of the American Indians when they first encountered the Europeans. We are no longer resistant to diseases widespread in the Old World."[51] Haseltine had good reason to emphasize these facts. But they did not explain how African populations seemed to resist HIV-1 infection no better than the Americans; how the conquistadors had also received infectious diseases; and how, finally, the rapidity of air travel could not prejudge the direction in which the virus might move.

The adversaries of the African hypothesis fell into two groups. Some opposed it on scientific grounds, others for political reasons. A fair number of eminent investigators today believe that the early clinical descriptions, presented here in chapters 11 and 12, sufficed to prove that AIDS existed sporadically in America as well as in Europe, well before the beginning of the current epidemic. According to Harold Katner, George Pankey, David Huminer, and several other physicians, the AIDS agent existed for a long time in the Western world and it was unnecessary to invoke its introduction from Africa to explain an epidemic whose wildfirelike spread depended exclusively on certain lifestyle changes.[52] Certain African leaders, meanwhile, struck positions dictated by the political situation and the emotional needs of black people.

Artful Disinformation: AIDS As a Biological Weapon

In a complex disinformation operation launched abroad, the lay press insinuated that the AIDS virus was an American biological weapon. In this account, the epidemic would have started in Zaire, but its true origin was not African. The virus would have been brought in 1978 from the United States. American virologists inoculated it in Africa into black subjects either intentionally or inadvertently. This murderous virus would have escaped from the laboratory, moreover, on the very spot where it was created.

A Soviet magazine, the *Literaturnaya Gazeta* of October 30, 1985, announced the news, citing as its source a report published in a New Delhi newspaper. (It was learned later that this Indian paper, despite its reputation for pro-Soviet views, had not published the report in question.) The accusation took on a more serious form in September 1986, when a report was distributed at the Harare, Zimbabwe, summit of nonaligned nations, bearing a serious appearance and the signatures of Jakob and Lilli Segal, "researchers at the Pasteur Institute." The report concluded that the "AIDS virus, in our current state of knowledge, could have been made solely through genetic engineering. The first appearance of AIDS coincides exactly with the opening of the P IV lab at Fort Detrick, Maryland, taking into account the incubation period; this is suggested also by the fact that the spread of AIDS in the population began in New York, neighboring city to Fort Detrick. The thesis by which AIDS is a product linked to the preparation of biological warfare can thus be advanced with certainty."[53]

After investigation it appeared that the two signatories were not researchers at the Pasteur Institute in Paris, but teachers in East Berlin. The report was an unbelievable tissue of suppositions, lies, and scientific impossibilities. The thesis that their report advanced "with certainty" was politically motivated and satisfied the wishful thinking of certain African attendees.

Fort Detrick is not far from Gallo's laboratory. According to the report's calumnious logic, he was accused of posing as the "discoverer" of the agent of which he would in fact have been one of the creators. Taking off from the Soviet Union and East Germany, the speculative lies were adopted and elaborated in the West, especially in an editorial by the London physician John Seale in the *Journal of the Royal Society of Medicine*,[54] then in an interview with the same author in the October 26, 1986, *Sunday Express*, and finally in a book by the French journalist Rolande Girard, published in Paris in November 1987. Soviet radio and television relayed and commented on these allegations. Seale responded by specifying that in the end he did not know whether the new virus was created by American scientists or by biologists at Moscow's Ivanovski Institute.[55] No doubts of this sort troubled Rolande Girard. She was convinced that HIV "is a genetic montage," made by American virologists with funding from the CIA and the Pentagon. The virus was fabricated at the Fort Detrick P IV laboratory by combining the visna virus with fragments from either the bovine leukemia or Gallo's HTLV-I virus. This military laboratory was not operational before September 1977; therefore Girard concluded that the new virus was fabricated "at the very earliest in the fourth quarter of 1977."[56]

None of these formulations held water, for several reasons, of which three will suffice: (1) the AIDS virus existed in nature before 1977; (2) no scientist in the world at this time possessed biotechnology sufficient to "create" this virus; and (3) if the HIV-1 was, in fact, morphologically close to the visna virus, it could not have been derived from it by means of an induced mutation or a genetic recombination.

The representatives of the scientific and medical institutions of the Soviet Union and East Germany carefully guarded against acceptance of the unofficial accusations cited above. If the disease was but a phony as a biological weapon, it nonetheless served quite successfully as a veritable psychological weapon.

Some Scenarios for the Worldwide Spread of AIDS

If a consensus has now been reached for the most part as to the place of origin and path of initial spread for the epidemic of minor AIDS, that is, the epidemic due to HIV-2, diametrically opposite views persist on how best historically to explain the geographical distribution of HIV-1 infection. Specialists agree on one point: whatever the origin of the causative virus, the disease spread from three distinct centers. The two American primordial areas, New York/Miami and San Francisco/Los Angeles, were certainly linked and formed a single epidemic ensemble. The best proof of this unity of origin was furnished by the initial confinement of the illness to the gay community. Early on, the geographical distribution of AIDS in the United States could be superimposed on a network of homosexual contacts of a particular type (organized group sex). The prevailing view is that the epidemic spread from east to west, but this is not proven. The only thing certain is that New York was the most important relay station in this worldwide spread.

The main historico-epidemiologic enigma resides in the relationship between African AIDS and American AIDS. In theory there are only three possibilities: either one of the two continents touched off the other, or else the epidemic started independently on both sides. Until now the epidemiologists have neglected the third of these possibilities. It seemed to be excluded by the belief that this new disease was born by means of the biological mutation of a nonpathogenic virus or by its recent passage from monkey to human. The African origin seemed to be a necessary consequence of this genetic hypothesis. The discovery of HIV-2, however, compels us to admit a double and even a simultaneous outbreak of the AIDS agents. Such a coincidence is extremely improbable, even impossible, if held to be the result of chance biological mutations. Particular factors must have favored such a double emergence of the recent pandemic. If so, these same factors could well have stimulated the independent appearance in disparate locations of two virulent strains of HIV-1.

For reasons given above, it is tempting to postulate a single place of origin for the HIV-1 epidemic, and to situate it in Africa. But it remains to be shown how the virus escaped. And it is as easy to imagine plausible scenarios as it is difficult to demonstrate their actual occurrence. Three pathways dominate the speculation: Haiti, Cuba, and the Peace Corps.

American specialists have a weakness for the "Haitian connection." According to Robert Gallo, at the beginning the AIDS virus was present in only quite limited areas of central Africa. He proposes that the virus at first remained "localized for some time, then began spreading to central Africa during the early 1970s. Later in that decade it reached Haiti and may have reached Europe and the Americas from there."[57]

Here the question posed in another chapter pops up again: why Haiti? In that part of the Caribbean an AIDS epidemic had actually exploded at roughly the same time as in the United States. There was no AIDS in Haiti before 1972: until that date, the blood trade, directed by the lugubrious Papa Doc's brother-in-law, was a national industry. Haitian blood was exported to the United States, but retrospectively it seems no recipient of it was ever infected. It was noticed in 1983 that an AIDS epidemic had in the interval moved into Port-au-Prince, important with respect to the percentage of affected individuals, but still very localized.[58]

For Haiti, those were the years of great economic misery and terror dealt at the hands of Papa Doc's *tontons macoutes*. Americans stopped buying Haitian blood but were still interested in the human resources of this island. In Port-au-Prince, female, male, and child prostitution took on frightening proportions. Tourists came in search of pleasure while the Haitians fled elsewhere in search of work and political asylum.

Undeniably, the Haitians contributed to the worldwide spread of AIDS. Haitian immigrants to the United States, to Europe, and to French Guyana exhibited a high degree of seropositivity.[59] But whence did this disease come to their island? According to the most popular hypothesis, it should have come from Africa. At the very beginning of the 1960s, numerous Haitians had served as workers in Zaire, especially in Kinshasa. This African nation had just gained its independence. To fill the gap left by the vacating colonialists, they called in cadres of Haitians, valuable because they were French-speaking, black, and without ties to Belgium. Returning to their own country, more than ten thousand Haitians would have been able to bring back the fateful virus. Arrived in Haiti, the virus would have continued its expansion in moving to the United States.[60]

The first step in this pathway is possible but not demonstrated. The second is questionable. The emergence of the Haitian epidemic occurred more recently than the earliest cases recognized retrospectively in the United States. The Haitian HIV isolates are more distinct from the African strains than they are from the American.[61] The epidemiologic profile of Haitian AIDS was of the Western type from the outset, with a preponderance of bisexuals and addicts, to be "Africanized" only in a later period.[62] Quite possibly, HIV-1 may have been introduced on the island of Haiti by American "homosexual tourism."[63] The question is not settled, but I am more and more convinced that Haitian AIDS represents a secondary center started by the American epidemic and not the African.

The Cuban pathway was detected by Jacques Leibowitch. Fidel Castro's soldiers and technicians had participated since 1972 in the nationalist rebellion in Angola. In 1977 Cubans were sighted on the Zairean border, in the tropical rain-forest zone. Brought back to Cuba by these former combatants, the virus could have penetrated the United States when, in 1977–1978, the Cuban government expelled a large number of undesirables among whom were homosexuals and Angola veterans.[64]

According to the third hypothesis, the exporters of African AIDS could have been members of the Peace Corps who came in massive numbers to Zaire and other African countries during the decade preceding the epidemic.[65]

Looking through a different geopolitical prism, one might reverse directions and accuse these same Americans of having brought the "white plague" to Africa.[66] Such a hypothesis is purely in the realm of speculation. Several American groups spent time in Africa in the 1960s and 1970s. White European and American mercenaries participated in the bloody events of central Africa. Some of them were homosexuals.

The Need for a Different Historical Approach

Even if AIDS originated in Africa and the African source predated the American, that does not exclude the possibility of the reintroduction into Africa of a non-autochthonous and particularly virulent strain. It is important not to forget two key epidemiologic facts: (1) AIDS in its epidemic form was as new in Africa as in America; and (2) in the second phase of the current epidemic, the whole world has essentially been infected by spread from the American strains. Before the emergence of AIDS in American homosexuals, the African strains of AIDS were introduced into Europe on several occasions, but gave rise only to sporadic cases.

It is possible, even probable, that there was never either a special animal reservoir for HIV-1, or a human reservoir in the form of an isolated and largely infected population. Perhaps for some centuries the virus existed throughout the world, scattered and manifest only at a low level, in sporadic cases and mini-epidemics invisible to medicine before 1980. In the past, such a virus would have been less virulent and the routes for infection less wide open.

CHAPTER 14

The Biological and Social Conditions of the Pandemic

The infectious diseases replace each other, and when one is rooted out it is apt to be replaced by others which ravage the human race indifferently whenever the conditions of healthy life are wanting.

—William Farr, epidemiologist

A PANDEMIC is a catastrophe in the mathematical sense of the term. It is a brutal departure in a new direction occurring as the unpredictable result of a series of seemingly minor events. Continuous quantitative changes in certain factors trigger a discontinuity and induce the appearance of a new phenomenon. The rupture of an equilibrium results in the dynamic search for a new one.

A pandemic always results from the convergence of biological and ecological factors. Certainly no one can explain the origin of an epidemic of an infectious nature without beginning to take into consideration the biological properties of the infectious agent. But that is only the first step along a path that leads to full historical comprehension. It is imperative to take human biology into consideration as well. And to grasp the genesis of an event that is essentially historical, we cannot fail attentively and critically to examine the sociological circumstances.

The leading specialists explained the recent expansion of AIDS either by means of a viral mutation rendering it suddenly more virulent, or by social changes characterizing the second half of the twentieth century: be it the mingling of populations; the multiplication of modern means of rapid transport; the liberalization of morals, notably among homosexuals; the massive use of intravenous drugs; the generalization of blood transfusion; and so on. It seems to be perfectly legitimate to invoke these social factors: legitimate, but not sufficient. For my own part, I would insist on another heretofore neglected factor: the role played by what I shall call "pathocenosis," which is to say the equilibrium in the frequency of all the diseases affecting a given population. The history of each disease thus contributes to the history of all the others.

A New Biological Explanation

One of the biological peculiarities of the retroviruses is their great genetic variability. Retroviruses evolve more quickly than DNA viruses.[1] They have an immense capacity to adapt. Retrovirus infection corresponds to the most elementary biological realization of what Manfred Eigen defines as a "hypercycle":[2] the speed of replication of the viral genome is influenced not only by the activity of the genetic matrix determining its structure but also by the concentration of the particular enzymatic subunits coded into the genome and thereby dependent in turn on the quantity of nucleotide strands. An efficient feedback circuit is superimposed on the replicative cycle. Natural selection can exert an especially great degree of pressure on this type of "replicator."[3] HIV is, moreover, a diploid virus, which further facilitates its genetic recombination and accelerates its evolution.

The AIDS agent is extremely variable.[4] It can as a result often produce highly virulent strains. Hence the recent appearance of such strains is no extraordinary historical accident. In previously prevailing conditions of life, however, a powerful strain had no tomorrow. Natural selection eliminated it because it killed its host before it could be transmitted to other individuals.

Such enhancement of pathogenic strength poses a grave handicap for a microbe to the extent that it undermines the health of its supporting medium, the host. This might be counterbalanced by the fact that its virulence is often associated with enhanced transmissibility, a property favored by Darwinian natural selection. A simple mathematical formula clearly shows that the relative importance of each element in the couplet of virulence and transmissibility changes as a function of the number of individuals actually exposed. When the number of susceptible people is high, the agent's rate of spread increases with the growth in the transmissibility even if the lethality is great. By contrast, greater lethality, an expression of enhanced virulence, becomes decisively unfavorable for the agent's spread in a population with a low transmission rate. From the microbe's point of view, the strategy that assures it maximum survival depends on the probability of infecting new hosts. Aggressiveness is indicated when the opportunity to infect other hosts is frequent; sweet conviviality is in order if a significant number of those not yet infected carry a strong resistance or if the routes of transmission are tenuous.[5]

In the past, only the strategy of silent parasitism could assure HIV's survival. Hardly a redoubtable enemy, it was a sneaky little devil. Since the particular routes by which it spread limited the number of persons actually exposed, a highly virulent strain had no chance of perpetuating itself across numerous successive host-passages and thereby causing a murderous epidemic. All that changed suddenly in the second half of our century as the result of considerable expansion of its former routes of transmission, the simultaneous opening up of new routes, and the longer survival of individuals already infected by a virulent retrovirus.

The explosion of such an epidemic in several aspects resembles that of an atom bomb. An atomic explosion is produced by the release of a nuclear chain reaction propagated by fast-moving neutrons in a critical mass of concentrated fissionable matter. We know that the initial bombardment of some atomic nuclei with neutrons (i.e., the ''infection'') is not sufficient. The matter will only explode if it is composed of a critical mass of heavy atoms (the ''vulnerable population''), the dimensions of which depend upon the mean distance covered by emitted neutrons (''transmissibility''). One might say that ignition occurs ''spontaneously'' once certain ''supercritical'' conditions are met. Natural radioactive fission continually throws off fast-moving neutrons, but these scatter without producing dramatic effects. Similarly, virulent infectious agents trigger an epidemic only once the threshold of certain conditions is exceeded.

David Durack, in a remarkable editorial in the *New England Journal of Medicine* (December 1981), posed the crucial question: ''Why now, and why not before?''[6] No one could then advance a scientifically well founded response. Today, a major part of the enigma seems resolved: the current AIDS pandemic was released when a series of circumstances coincided, facilitating the transmission of the highly virulent strains of an old virus, namely sexual contacts of a quantitatively new type (organized homosexual promiscuity, greater liberty in amorous behavior, mixing of diverse populations, travels that significantly expanded the choice of sexual partners); transfusion of blood and blood products; and rupture in the pathocenosis, particularly the great falloff in the incidence of other infectious diseases. Most of these events are quite recent cultural artifacts.

The Concept of Pathocenosis: Relationships between AIDS and Other Diseases

The frequency of all diseases affecting a population conforms to certain rules and can be studied using mathematical models. Until very recently, historians of medicine and epidemiologists almost always studied single diseases or, at best, groups of related diseases in isolation from one another. To facilitate a synthetic approach, I have defined the concept of ''pathocenosis'' (a neologism based on the term ''biocenosis''). The study of the distribution of diseases according to their frequency presents a problem similar to that of determining the distribution of animal and plant species according to the number of individuals living in a biotope. Pathocenosis, in its state of equilibrium discernible only in a relatively closed and ecologically stable population, presents a mathematically regular structure. That structure corresponds to the conjunction of linear, logarithmic, and normal log distributions. The log normal series expresses the probability of the distribution of variations whose classes are characterized by a geometric progression, as a Gaussian curve expresses the probability of the distribution of variations in an arithmetic progression. This sort of series predominates in a setting of pathocenosis, and determines its general aspect. It follows from my concept of pathocenosis that the frequency and overall distribution of each disease, above and beyond various endogenous and ecological factors, depends on the frequency and distribution of all the other diseases in the same population.[7]

A sort of congruence unifies not only all the diseases in a given population, from now on in almost all the populations of the world, but also the totality of microbes. Between these tiny and seemingly so simple organisms there are subtle equilibria, exchanges of information, and adaptive potentials whose existence we have scarcely begun to suspect.[8]

What we know about the historical dynamic of pathocenoses can thus be applied to the current epidemic.[9] As a general rule, a pathocenosis changes and ''new diseases'' flourish after major demographic upheavals. They often strike selectively in some more fragile groups. Four great ruptures of the pathocenotic equilibrium have occurred in the history of the Western world: in the Neolithic, with the shift to a sedentary lifestyle; in the High Middle Ages, with the migrations of the Asian peoples; in the Renaissance, with the discovery of America; and, finally, in our own epoch, with the worldwide unification of the pool of pathogens and the spectacular decline of most infectious diseases.

Each historical population has suffered a half-dozen often-lethal diseases, but not always the same ones. Once a pattern of morbidity disappears, another appears.[10] Over the past two centuries the advantage of these changes consisted in the fact that the new dominant diseases struck more and more the older part of a population. AIDS has evaded this rule.

For the past one hundred years or less, successes in the struggle against infectious diseases have practically doubled the average life span in the Western nations. On the eve of the AIDS epidemic, statisticians had calculated that by eliminating all the remaining infectious diseases, the life expectancy at birth of a newborn child in some European and American economically developed countries would not even be increased by a single year![11]

The phenomenon that most clearly marks the change in twentieth century morbidity has been the spectacular regression of tuberculosis. At the beginning of the century, pulmonary phthisis and other forms of tuberculous infection were still highly lethal and widespread, despite the fact that a general improvement in living conditions had begun its moderation since the beginning of the nineteenth century. In the first half of the twentieth century, the falloff in the specific rates of morbidity and mortality from tuberculosis were nearly constant, with a transient recrudescence at the time of the First World War. The Second World War also marked a retrograde step, but the gap was soon filled: pharmacotherapy, early detection, and the general acceptance in Europe of the BCG antituberculosis vaccine accelerated its decline during the 1950s and 1960s. Until the midcentury, deaths from tuberculosis fell briskly without the infection itself being eradicated: medicine transformed lethal forms into chronic forms. Beginning in the fifties, vaccination and antituberculous drug therapy also reduced the morbidity. By the 1970s tuberculous primary infection was relatively rare, probably for the first time since the Neolithic. In the United States, in England, and in the Scandinavian countries, tuberculosis was the stated cause of death in about two hundred per one hundred thousand cases in 1900, about fifty in 1939, and less than three cases in 1960 and at the moment when the current AIDS epidemic began. The situation is less favorable in France and Italy, where the rates were about twice as high.[12] In most countries, the prevalence of tuberculosis today is a hundredth what it was at the beginning of this century.

The agents of a large number of diseases persist in a practically invisible manner. Thus, for example, in the poor hygienic conditions generally found in war, exanthematous typhus could appear even in the midst of a population in which previously no cases had been noted.

More than any other disease, AIDS, or an analogous viral infection acting on the immune system, could have existed unsuspected in the past, especially in the period when other infectious diseases were the predominant cause of death. The AIDS virus hides behind other diseases. Numerous authors have underscored this invisibility of the agent in equatorial Africa;[13] before the twentieth century, the situation would not have been a bit different in Europe and America. The introduction of HIV or a retrovirus with similar pathogenic consequences would have been translated into a perception of illness only when it might cause the resurgence of certain other diseases.

Even after the outbreak of the present epidemic, AIDS was not always recognized. In a university hospital in New York, for example, this disease was not correctly diagnosed before autopsy in more than half of the one hundred or so patients dying between May 1981 and May 1987. Most such lapses date back to the period before the screening tests were available, but even now diagnoses are missed.[14]

The direct relations between AIDS and other infectious diseases are complex. On the one hand, AIDS favors the emergence of the so-called opportunistic diseases. On the other hand, certain local infections of the genitalia facilitate HIV infection. The most remarkable interactions concern the evolution of the disease on the individual level. It certainly seems as though the period of latency can be shortened by the stimulation that various pathogenic factors exert on the immune system. Chronic exposure to viral, bacterial, and parasitic antigens accelerates the progression of AIDS.[15] The association with tuberculosis is doubly unfortunate: each agent potentiates the effect of the other.[16]

The infectious diseases thus disguise the picture not only because they hide the ill effects of the HIV virus but also, and especially, because they hamper its epidemic diffusion. Introduced into a population in which tuberculosis and other infectious diseases are highly pervasive, the virulent strains of AIDS must have become rapidly eliminated or at least circumscribed. AIDS could only persist in the form of sporadic cases or quite small outbreaks: the preponderance of the infectious diseases reduced patients' survival and hence occasions for the virus to expand. Its dissemination was not possible before modern medicine's successes breached the bulwark that other common infectious diseases had formed against it.

The Transfusion Gap

The discovery of the blood groups at the very beginning of the twentieth century opened the way to blood transfusion. Its utility was demonstrated during the First World War. It was then rapidly developed and became one of the most effective and frequently used therapeutic methods. Still, it was only toward the middle of the century that the practice of transfusion opened a gap in the barrier which, from an epidemiologic point of view, separates the blood of one human being from that of others. Over the past few decades, important qualitative and quantitative changes have occurred in blood transfusion. New procedures for blood preservation and extraction of its constituents replaced the former system of transfusing fresh blood directly from donor to recipient with a complex chain, in which the first links are the removal and preparation of blood in specialized centers or blood banks. Road accidents and the extraordinary rise of surgery greatly increased the exchange of blood between individuals and, this time, provided some viruses with opportunities to spread that were incomparably greater than in the past. For the microorganisms, blood transfusion had formerly been a narrow path, used only in exceptional occasions for transmission of some sporadic infections. Today it has become the royal road requiring delicate and difficult monitoring.

In 1977 the AIDS agent contaminated American blood banks. Suspicions to this effect started in summer 1982; their correctness was demonstrated in the fall of 1983, but no effective countermeasure was taken before spring 1985. At New York's Bellevue Hospital, AIDS was diagnosed in 1982 in a transfused patient who had no other history of risk factors. Several medical journals, including the *New England Journal of Medicine* and the *Annals of Internal Medicine*, rejected the manuscript reporting this case. The editors feared a faux pas and the wrath of powerful institutions. So the New York case was not published until 1984, after much delay and only after the publication of the Mayo case (November 1983) and the official recognition by the CDC epidemiologists of the transfusion danger.[17]

Until the end of 1984, blood bank authorities sought to interpret observations on posttransfusion AIDS as minor accidents and refused to draw appropriate practical inferences from it.[18] Some even criticized the publication of posttransfusion infection cases in the medical journals. In 1984 the editors of the *Annals of Internal Medicine* were reproached for "hasty publication of every item relating to this syndrome" and for exhibiting "anecdotal information" injurious to the blood banks' reputation.[19] "You shouldn't yell *fire* in a crowded theater, even if there is a fire, because the resulting panic can cause more deaths than the threat," said Aaron Kellner, head of the New York Blood Center, trying to justify this attitude.[20] The CDC moved with a great deal of consideration for the institutions under question. A screening program was put in place only in March 1985. Thus for eight years a path of infection remained mostly open for the AIDS virus; a similar occasion could have never arisen in the past.[21]

In the United States, the percentage of AIDS cases from blood transfusions remained remarkably constant over four recent years—1.5 to 2.5 percent of the total number, and about 10 percent in women. Its increase was thus parallel to that of all AIDS cases: in other words, the gap was not filled. Taking the latency period into account, this situation was probably to last two to three years longer. By contrast, between 1986 and 1988 the percentage of seroconversion after transfusion was clearly reduced.[22] With the new measures for donor screening, the infection risk by blood transfusion fell rapidly.

In most European countries, blood cannot be commercially bought and sold. It is offered by volunteer donors and collected in special centers. Contamination of blood in European establishments arrived after a bit of delay in relation to the United States, but its immediate impact was just as great. In the course of the summer of 1985, France, West Germany, and several other European countries introduced mandatory screening at the time of each blood donation. This procedure is now universal. It offers security of a very high degree, but not absolute.[23] There are seronegative carriers of the HIV virus (about one half to one percent of all carriers). In the United States and in Western Europe today the risk of infection is estimated to be about one in fifty thousand to one hundred thousand. That is low but presses us nonetheless to strive to cut back on transfusions whenever possible, and, failing that, to encourage reinjection of the patient's own blood in cases where elective surgery allows earlier collection and freezing of specimens.

Curiously, there is a risk of infection for blood donors, not in the case of simple collection of their blood, but rather in the case of plasmapheresis, that is, donation followed by reinjection of the blood's formed elements. In 1983, in a Valencia, Spain, center that bought its plasma in a commercial operation, several donors were infected, no doubt as the result of a contaminated plasma-pheresis apparatus. Frequented by penniless travelers, this center contributed to the spread of AIDS not only in Spain, but also in several European countries and even as far away as Australia.[24]

The Ambivalence of Medicine: The Hemophilia Tragedy

Hemophilia is a hereditary malady, transmitted by women but, rare exceptions aside, affecting only men. The genetic defect consists of the body's inability to synthesize plasma proteins required for clotting. Affected children bleed interminably after the smallest cut. Until the middle of this century hemophiliacs died young, usually before the age of twenty. Their fate was changed by transfusion treatment. Transfusing fresh whole blood or preserved whole plasma already yielded good results but required frequent hospital stays and eventually caused immunologic complications. Decisive improvement in the late 1960s came from the use of clotting factor-rich plasma fractions. Between 1968 and 1979, the life expectancy of a hemophilia patient doubled.[25]

In barely twenty years, modern medicine had thus transformed hemophilia patients' lives and made them bearable. But what followed showed that this boon of biotechnology could be vitiated. Simple cryoprecipitate was derived from a single donor, but freeze-dried cryoprecipitate and, especially, concentrated factors VIII and IX are derived from a mixture of donor plasmas. The commercial concentrates are made industrially and distributed internationally. Each lot of such concentrates contains the clotting factors from the blood of twenty-five hundred to twenty thousand donors. With the introduction of this production method, the risk of viral contamination became enormous. Each multiply transfused hemophilia patient found himself exposed to the blood of dozens to thousands of donors, and each donor carrying the virus theoretically could infect about one hundred hemophiliacs with each donation.[26]

The AIDS virus did not miss this opportunity for expansion. Immunologic analysis of frozen specimens of multiply transfused hemophilia patients prove that the first case of AIDS seroconversion goes back at least as far as 1979 in the United States, and to 1980–1981 in England and Denmark.[27] The clinical disease emerged in American hemophilia patients in December 1979, but was not recognized until January 1982.[28] Until July 1982 the CDC had registered three cases and issued a warning, cautious in its wording but full of somber omens.[29] In 1983 there were already twenty-one known American cases, as well as eight in Europe.[30]

Although unimpeachable proof was not yet available, the evidence for contamination in the blood concentrates was so compelling that it became mandatory to respond immediately and to take security measures, notably by using simple cryoprecipitate whenever possible. In the January 13, 1983, *New En-*

gland Journal of Medicine, associate editor Jane Desforges claimed that "physicians involved in the care of hemophiliacs must now be alert to this risk. Preventing the complications of the present treatment may have to take precedence over preventing the complications of hemophilia itself."[31]

At that time, however, this cry of alarm produced no immediate effects. An editorial in the *Lancet* for April 2, 1983, reflected the reticence of the medical community. Its conclusions were at one and the same time correct theoretically and yet dangerously wrong in practical terms: "The recognition of disease in a few hemophiliacs does not necessarily reflect the tip of an iceberg. . . . The links (between factor VIII concentrate transfusion and AIDS) suggested by the American workers must be regarded as not proven."[32] This gave a clear conscience to the blood banks, which continued imperturbably to sell their products. Experimental investigations of ways of sterilizing blood derivatives by heat or radiation suffered from the fact that there were no convenient animal models at the time, and indeed the causative virus itself was not yet known.

The percentage of infected hemophiliacs increased at a frightening rate during the years 1983–1984. This was recognized thanks to the serologic screening that had begun precisely in those years. The first serial serologic studies showed that the percentage of seropositive hemophiliacs in 1984 had reached 33 percent in England, 64 percent in Denmark, and over 70 percent in the United States.[33] In New England, 53 percent of thirty-four hemophiliac sera collected in 1983 were seropositive; the following year, fifteen of sixteen sera tested (94 percent) already showed evidence of AIDS infection.[34] In California, it exceeded 85 percent, most of the seroconversions having occurred in 1983–1984.[35]

In France infection began in 1981, escalating dramatically in 1983–1984. In 1985 Christine Rouzioux, François Brun-Vézinet, and their colleagues studied the blood of three groups of patients: (1) in 128 hemophiliacs, treated routinely with large quantities of factors VIII or IX, the seropositives reached about 59 percent; (2) in fifty-eight patients treated at another Paris center with occasional, reduced quantities of blood derivatives, there were 10 percent seropositives; (3) fifty-nine Belgian patients treated with locally made products had a rather low rate, below 4 percent. Earlier samples of their blood were studied: in fifty patients from the first group, samples dating from 1980–1982 yielded fifteen positives for 1981, with three more converting by 1982.[36] Dominique Mathez, Jacques Leibowitch, and their collaborators, in another retrospective study screening French hemophilia patients' blood, showed that none of eight specimens from 1981 were seropositive; by 1982 the proportion was already disquieting (18 percent of thirty-three samples); by 1983 the majority (55 percent of forty-nine samples) had converted.[37]

In February 1986 the French National Center for Blood Transfusion conducted a study of nearly two thousand hemophiliacs living in France, almost half of the estimated total number of these patients. The prevalence of seropositivity was 50.5 percent (51 percent for hemophilia-A and 46 percent for hemophilia-B). The geographic distribution was not uniform: in Paris the prevalence was 71 percent, while it was 60 percent in the south and 16 percent in the north. After 1980 French patients with hemophilia-A were treated with products made within the country (80 percent) or abroad (20 percent), while those with hemophilia-B used exclusively the French product.[38]

The American-made plasma was more dangerous than that collected in Europe. Most European manufacturers of blood concentrate used, at least in part, plasma purchased from American blood banks. It was the international plasma trade, supporting blood derivative preparation, as well as the trade of already fabricated products, that led to the worldwide spread of AIDS. In the United States, by this means, AIDS penetrated into the central valley of Ohio, into Colorado, and even into Alabama.[39] Some early Japanese cases of AIDS in hemophiliacs were attributed to the international blood trade. In Europe, through blood products AIDS reached Spain, Greece, and, in parallel with the homosexual route, Italy.[40]

Although the danger of blood derivatives had been pointed out as early as 1983, and recognized clearly with the screening tests implemented in 1984, it was only in 1985 that efficient control measures were begun. Since the end of 1983, heating antihemophilic concentrates above 60°C (140°F) for several days was known to inactivate the virus while conserving the clotting power of the material. But time was needed to establish the reliability of different ways of carrying out the process. In 1984 the CDC recommended the use of heated products, but other specialists differed. Manufacturers found themselves faced with economic problems posed by their backlog of stocks already on hand and by the cost of the new techniques. In the United States production was in the hands of private companies, subject therefore to the laws of the marketplace and of competition. In France it was in the monopoly hands of a national foundation, nonprofit but subject to bureaucratic delay. Faced by the challenge of AIDS, neither system reacted in a very satisfactory manner: in retrospect, the heel-dragging and neglect seem scandalous. The years 1983–1985 were tragic for hemophilia sufferers. The statistical data cited above clearly show that the danger was known but not avoided. Most of the unscreened blood product stocks on hand were not retired. Certain banks continued to distribute them until the end of 1985. In France, for example, the minister of health decreed in July 1985 that beginning in October the use of unheated products would not be reimbursed by the state health insurance agency. It would be hard to come up with a better way to stimulate rapid distribution of the old stocks. Beginning in 1985, France imported heated products; even so, several regional centers handed out dangerous lots until October 1985, in some cases even until the beginning of 1986.[41]

Today this route of infection is blocked, but the tragedy continues for those already infected. Paradoxically, the blood concentrate made from numerous donors now presents less of a risk than single-donor transfusion. Recent estimates suggest that a third of European hemophiliacs and three-quarters of their American counterparts are seropositive. In France their number has passed the 50 percent mark. The situation in Paris is comparable to that in the United States. Only 2 percent of these patients so far have developed overt AIDS. It seems therefore possible that hemophiliacs either have an unusually long latency period or else possess some as yet unidentified protective factor.[42]

Seropositive hemophiliacs can transmit the virus to their sexual partners. About 7 to 10 percent of their spouses have seroconverted, a tragically high number that will contribute to the agent's spread outside the medical and homosexual routes. At the same time, this percentage is moderate and shows the low epidemiologic effectiveness of the heterosexual route, unless we are currently deceiving ourselves about the number of individuals infected without seroconversion.

Substance Abuse: Injection Replaces Oral and Inhaled Drugs

Drug addiction has played no small part among the factors facilitating the worldwide spread of AIDS. If the use of euphoric substances is very old, their routes of administration have changed enormously since the middle of this century. No civilization has been able to pass up its intoxicants, but in the past they were eaten, chewed, snorted, smoked, or drunk. Injecting our path to artificial paradise is a recent phenomenon.

The hollow needle and syringe for drug injection have been known since the seventeenth century, but the construction of the first convenient model, by the French physician Charles Pravaz, only goes back to 1853. Its therapeutic use began to spread at the beginning of the present century and was not widespread until after the Second World War. Early injections of medication were subcutaneous, then intramuscular, and finally, intravenous as well. This last form of drug administration only truly met with approval after the striking successes of syphilis therapy by Paul Ehrlich and Sahachiro Hata using salvarsan (1910).

The risk of transmitting infectious diseases by therapeutic injection became negligible with the introduction of proper methods of sterilization. The AIDS virus, for example, is itself easily destroyed by normal procedures for instrument sterilization. The general use of techniques that introduce therapeutic substances directly into the blood have not contributed to the spread of the disease.

This state of affairs nonetheless changed starting in the middle of this century. Rather suddenly the syringe became a dangerous vehicle for pathogenic organisms, not through its conventional, well-defined medical use but as it spilled over into the hands of addicts in rich countries and of healers in poorer countries. Technical progress in this case played an unexpectedly mean trick.

Beginning in 1970, metal and glass syringes, easily sterilized, were replaced by supposedly disposable plastic ones. The relatively straightforward preventive measures of years gone by were cast out, while the addicts and the quacks treating the dispossessed could rarely resist the temptation to reuse their precious, indispensable "works."

In several industrial countries, the sale of medical syringes and needles is subject to regulation. It is sometimes hard to say if these legal measures achieve their aims, that is, to slow the distribution of "hard drugs," but there is no doubt about their unhappy effect on the systematic reuse of syringes and, consequently, on the spread of AIDS.

The main intravenous narcotic used in the United States and Europe has been heroin. Although this substance has been known for over a century, having been synthesized in 1874 by the acetylation of morphine, its abuse remained limited for a long time. In 1934 Emanuel Apfelbaum and Ben Gelfand, studying three New York heroin addicts who had never traveled in malaria zones, demonstrated infection with the malaria plasmodium, acquired through the use of syringes borrowed from other affected addicts. In the 1950s the first deaths following heroin overdose were confirmed. Toward the end of the 1960s heroin use soared to an unprecedented degree.[43] Between 1965 and 1975 a new form of juvenile addiction appeared in the large cities of Europe and America. After the "hippies," who sought escape from the ordinary life or a "trip" in smoking marijuana and dropping the hallucinogen LSD, came the "hard-core," the "junkies," the "shooters," injecting heroin directly into their veins to experience the stupefying "flash." Only very recently did some people start to use intravenous injections of cocaine and similar drugs.

Several factors came together to expose heroin and other drug addicts to the ravages of AIDS, notably frequent daily injections, group living, needle sharing, the absence of personal hygiene, promiscuity, prostitution both homosexual and heterosexual, chronic debilitation, and, finally, their disregard for danger. Always in need of money to procure their drugs, and rarely capable of regular remunerative work, addicts often resorted to prostitution and, in countries where it was possible, sold their blood. All these circumstances had serious consequences and facilitated the spread of AIDS.[44]

In several countries prostitution in bisexual addicts was one of the paths by which the virus passed from homosexual networks into the general population. In some parts of the world, for example on the French Riviera, in Milan, and in Rome, addict groups were larger reservoirs of infection than the homosexual community.[45]

In America the AIDS brushfire was touched off among the addicts beginning around 1982. In Europe the critical turning point was toward the end of 1984. In October 1984 heroin addicts represented 2 percent of the AIDS cases reported in three European countries; by September 1985 they accounted for 8 percent of the cases reported in nine countries.[46] In Italy, for example, there were in 1984 only 11 addicts with overt AIDS; a year later there were already 87, then in 1986 the number exceeded 250, reaching 639 in 1987. More than half of American, French, and Italian addicts are seropositive today—the figure is above 70 percent in New York, Paris, and Nice. Their number doubles every six months, much more rapidly than the number of seropositive persons in the general population.

In contrast to homosexuals, who carefully heeded new data, the addicts were refractory to education campaigns. Their fundamental problem was psychological. A Paris psychiatrist stated it well: "In shooting up, they already play with their own lives and mock others'."[47] Too often the act of taking drugs is no more than acting out their desire to destroy themselves. Add to that the action of the narcotic on the central nervous system: the uncaring victim becomes a peddler of death.

The Liberalization of Morals

Anthony Pinching, immunologist at St. Mary's Hospital in London, says that "it is merely an accident of social history that we initially regarded AIDS as a homosexual disease."[48] This statement contains an unmistakable truth, but the word "accident" suggests a historical judgment that could easily be misinterpreted. It is certainly true that the epidemic had broken out in American homosexuals not because they had "sinned against nature," but because, as a group, they had been more prone to promiscuity than heterosexuals. However, it would be a methodological fallacy to consider this event as an accident in the strict sense, that is, as the fortuitous result of "playing the odds." American homosexuals created the conditions which, by exceeding a critical threshold, made the epidemic possible. They were a sort of "culture medium" that permitted virulent strains of HIV to emerge.

In the nineteenth and early twentieth centuries, homosexuality was socially repressed in most countries of the world. The famous Kinsey Report well demonstrated that by 1948 it was still poorly tolerated by American society. Toward the middle of the 1960s a profound change of mind began in the United States, translating into a sort of sexual revolution. In the course of the sixties, this phenomenon became commonplace. The general liberalization of morals and contraception promoted early sexual relations among adolescents and multiple partners. In the wake of the social struggle for their rights, the homosexual community began to organize and became a factor in American political life.

The homosexual community announced its presence on the social scene with the riot at the Stonewall, a New York City bar where, in summer 1969, the customers barricaded themselves to defend against a police raid. It was their storming of the Bastille. In the 1970s an extraordinary proliferation of clubs, bars, discotheques, bathhouses, sex shops, travel agencies, and gay magazines allowed the community to "come out" and adopt a whole new repertoire of erotic behavior, out of all measure to any similar past activities. The first citadel of new rights was New York, but soon two major California cities took up the baton. They were part of a new Gold Rush: between 1969 and 1973, at least nine thousand homosexuals arrived in San Francisco followed, in the 1974–1978 period, by twenty thousand others. Each year between 1979 and 1982 about five thousand homosexuals settled there. It was estimated that by 1982 there about ninety-eight thousand homosexuals in San Francisco, of whom almost half lived in a particular part of the city center.[49]

Never in human history had one city known such a concentration of homosexuals, nor such promiscuity. The search for physical pleasure and multiple partners passed for fundamental expressions of individual rights. Meeting places made room for those who wished to have sex with several anonymous partners in a single day and to play both the active and receptive roles. Studies showed that, in male homosexual relations, receptive anal intercourse is by far the most important factor of risk for HIV infection and that insertive anal intercourse is not more conducive to seroconversion than insertive vaginal intercourse.[50] Epidemiologic analysis by mathematical models shows the capital importance of the nonseparation of roles in a population of male homosexuals. The spread of AIDS is facilitated and increased in a critical way if a considerable number of homosexuals adopts neither the active nor passive role exclusively but combine the two. But if the polarity of the roles was the rule of homosexual relations in antiquity, and if it dominates in Eastern countries, one of the characteristics of the behavior of gay Americans is precisely their refusal. Among Western homosexuals in our era, ambivalence has become the new rule of proper homosexual conduct.[51]

The new way of living required promiscuity at times even in those who had entered into a couple. Studies showed that most American homosexuals living in large cities had several dozen sex partners each year; mean figures of eighty to one hundred partners were not rare and some mounted into the hundreds. About 10 percent of homosexuals interviewed had had sexual contact with over five hundred persons during their lives. In medical terms the almost immediate result was an increase in the "classic" sexually transmitted diseases, notably syphilis and gonorrhea; of certain viral diseases, such as hepatitis, herpes, and cytomegalovirus; and intestinal parasites such as amebiasis. Skin disorders of an otherwise relatively rare nature, and chronic diarrhea, become the daily lot of homosexuals. The rise in these disorders preceded the AIDS outbreak, and already indicated the point at which the epidemiologic situation was ready to explode. In San Francisco's Castro district and New York's Greenwich Village, the spread of AIDS in 1981–1982 was catastrophic, faster than anywhere else in the Western world.[52] It was thus in the crowded ranks of the American homosexual community that the AIDS virus finally passed the point of no return in its epidemic spread.

French physician Jean-Paul Escande characterizes the situation as follows:

AIDS is not a divine lightning bolt, but its advent shows that, when a community profoundly changes its life-style, a certain number of diseases will crop up without fail; the excesses of sexual liberalization among homosexuals are probably responsible for the biological modification that fostered the rise of AIDS. . . . AIDS mushroomed not because they transgressed certain sexual taboos, but rather certain rules for living which, until then, had concurred to maintain a relative biological equilibrium.[53]

Numerous American homosexuals maintained broad cultural interests, bonds of friendship with the outside world, and the means to travel and offer hospitality to foreigners. From them the AIDS virus probably moved to Haiti and certainly to Western Europe and Australia. Europe's homosexual community followed the American example but formed a less homogeneous subpopulation.[54] About 25 percent of French homosexuals lead an "open couple" lifestyle, corresponding to the American profile. The AIDS agent was introduced in France on several occasions, as much from Africa as from the United States, but the epidemic that began to rage among Paris homosexuals clearly had its origin in the virus of the New York homosexual community.

If the homosexual community was the ideal "culture medium" in which, as though in a laboratory experiment, the virus could multiply during its critical phase, it propagated equally well later in heterosexuals. Two factors helped: the increase in the mean number of sexual partners and, it would seem, the practice of anal coitus. These days a quarter of American women occasionally practice sodomy, and about 10 percent practice it regularly. According to French studies, the practice is less widespread there, but it is noteworthy that it is clearly more frequent among young women.[55]

CHAPTER 15

The African Source

Ex Africa semper

aliquod novi.

—Pliny the Elder,

polyhistor

BY THE TIME of the international conference on African AIDS, held in Brussels in November 1985, the World Health Organization (WHO) had been informed of no more than an insignificant number of affected Africans. Belgian and French physicians attending the meeting insisted that a true epidemic was under way on the Dark Continent. The representatives of the affected countries took offense and insisted on denying the problem—or at least on drawing a veil of chastity around it. The Africans' reaction was understandable: they stood on the dock of the accused alongside homosexuals and drug addicts, and they were objects of Western fantasies about their sexual behaviors. African tourism would suffer, blacks living in Europe would be mistrusted. But the reality of the danger soon modified their initial impulse to negate, quasi-magically, the epidemiologic facts. Today the inhabitants of equatorial Africa are desperately seeking aid since, from all evidence, the life force of these young nations has been threatened: they have been thrown into a crisis, menacing them both demographically and economically.

Three Epidemiologic Schemas

AIDS is now a pandemic disease. The agent has already spread onto every continent, ravaging some countries and insinuating itself little by little into others. It does not, however, propagate everywhere by the same means. We can distinguish three fundamental models or schemas.[1]

The first model can be used to characterize the epidemiology of AIDS in the United States, Canada, Western Europe and certain urban zones of Latin America. Here the epidemic began among homosexuals, only then to reach heterosexual hosts and thrive among the addict population. In these geographic loci, homosexual contacts and needle sharing among addicts remain the predominant route of transmission, while heterosexual contacts and perinatal transmission are both gaining in relative importance. Men are more often affected than women in this schema.

In the African model, AIDS spreads differently. Heterosexual transmission predominated from the start, and women have been infected as often as men. Prostitutes play an important role in disseminating the virus. The growing number of infants born infected poses a grave medical problem and a terrible demographic threat.[2]

At first it seemed that this second schema applied only to equatorial Africa, but the situation in the Caribbean and in parts of Latin America begins more and more to resemble it. The differences between the two schemata are determined by social factors such as promiscuity, lamentable hygienic conditions, poor nutrition, multiple intercurrent infections, and the resulting constant assault on the immune system. Thus, for example, in a poor area of the United States such as Belle Glade, Florida, the AIDS epidemic is proceeding according to the "African" model.[3]

The third schema takes into account the particular status of Eastern Europe, Australia, Oceania, and especially certain Asian countries. The disease is relatively rare there, primarily affecting persons with multiple sexual partners, be they heterosexual or homosexual. Even among prostitutes the disease prevalence here is low.

The first and third schemata tend to take the form of the second. This gives the impression that the African model may be a further phase of the epidemic and that, consequently, the disease developed in Africa much earlier than on other continents. Such reasoning is unjustified. It would have been applicable only if social conditions everywhere were similar.

AIDS Expands in Equatorial Africa

An African source was suspected on the basis of observations made in 1981–1982 in Paris and Brussels on patients from Africa. Then, in 1983–1984, in the heart of that continent, it was confirmed in the field. The center was situated in the western part of Zaire and Rwanda. HIV-1 infection radiated out from this central zone and seriously hit the Congo-Brazzaville, Rwanda, Burundi, Uganda, Tanzania, the Central African Republic, the western part of Kenya, Zambia, Malawi, and Nigeria.[4]

Although HIV-1 probably existed in Africa for a long time, its manifestations were relatively discrete, limited to sporadic cases and perhaps to one or more low-level endemic zones. For Africa, as for all other continents, AIDS in epidemic form is a recent phenomenon. Retrospectively, the beginning of the present flare-up can be suspected from the multiplication of aggressive Kaposi's sarcoma cases in equatorial Africa starting at midcentury. It became especially conspicuous in the early 1960s among the seasonal workers who came down to South Africa from the central regions with highly malignant Kaposi's sarcoma complicated by fatal meningitides and pneumonitides.[5]

Roughly from 1975 on, in Kinshasa (Zaire), cases of resistant diarrhea with severe weight loss were observed,[6] followed, around 1981, by a spectacular increase in cases of cryptococcal meningitis.[7] Also, in Zambia, at the beginning of the 1980s there appeared a new form of Kaposi's sarcoma,[8] and, in Kigala (Rwanda), a rise in serious cases of oral and esophageal thrush.[9] An AIDS-related enteropathy and the aggressive form of Kaposi's sarcoma were recognized in Uganda in autumn 1982.[10] It was then, too, that the number of African AIDS patients seeking medical attention in Europe increased. If, perhaps, the infection were previously confined to the rural poor until the 1980s, it certainly spread thereafter among the well-to-do of the major cities.

In July 1984 an international AIDS surveillance activity was inaugurated in Kinshasa. Toward the end of 1986, the truth about the African situation exploded into full view: it was a wildfire epidemic without precedent. WHO gave a new definition of African AIDS, adapted to the disease as it presented on that continent. Statistics began to emerge on the basis of serious sampling efforts. At the beginning of 1987, the number of deaths in all of Africa was estimated to be five thousand; experts spoke of two to three million seropositive individuals. The situation was considered extremely alarming—the rapidity of spread was even more striking than the actual number of affected individuals.[11] In certain regions of equatorial Africa the seroprevalence in the general population in fact rose from 1.2 percent to 10 percent or even 20 percent.[12] Jokes about An Imaginary Discourager of Sex (Syndrom Imaginaire pour Decourager les Amoureux) no longer sufficed to exorcise the collective fear. No one knew how to stop the progression of the disease. The Zairians hoped that a vaccine developed by Daniel Zagury, and in clinical trials conducted in their country under the direction of African doctors, might be effective, and that MM1, a medication developed by Zirimwabagabo Lurhuma, a local physician and professor at the University of Louvain, would be more successful than the white men's remedies.

The differences between the clinical pictures of AIDS generally seen in Africa and that habitually seen in Europe or the United States are best understood not in terms of different HIV-1 strains but rather of the particularities of climate, living conditions, and, especially, exposure to opportunistic organisms. In east African AIDS patients, *Pneumocystis carinii* pneumonia is relatively rare; by contrast, they suffer much more than Americans or Europeans from cryptococcal meningitis, esophageal candidiasis, cytomegalovirus chorioretinitis, herpetic ulcers, amebiasis, and salmonellosis.[13] In African patients, tuberculosis, malaria, and other parasitic diseases produce an antigen burden that modulates the natural history of HIV infection in a particular direction.[14]

The HIV-2 Epidemic

A second epidemic raged in Africa, independent of this first one since it was caused by a different agent. Its primary seat was the westernmost area of sub-Saharan Africa, namely Senegal, Gambia, the Cape Verde Islands, and, especially the Republic of Guinea-Bissau, from which it spread to the Ivory Coast, Mali, and the Central African Republic.[15] The disease was recognized in 1981 among these countries' refugees seeking medical care in Portugal and France, but its precise nature and the extent of its primary focus were not clear until somewhat later. Only after the HIV-2 virus was isolated at the end of 1985 were specific serologic tests available to perform systematic epidemiologic studies.[16]

Among certain patients with antibodies to HIV-2 at the Claude Bernard Hospital in Paris, the infection could be shown to go back to the beginning of the 1970s.[17] The virus no doubt existed for a long time in the Portuguese possessions in West Africa, but was manifest only at a low level and in a limited area. Its epidemic expansion was aided, if not actually initiated, by the disorder and the mingling of population groups in the independence struggles that upended normal life in Portuguese Guinea between 1966 and 1975. It is, we must recall, one of the world's ten poorest countries.

According to Venâncio Furtado, director-general of public health services in Guinea-Bissau, AIDS in his countries was "an old disease with a new name." For centuries people there died of persistent diarrhea and galloping tuberculosis. Around 1978–1979, at the Simâo Mendes Hospital in Bissau, an unusual increase was noted in serious cases of irreversible wasting with chronic diarrhea and pulmonary complications. Several of these patients were subsequently sent to Lisbon, where, in 1981, Wanda Canas-Ferreira and other physicians at the Egas Moniz Hospital made the diagnosis of AIDS.[18]

HIV-2 is primarily transmitted by means of heterosexual relations and blood. Infection with this virus evolves more slowly than that due to HIV-1, with longer survival and a higher incidence of non-Hodgkin's lymphoma. The relative benignity of HIV-2 is illustrated well by the case of a patient infected fourteen years ago in Africa, who, despite this long delay, has never exhibited the least problem clinically.[19]

The epidemiologic situations in the Central African Republic and in the Ivory Coast were especially instructive in that two epidemics, due to two different viruses, met and overlapped. In the first of these two states, HIV-1 predominated; its presence before that of HIV-2 seems not to have impeded the progress of the latter.[20] In the Ivory Coast, on the other hand, the seroprevalence for the two types of AIDS infection was about the same: about one percent of the general population (1987).[21] Infection by one of these viruses confers no protection against the other. HIV-1 and HIV-2 seem to be able to act synergistically rather than competitively, at both the population and the individual levels. Infection by a combination of the two is particularly serious; the two viruses are mutually potentiating in their cytopathogenic effects.[22]

According to the 1985 serologic survey conducted by Francis Barin and Souleyman M'Boup, most of the prostitutes of Dakar were infected by a virus subsequently identified as HIV-2. But none of these seropositive Senegalese prostitutes exhibited actual health problems associated with their specific infection.[23] That meant either there was a very weak strain of HIV-2, or the Senegalese possessed an unusually high resistance to this agent, or the introduction of the virus into Dakar was so recent that its pathogenic effects had not yet had time to manifest themselves.

Social Upheavals

Population movements and changes in certain ancestral customs were the major causes of the African AIDS epidemic. Such changes were certainly the cause of its expansive radiation across the continent, and perhaps also of its initial development. According to Alex Shoumatoff, *New Yorker* reporter and eyewitness to recent African upheavals, that continent has submitted to biological and cultural destruction on a previously unknown scale due to overpopulation and to the arrival of the accessories of modern life.[24]

In the middle of this century, rapid decolonialization added new social traumas to the old wounds of colonialism. Since the early 1960s, armed conflicts have jolted equatorial Africa, uprooting populations and shredding venerable social structures. The reckless behavior of an Idi Amin Dada, of a Tschombé, and of other bloody dictators illustrates the difficulty of grafting modern Western institutions onto tribal stock. The states particularly affected by war and its social backlash have been the former Belgian Congo and Uganda, namely just those countries where AIDS rages today.

On the eve of this epidemic, two sorts of human dislocation of unprecedented scale took place in Africa: an influx from the world beyond, and an internal mingling of populations concentrated in the urban agglomerations. From the outside world came both tourists and servicemen. The latter came en masse as members of expeditionary forces, as mercenaries, or as so-called technical advisers. The Africans accused them of introducing their countries to homosexual practices—behaviors traditionally heaped with opprobrium there.

Despite the convulsions shaking the new political regimes, international tourism grew exponentially: during the last quarter of this century more foreigners visited equatorial Africa than in all its prior history. In 1974 the Mohammed Ali–George Foreman fight attracted twenty-five thousand American fans to Kinshasa. The television series *Roots* prompted sentimental visits by thousands of African-Americans. Travel agents assured a constant to-and-fro of tourists, among whom some were keenly interested in local prostitutes.[25]

The main characteristic of the internal African population movements was a rush to the cities. At the beginning of the twentieth century Kinshasa (capital of the Belgian Congo, called Léopoldville until 1966) encompassed about 10,000 inhabitants; in 1960, at the moment of its independence, that number had grown to 400,000. At the beginning of the 1980s, the formerly alluring colonial town had grown into an enormous urban mass of some 2.5 million by official estimates; today the number of inhabitants is approaching 4 million. Small wonder, then, that today Kinshasa, Mombasa, Nairobi, Kigala, Kampala, Bangui, Lusaka—these megalopolises of the Third World where poverty and ghastly hygienic conditions reign over all—form the nurseries of the AIDS virus.

In the spread of AIDS over Africa, homosexuality, drug addiction, and hemophilia have played practically no role. Transfusion had a minor influence, at least at first. The two main routes were heterosexual relations and the medical (or paramedical) use of syringes. Pronounced promiscuity is the only attribute that African heterosexuals have shared with the homosexuals in whom the AIDS epidemic began in America.

In the cities of Africa, overpopulation and overcopulation grew together. Here prostitution enjoyed an extraordinary surge; a system of ''free partners'' replaced traditional polygamy. Since time immemorial there had been a great deal of flexibility in African sexual customs. Long-lasting unions had been unusual; in a lifetime women and men alike had multiple partners.[26] But sex life had nonetheless been regulated in a way that, if it corresponded to no strict Christian moral code, was still no less constraining and hence considerably limited the genital transmission of pathogenic organisms—the interdiction of prostitution, fear of the corrupting influence of foreigners, and so on. Liberated from the yoke of behavioral expectations imposed by the traditions of small village groups, the inhabitants of the big cities abandoned themselves heartily to elaborate sexual play. Urban prostitution, and still more the emergence of new categories of ''free women'' and single males, promoted a multiplicity of partners.[27] In such a new social situation the HIV virus found a propitious setting for its propagation. Moreover, instructive in this regard, the AIDS epidemic here was preceded, as it was among American homosexuals, by an outbreak of other sexually transmitted diseases.

By way of example take Kinshasa, where the epidemiologic situation has been relatively well understood as the result of an international surveillance program.[28] Syphilis, gonorrhea, herpes, and genital warts were on the increase there since the 1960s. Forerunners of AIDS, they heralded with precision the social and age categories that were to be at risk for AIDS. We still do not know when the first strain arose or where it came from. Since the mid-1970s, most infections occurred in the city itself. The main risk factor, for men as well as women, was the number of partners. Men were affected a bit less frequently than women, and became infected at an older age. There were three times as many seropositive young women (between fifteen and twenty-five) as young men their age. The seropositive women were most often single and without stated profession.

Prostitutes were the principal source of AIDS infection in African cities. Thus, for example, in Butare, site of both a military camp and the University of Rwanda, prostitution flourished—almost all the good-time girls in this region were infected. In 1984, twenty-nine of thirty-three examined prostitutes were seropositive (88 percent).[29] In Nairobi, Kenya, the increase in the seropositivity rate among prostitutes reflected the epidemic's progress: 5 percent in 1982, 12 percent in 1983, 22 percent in 1984, 54 percent in 1985, 65 percent in 1986, and 83 percent in 1987.[30]

Serologic studies pointed to the notion of the relative antiquity of HIV-1 infection in the rural areas of Zaire and Kenya.[31] It is possible, however, that a number of false positives may have been counted in these surveys. In any case, the seroprevalence in these zones has remained at a level of around one percent, that which prevailed at the beginning of the epidemic. A comparative study shows that the seroprevalence of the AIDS antibody in Rwanda is eight times greater in the cities than in the rural areas. HIV infection hence spreads essentially in the cities and along the merchant routes of Africa.[32]

"Slim" in Uganda

The history of the AIDS epidemic in Uganda is exemplary. Uganda is a very poor country. Decolonialization was a painful process, with civil war and a collapse in the infrastructure, especially in the health services. Traditional society was composed of polygamous rural families living in closed groups and never venturing more than a few dozen kilometers from their homes. All this began to change in the 1970s.

During the autumn of 1982 a new epidemic disease in Kasensero, in the Rakai district, was reported to the Kampala public health authorities. It is a village of about five hundred inhabitants on the shores of Lake Victoria, near the Uganda-Tanzania border. Seventeen people from the village were complaining of intestinal troubles and rapid general decline. They were smugglers. This quickly led to explanations not dissimilar from those invoked in a more distant past at the start of nearly every epidemic: first, the disease came from foreigners (Tanzania), and, second, it was divine retribution for sins committed (robbery, smuggling).[33]

The *vox populi* at first spoke of the "robbers' disease." Then, when the infection struck down women and other individuals whose honesty was not in doubt, it was dubbed "slim," from the English word connoting a slender or emaciated habitus. Men were first affected, but then their women followed them down the suffering path until rapidly all quantitative gender differences vanished. Leaving the Tanzanian frontier, the disease moved north along the road bordering Lake Victoria. In 1985 it arrived in Kampala, the capital city. The disease was then brought into relationship with the AIDS epidemic in the neighboring states of Rwanda and Zaire. Its direct relationship to the AIDS complex was confirmed by the finding that almost every Ugandan slim patient had antibodies to HIV-1.[34]

Slim presented as a syndrome with three separate phases: first, spiking fevers with general malaise; some months later, intermittent diarrhea with rash, thrush, and significant weight loss; and finally, generalized weakness with respiratory distress and hyperpigmented scars. These patients, voiding frequent stools as though their flesh was liquefying, came to resemble living skeletons, dying in a state of total debilitation.[35]

In 1987 the CDC modified the definition of AIDS, including the slim syndrome within it, as a clinical variant of infection with HIV.[36] By that time this was no longer a curiosity of local pathology in Uganda, but a veritable national catastrophe. The village of Kasensero was depopulated, as were many other villages in the Rakai and Masaka districts. In 1988 a little more than five thousand Ugandans were officially stricken by the new disease, but the real figure was surely much higher: about 40 percent of individuals examined for a variety of reasons in Ugandan hospitals are seropositive. The seropositivity rate has reached 70 percent in Kampala prostitutes, and 33 percent in truck drivers. About 10 percent of the registered cases are infants infected before birth.[37]

Like the proverbially mysterious sources of the Nile, can the cradle of AIDS be found in this part of central Africa? This is the opinion of some American scientists, notably Robert Gallo, in emphasizing that the uncultivated and wild areas along Lake Victoria's border represent the only rural part of Africa in which AIDS is rife in epidemic form.[38] In my opinion, this is rather an argument for the opposite theory: the violence of the south Ugandan epidemic suggests the virus's recent introduction there.

According to recently obtained epidemiologic data, Uganda was hit by two successive waves of HIV-1 infection: the first was manifest by the appearance of an aggressive form of Kaposi's sarcoma and by the considerable growth of this form of Kaposi's sarcoma since the beginning of the 1970s; the second by the advent of slim disease and its expansion during the 1980s. The two waves seem to have different points of departure: the first was initially found in the north, in the Nile region; the second in the south, on the Uganda-Tanzania border. The difference between their clinical pictures suggests the existence of two strains of the HIV-1 virus: the first autochthonous or introduced from either Kenya or the Central African Republic; the second certainly new to Uganda and brought either by Kasensero smugglers or by Tanzanian soldiers during their Ugandan raids in 1980. Retrospective serologic studies show that the HIV-1 virus did not exist in epidemic form in this country before the 1970s. Test results for the blood samples collected after 1970 are contradictory, but it seems nonetheless certain that the explosive augmentation of the disorder did not begin before 1982. The absence of seropositivity in elderly people, and the relatively low seroprevalence seen in the last year in the Nile region, speak in favor of the recent introduction of AIDS into Uganda.[39]

Cultural Incompatibilities

Certain ancestral African customs may have contributed to the transmission of AIDS: clitoral circumcision, infibulation, scarification for esthetic and ritual purposes, tattooing, ceremonies establishing "blood brotherhood," and so on. That these practices continue is sometimes invoked to help explain the particularities of the African epidemic. Bloody operations on the female genitalia are thus invoked, for example, as one of the factors responsible for the uniform distribution of AIDS between the sexes. No correlation could be established, however, between the frequency of such ancestral practices and the spread of the AIDS epidemic. They represent possible modes of transmission but of only secondary importance.[40] The same holds true for the small skin incisions made by local healers in order better to instill their traditional balms, since they operate on several people with the same instruments.

A major role must be accorded to sexual promiscuity. It existed in the tropics since time immemorial but recently took on new forms. In "modernizing," Africa tried to reconcile very different, and in many respects incompatible, cultural traditions. Urban poverty, a new phenomenon in the extent it reached only after the middle of this century, was accompanied by the expansion of prostitution and the range of possible sexual contacts.[41] Those who threw off the moral and material shackles of the old rural milieu and tribal customs now fell into the trap of a relentless new social system. One of the results of this release was a wildfire of classic sexually transmitted diseases. They created the medium for AIDS and—everywhere—preceded the new epidemic.[42]

Modern Western medicine had brought a great deal of benefit to the Third World, much of which had at first been placed in aid of controlling the most lethal infectious diseases. But even with regard to this benevolence, the grafting of one civilization's achievements onto another's ancient rootstock posed major problems and ultimately bore bitter fruit. We might bypass those examples of incompatibility over food hygiene and other medical domains not immediately linked to the AIDS epidemic, and remember two problems linked essentially to the disease's expansion in Africa: the use of syringes and vaccination.

The spectacular successes of modern medicine in Africa are due to antibiotics and vaccination. In the eyes of Africa, the white man's medicine consists essentially of giving injections. The physician's syringe is a quasi-magical instrument. The massive reutilization of syringes and of poorly sterilized used needles should therefore come as no surprise. Sterilizing these materials is quite difficult in any case, since they are mostly designed to be disposable. But in a poor country everything is reserved and reused as much as possible. So the disposable syringe, an undeniable technological advance in one cultural milieu, becomes a disadvantage in another. African nurses and practitioners freely utilize old syringes. Even village witch doctors have added them to their professional armamentariums.

It seems that the reutilization of syringes and needles has been a significant path for the transmission of the HIV virus in Africa.[43] But some experts well versed on African epidemiology, for example Robert Biggar, believe we must guard against putting too much stock in the syringe-induced diffusion hypothesis. Indeed, traditional medicine men practice injection without preference on subjects of all ages, while the majority of seropositive and full-blown AIDS patients are young adults.[44]

The improper implementation of preventive medical procedures, or modern therapeutic maneuvers, can have unfortunate consequences. According to the official report of Raf Mertens of WHO, at the time of the Zairian plague-vaccination campaign, between November 1986 and March 1987, 165,000 inhabitants of the country were vaccinated by five teams lacking elementary medical training and without a bit of scientific supervision. One such team, whom Mertens encountered himself in the field, had available a mere seven needles and four syringes. The vaccinators systematically reused the same syringe from one subject to the next without aseptic precautions.[45] This happened when the AIDS danger was already appreciated. One shudders to think of everything done in good faith in the preceding decades.

Needle-free injection apparatuses probably carried risks of their own; we now know that they could transmit the hepatitis-B virus.[46]

According to some investigators, the geographic distribution of the peak incidence of African AIDS may well have corresponded to that of countries in which the final effort to eradicate smallpox was made. Might the massive introduction of vaccinia virus, into the heart of a seropositive but disease-free population, have "awakened" the HIV and triggered the epidemic? Would the vaccinia virus not have heightened the virulence of a simian precursor of HIV? In one case report a seropositive American soldier experienced acceleration of his AIDS, fatal in a matter of weeks, after his smallpox vaccination. The problem remains delicate and unresolved despite the energetic denials issued by WHO.[47]

A historical aspect of this relationship between the poxviruses and lentiviruses has been neglected: the competitive synergy of combined infections at the individual level becomes a most effective antagonism at the level of the pathocenosis.

We are still quite poorly informed about the epidemiologic relationships between AIDS and the other endemic diseases, notably those capable of producing chronic immune depression. A pediatric service team from the Mama Yemo Hospital in Kinshasa, studying the links between malaria and AIDS among Zairian children, has just confirmed the existence of a positive correlation between malarial plasmodium infection and HIV seropositivity, but with an important caveat, namely, in the recent situation the link has been indirect: more frequent blood transfusion of malaria-infected infants is mainly and perhaps even solely responsible.[48] Hence malaria may have recently interfered in the ecological setting of Africa by "preparing the ground" for HIV infection. It seems most likely to me that, before the advent of antimalarial compounds and modern insecticides, it played an opposite role by holding back the epidemic expansion of the most virulent forms of the AIDS virus.

CHAPTER 16

Modern Medicine: Its Highs and Lows

S'il est terrifiant de penser

que la vie puisse être à la

merci de la multiplication

de ces infiniment petits

il est consolant aussi

d'espérer que la science

ne restera pas toujours

impuissante devant de

tels ennemis.

—Louis Pasteur,

chemist, founder of

medical microbiology

IN A DECEMBER 7, 1987, interview in the magazine *Le Point*, Luc Montagnier characterized the AIDS battle in this way: "We're more or less up to our knees in the middle of it. We've identified the enemy, we know how to avoid infection from blood products, we've got the prevention campaigns rolling. And we have a little hope, on the therapeutic side, thanks to a drug, AZT, which, while it doesn't cure, slows down the disease's progress and prolongs patients' lives. . . . What we haven't managed is either a complete recovery from AIDS by means of medication, or its prevention by means of a vaccine."

In the AIDS battle there is in fact a terrible disproportion between the theory and practice, between the rapid headway we have seen in scientific knowledge and the stagnation of attempts to achieve progress in therapy or prevention.

Worldwide Mobilization

The first international conference on AIDS took place in April 1985 in Atlanta, headquarters of the Centers for Disease Control. This sort of international collaboration, furnishing an opportunity both for an exchange of viewpoints between specialists and for raising public awareness, was continued with follow-up meetings in Paris (1986), Washington (1987), Stockholm (1988), and Montreal (1989). The United States remains one of the most heavily AIDS-ravaged countries, and one of the best organized for its surveillance; but international efforts are now centered in Geneva, where the Global Program on AIDS operates under the aegis of the World Health Organization (WHO). According to an official declaration of the director-general of WHO, AIDS is "the world's chief public health problem."

At the Stockholm meeting, the WHO program's director, Jonathan Mann, presented a chart of AIDS worldwide, dividing the epidemic's history into three periods: the silent period (ca. 1970–1981), the initial discovery (1981–1985), and worldwide mobilization (1985–1988).[1]

The current pandemic has prompted violent social reactions in some countries and in the international arena. Some people are disturbed by the idea that the epidemic should become an occasion for reinforcing state control over individuals, leading to abuses by totalitarian political systems. Managers and citizens alike in the equatorial African nations manifest ambivalence when confronted with American and European medical teams. On both sides in the game of medical aid furnished by the great powers to the Third World, there are elements of exploitation that have nothing to do with their announced humanitarian ideals. Speculations about the origin of AIDS collide with national sensibilities. The Africans have felt themselves accused and scorned.

In an atmosphere where mistrust, irrational fears, and political intrigues subtly mingle and interfere with the desire for an effective collective effort in the battle against AIDS, this disease, in October 1987, found its way onto the agenda of the General Assembly of the United Nations. It was the first time that a disease formed the object of a debate at this level of international political collaboration.

Looking for Treatment

Three strategies have guided the treatment of AIDS and inspired researches aimed at its amelioration: medication of the opportunistic infections, restoration or enhancement of immune activity, and antiviral chemotherapy (drugs that disrupt the life cycle of a virus).

Until 1983, before any precise understanding of the etiology of AIDS, treatment had been limited to specific therapy of the opportunistic infections and to palliative measures directed against various secondary symptoms. Successes were obtained in combatting with antibiotics certain well-known opportunistic microbial agents. Kaposi's sarcoma and lymphomas could be treated with radiation therapy, chemotherapy, or surgery, thus providing at least local and symptomatic relief.[2]

At first, immunostimulants were assayed as potential treatment modalities, since an immunologic deficit was one of the principal characteristics of AIDS. To this end, biological modifiers of the T-lymphocytes, such as interleukin-2 (IL-2), hormones derived from the thymus gland, or thymomimetic drugs (DTC, commercial name Imuthiol), were tried, as well as transfusion of HLA-matched lymphocytes or even bone marrow transplantation. But the efforts were disappointing. Numerous physicians remain convinced nonetheless that the therapy of the future will consist of a combination of immunomodulation and antiviral drugs.

In October 1985 Jean-Marie Andrieu, Philippe Even, and Alain Venet, through the unorthodox route of a ministerial declaration and a sensational press conference, announced that three patients treated at the Laennec Hospital in Paris (two with AIDS and one with "pre-AIDS") had displayed an increase in lymphocyte count and clear-cut general improvement after receiving the drug called Cyclosporin A. This substance is a powerful immune suppressant; the apparently paradoxical idea of using it to treat AIDS derived from the hypothesis that T-lymphocyte destruction was not a result of direct viral action but rather an autoimmune reaction on the part of the host organism. The Paris trial quickly ran into a stunning reversal: the first patient died scarcely fifteen days after beginning the treatment. Five other patients experienced worsening of their symptoms or at least got no better. Although Cyclosporin had possible antiviral properties, its use was abandoned in the struggle against AIDS.[3]

Any reasonable hope of finding a miracle cure had to be founded on research on drugs capable of blocking viral replication or cellular entry. To this end various antiviral nonspecific physiologic substances with antiviral properties and specific synthetic drugs were studied in hopes of preventing the retrovirus from multiplying.[4]

In the first group, there was at first glance only one potentially valuable candidate: alpha interferon. Its effects were limited and judged insignificant. Also now in trial is an interferon inducer called ampligen. In the second group, investigators undertook clinical trials in 1983 with HPA-23 and, in 1984, with Suramin, phosphonoformate (foscarnet), and ribavirin.

The first of these products, antimoniotungstate or HPA-23 (so named because it was the twenty-third heteropolyanion synthesized by chemists Gilbert Hervé and André Tézé), was known ever since the 1974 work of Claude Jasmin and Jean-Claude Chermann as an inhibitor of reverse transcriptase in the retrovirus responsible for murine leukemia and sarcoma. Chermann studied its action on the AIDS virus. HPA-23 inhibited the activity of LAV reverse transcriptase in vitro. In collaboration with clinicians Willy Rozenbaum, Dominique Dormont, and others, between July 1983 and June 1984, the Pasteur Institute investigators showed how administering this substance to patients reduced viral replication in humans, making it impossible to find the virus in lymphocytes. A thirteen-year-old hemophilia patient with cerebral toxoplasmosis was the first AIDS patient who, on July 26, 1983, in a Paris hospital, received a synthetic antiviral compound.[5] HPA-23 had its hour of glory when Rock Hudson came from the United States to Paris in search of it.[6] Produced by the Rhône-Poulenc company, this medication is still the object of therapeutic trials, but today we are quite sure that it is both highly toxic and ultimately of little benefit to patients.

In the summer of 1984, Hiroaki Mitsuya and Samuel Broder, investigators at the National Cancer Institute (NCI), obtained a strain of HIV-1 from Robert Gallo and began systematically testing it in vitro against all compounds previously reported to inhibit murine retroviruses. In one year they tested three hundred chemical products and found that fifteen arrested the replication of

HIV in the test tube. Of these fifteen substances they chose one for clinical testing: 3'-azido-2',3'-dideoxythymidine, also called zidovudine or azidothymidine and hence given the acronym AZT. It had been synthesized in 1964 by Jerome Horwitz and manufactured by Burroughs Wellcome Laboratories as an anticancer drug. According to in vitro tests done in February 1985, AZT powerfully inhibited the AIDS virus in lymphocyte cultures without being particularly harmful to the cells themselves.[7] On July 3, 1985, a patient was started on AZT treatment, and toward the end of the year Robert Yarchoan, Samuel Broder, and their collaborators had collected auspicious data on thirty-three patients with AIDS or related syndromes.[8]

In February 1986 the NCI in Bethesda inaugurated a double-blind therapeutic trial in twelve American centers, directed by Margaret Fischl of the University of Miami and Douglas Richman of the University of California, San Diego. They divided 282 patients into two groups matched for age, weight, symptoms, and hematologic status. The first group got AZT, the second a placebo. Neither the patients nor the physicians treating them knew who was getting the real drug. By the fourth week the general physical status of the groups was already beginning to diverge: the AZT-treated patients regained weight while the others lost. At the end of six months only one patient in the first group was dead, while there were nineteen deaths among the 137 patients in the control group. In September 1986, before the end of the period initially anticipated for the study, its ethical oversight committee stopped the trial. They deemed it morally unjustifiable to further deny the patients in the second group a better chance of survival.[9]

In the spring of 1987 Wellcome was authorized to market AZT, commercially named Retrovir. It has today become the drug of choice in treating AIDS. But the more time passes, the greater the disappointment becomes. On the one hand, we now know that AZT quite effectively inhibits reverse transcriptase: it "tricks" the virus and prevents its replication by competing biochemically with the nucleoside thymidine, a normal component of the genetic material. The drug probably acts also by stimulating the immune defenses. But on the other hand, it does not cure AIDS and, through various secondary effects, injures the cellular elements in the bone marrow that produce red blood cells as well as white blood cells. While its action is clearly beneficial early in the course of treatment, the therapeutic effects later begin to taper off and toxic effects take over. In the long run the condition of those treated with the drug begins to approximate that of patients who never took it. The HIV strains exposed to AZT progressively acquire a specific resistance.

The patients in the pilot study were followed up: eighteen months later, 30 percent had had to abandon the treatment because of its toxicity. The probability of survival of patients treated early in the trial was 69 percent, against 59 percent for those from the control group who began treatment later. Some of the results obtained with AZT improved gradually over time, notably as a consequence of better dosing; they are encouraging but far from satisfactory.[10]

No one of the paths taken thus far is clearly good. Hundreds of laboratories across the world labor feverishly. Animal and in vitro tests on fifty products are currently under way. But serious difficulties arise from the fact that no adequate animal model is yet available for such pharmacological experiments.

Hiroaki Mitsuya and Samuel Broder are now working on other chemical compounds, notably dideoxycytidine (DDC), a reverse-transcriptase inhibitor which is more effective in vitro than AZT but which induces serious toxic effects on peripheral nerves. There is a great deal of discussion of peptide T, a molecule believed to mimic a segment of the viral envelope protein. It was created in 1986 by Candace Pert in Bethesda. By latching onto the CD4 receptor, this molecule was reported to compete with the viral gp120 antigen and thus block viral entry into the cell. Other attempts to inhibit viral binding to the target cells consisted of inundating the blood with free CD4 receptors by using a soluble form of CD4 protein obtained by genetic engineering; using a recombinant of the receptor molecule with a bacterial exotoxin; or even simply eating dextran sulfate. Meir Shinitzky in Tel Aviv and Arthur England in New York claim to have gotten encouraging results with a lipid extract of egg yolks (AL721). In their despair the afflicted resorted to miracle drugs, obtained from underground sources and scorned by scientific medicine, such as Compound Q. Derived from a cucumberlike Chinese plant, this compound was to have been subjected to clandestine clinical trials in four American cities. But all these recent efforts must await their own historian.[11]

Toward the end of 1988 a new concept appeared in the general strategy of the AIDS campaign: chemoprophylaxis. With malaria prevention as the model, the hope is to find chemical products able to prevent specific infection in exposed individuals.

Chimeric Vaccines

Prevention is better than cure. Our victory over most infectious diseases owes more to vaccination than it does to drugs. We may be forgiven for harboring the same hopes with respect to AIDS. As soon as cell culture of the virus furnished quantities of its antigens for research, a number of investigators proceeded to develop and purify vaccines. The hope was that such vaccines should be able to stimulate the production of specific antibodies in healthy individuals and thus render them immune, resistant to infection by a virulent virus. But difficulties arose immediately. The usual methods of vaccine preparation were of no avail. This virus attacked the immune system itself. In its proviral intracellular hiding place, it was out of reach; in its free state it defended itself with great effectiveness: it changed its antigenic structure continually, thus escaping attack by preformed antibodies; it used part of its own structure as a sort of decoy against the host's antibodies; it hid its immunologically sensitive external parts in a particular sort of furrow.[12]

Preliminary experiments on chimpanzees showed that immunization by inactivated HIV or by purified viral glycoproteins conferred no protection against actual HIV infection. Various viral recombinants were therefore tried, introducing, for example, certain HIV viral proteins into vaccinia virus. Chimpanzees vaccinated with these products were not protected against HIV infection. In fact, no convenient animal model was available to test the effectiveness of a vaccine against human AIDS: infected chimpanzees did not get sick.

In humans, vaccination might attenuate the course of the illness in cases in which it failed actually to prevent infection. It is very difficult to test this sort of vaccine in man. On top of the ethical difficulties there are technical problems, especially those tied up with the remarkably long latency period. An important human trial was undertaken in November 1986 in Zaire under the direction of Parisian immunologist Daniel Zagury and Kinshasa physicians Zirimwabagabo Lurhuma and Jean-Jacques Salaun. They tried a genetically engineered vaccinia (cowpox) virus vaccine, containing the gp160 HIV protein, on a dozen volunteers as well as on Zagury himself. This time the effort resulted in an immune response followed by seroconversion.[13] In an extraordinary act of courage, Zagury proved that this type of vaccination was not dangerous and that it could artificially stimulate anti-HIV antibody production. The protective potential of this vaccination remains to be demonstrated. Since 1987 several clinical trials of AIDS vaccines have been begun both in the United States and in other countries.[14] Most specialists look on this with growing skepticism. Whether stimulated naturally by viral infection or artificially by a vaccine, seropositivity, namely the presence of anti-HIV antibodies in the bloodstream, clearly confers no protection against the retrovirus. Biological chimeras in the literal sense, these recombinant vaccines risk becoming chimeras in the figurative sense as well. If the virus itself does not induce a good immune response, remarked David Baltimore, how are we supposed to do better than the virus does already?[15]

The Social Dimension of AIDS

The grandeur of modern medicine—its highs—may be displayed in the rapidity with which some complex problems of AIDS are resolved: its semiotics and pathology, the nature of the causal agent, its routes of infection and epidemiologic surveillance. But miseries of modern medicine—its lows—are no less evident at the moment when we pass from understanding to action, from knowledge to power.

Treatment is still disappointing. We can only strive to assure our patients a proper palliative treatment in a dignified setting supported by the community, and without discrimination. Lacking any means of biological prevention as yet, the battle against the spread of AIDS comes down to serologic screening of blood donors and adjustment of sexual mores. No effective prophylaxis exists outside of serologic detection and information campaigns covering risk and prevention. That is precious little.

Screening of blood donors and heat treatment of blood products have reduced iatrogenic infection, but it is difficult to evaluate the real impact of other preventive measures. The extent of administrative measures varies from one nation to the next: relatively coercive and repressive methods in Scandinavia, in certain parts of West Germany, in Cuba, in India, and in certain eastern European countries; quite liberal attitudes, for example, in France, Italy, and the United States. It is generally conceded that screening tests should be used for all blood, sperm, and organ donations, and, with informed consent, for patients hospitalized on surgical, trauma, and obstetrical-gynecological services. Opinion is divided, however, with respect to the utility of mandatory testing in all patients treated in a medical institution or, propositions and practices still more controversial, in nonmedical social categories such as foreigners, premarital couples, prostitutes, prisoners, soldiers, students, new hires, or employees. Until 1989 no nation had implemented systematic screening of a very large segment of its population, or a significant proportion of a city or region, for the cost was considered too high in relation to any potential benefits. In 1987 the foreign ministers of twenty-one European countries had adopted a common declaration stating that no mandatory testing should be undertaken by the signatories either for their general population or for any special groups.

The solemn appeal issued in September 1988 by three renowned French physicians, Léon Schwartzenberg, Paul Milliez, and Jean-Claude Chermann, reflected the ethical impasse of recent events: they asked the citizens to "accept general but voluntary screening tests." But the two adjectives are contradictory. To be truly significant from an epidemiologic point of view, any screening must be "general" in the strict sense of the term, and hence obligatory. Sampling methods cannot depend on the good will of those examined. This has been well demonstrated in the past in systematic campaigns of detection for syphilis and tuberculosis. But given the impotence of present therapeutic approaches, how can we make a duty of a test whose results promise those concerned no more than the most somber of outlooks?

Feelings of rejection, fear, and stigmatization follow in the wake of this plague in part of the population of every country. Such feelings do nothing to help in the struggle against its spread, and often make for perverse effects. Some have conceived of a plan, and in a few exceptional instances even begun implementing that plan, to segregate AIDS patients as well as to isolate seropositives. These vexatious measures arise from minds obsessed with impurity and sin, crime and punishment. They bear witness to the persistence of magical thinking in the world, and, despite appearances, have no medical justification.

After early detection, eyes next turned rapidly to condoms as a way of protecting against transmission of the HIV virus in homosexual and heterosexual relations. Only as recently as 1986, however, were such measures shown to be effective.[16] A goodly number of such products on the international market were of low quality. Public relations campaigns praising the use of the condom as a ''new gesture of love'' intensified in 1987. It is noteworthy that in France and several other countries, publicity about condoms was previously prohibited. The Vatican reacted in a conservative way: it took care to invigorate the formal condemnation of their use by Catholics. But in any case, it seemed that neither publicity sponsored by the civil authorities nor interdiction by religious authorities would have a decisive effect on the behavior of the affected populations. Everywhere, condom use hovered at a relatively low level, effectively competing with neither the contraceptive pill in industrialized states nor the ancestral habits of people in developing countries.

Finally, we must recognize that public-relations campaigns are most often appreciated only by those already forewarned, and that the obsession with safe sex will do more to assist the spread of telephone obscenity than it will to rein in the spread of AIDS.

This book leaves in shadow the unspeakable suffering of the patients, the family dramas, the psychological aspects, the repercussions of AIDS in the collective imagination, its effects on social and political activity.[17] Among the innumerable subjects that future historians will have to consider will be the progressive social construction of the disease, notably the role played by the mass media;[18] the anguish, panicked reactions and justified fears of the gay community, the medical corps, the caretaking personnel, and every one of us;[19] the changes in the daily routine of the dentists, surgeons, and nurses;[20] the economic consequences;[21] the new ethical conflicts and the legal problems, often inextricably interwoven;[22] the relationships between AIDS, criminality, and incarceration (prisons in which homosexuality and drug addiction have become important sources for the spread of AIDS);[23] the reflections of AIDS in belles lettres and plays;[24] the pathography of famous individuals and the social echoes of their affairs;[25] and so on.

The Epidemiology of HTLV-I

Research in the past six years has clearly exonerated the adult human T-cell leukemia virus (Gallo's HTLV-I or Miyoshi and Hinuma's ATLV) as the putative agent of AIDS. But it has also been shown that the pathogenic action and geographical distribution of this virus are a great deal more complex than initial observations suggested.

Just like the AIDS virus, HTLV-I attacks more than just lymphocytes. It also affects the central nervous system. This neurotropic effect is so slow and insidious that it becomes very difficult to detect it. HTLV-I was implicated as the causal agent of multiple sclerosis, then exonerated only to be implicated more successfully as the etiologic explanation of tropical spastic paraparesis. Long known in certain regions of the world, this syndrome of quadriplegia with spasticity of the upper limbs remained enigmatic. In 1985 Lyons virologists Antoine Gessain, Francis Barin, and Guy de Thé, and Fort-de-France (Martinique) physician Jean-Claude Vernant, shed light on the causal link between the insidious appearance of this neuromyelopathy and prior chronic infection by the HTLV-I virus. Their demonstration was based on serologic findings. In 1988 Steven Jacobson, Cedric S. Raine, and their collaborators in Bethesda and New York isolated an HTLV-I-like retrovirus from such patients. In endemic regions, the prevalence of this spastic paraparesis was between ten and one hundred per one hundred thousand persons.[26]

The HTLV-I virus is less infectious and even much less pathogenic than HIV. Their routes of transmission are similar; combined infection is not uncommon. HTLV-I remained confined to certain endemic regions and did not start spreading outside those zones until the 1960s. Until then it was limited to three classic foci: black Africa, southern Japan, and the Caribbean. It was found in people of color in the United States and in Latin America, next turning up in an endemic pocket in England among black immigrants from the Caribbean, as well as in southern France among people of north African origin.[27]

The discovery of viral carriers among the native inhabitants of southern Italy was therefore a great surprise. The first suspicion arose in September 1984, when Vittorio Manzari, Paola Verani, and their collaborators at the University of Rome isolated a virus of the HTLV type in a patient who had since 1982 suffered from T-cell lymphomas. The patient, a sixty-four-year-old heterosexual from a small western Sicilian village, denied any intimate contact with foreigners. The isolated virus was probably HTLV-I, despite the fact that the strain was notably different from the prototype. The Italian investigators, however, beguiled by Gallo's hypothesis, were mistaken in believing they had isolated HTLV from a second patient as well, hospitalized in Rome and clearly afflicted with AIDS (weight loss, T-lymphocyte depression, opportunistic infections, and Kaposi's sarcoma). This case was typical not only for the symptoms but also for the history: aged thirty-nine, the patient had spent time in New York and Miami and had had homosexual contacts since 1981. In September 1984 Manzari and his colleagues in fact succeeded in isolating the true agent of AIDS but confounded it with Gallo's HTLV.[28] This virus failed to survive in lymphocyte cultures, rendering still more plausible its identification with HIV. According to Manzari's unpublished data, this patient's frozen serum, studied by retrospective serologic techniques, would have been as positive for antibodies to HTLV-I as it would for anti-HIV antibodies.

In 1985 Vittorio Manzari and his Roman team, in collaboration with Gallo's Bethesda laboratory, undertook a systematic survey to look for

HTLV-I among sixty-eight lymphoma patients from all around Italy. Only two patients were seropositive. They both lived in the county of Lecce: a man, aged thirty-five, and a woman, aged twenty-seven. They also denied both any trips outside of southern Italy and any sexual contact with foreigners. Alerted by the potential common source for these two patients, Manzari's team tested 275 sera from persons living in Apulia with no sign of blood disease. Among these, the team found twenty-three cases of anti-HTLV-I antibody carriers, of whom twenty-one were over fifty years old. There was not a single case of seropositivity in the control group consisting of inhabitants of various other parts of Italy. The seropositives came from a well-circumscribed area: a dozen villages on the Salento peninsula. Nearly 10 percent of the region's inhabitants were HTLV-I carriers. Thus the first endemic focus for this virus was discovered in a white European population.[29]

How far back can we date the Lecce endemic? For clear historico-geographic reasons, Italian scholars have thought immediately of Africa as the source of the HTLV-I infection. This hypothesis would be the best one if we can prove that the introduction of the virus in Italy is quite an old event. According to the immunologist Franco Pandolfi, HTLV-I could have been brought to Sicily and into Apulia by the Saracens in the ninth century, or by the Normans some centuries later.[30] In my opinion, this was a recent introduction, going back no more than thirty years. How else to explain the concentration of the endemic in a territory with more administrative than natural borders; or the mean age of the seropositives; or, especially, the paucity of distinct cases of T-cell lymphomas and spastic paraparesis? Iatrogenic importation of this virus would account for certain characteristics of the endemic. There are multiple possibilities: transfusion; contaminated medications; vaccination, notably the preventive campaign during the cholera in Naples; and so on. If the introduction of the virus was truly recent, its adverse consequences have not yet had time fully to manifest themselves. A quite lengthy latency period (several decades) separates primary HTLV-I infection from the emergence of clinical disease.

Further research showed that this virus had vaulted past the previous endemic zone's limits by means of the drug-addict population. Toward the middle of the 1960s, even before the AIDS virus arrived in Italy, HTLV-I had already started to spread among the heroin addicts in large cities such as Rome, Milan, and Genoa.

The Soviet Union's "Patient Zero"

How the AIDS virus infiltrated the Soviet Union is instructive. The first known patient, citizen K, aged thirty-five, lived in an east African country in 1981 and over a period of several months had homosexual contacts with a native. Vacationing in his own country and enjoying a brief liaison with a Russian in November 1981, K had passive anal sex with a bisexual African in March 1982. That summer he began to experience mild fevers accompanied with headache, insomnia, and respiratory distress, followed by blood-tinged diarrhea. When routine examinations failed to explain his clinical picture, K was repatriated and spent five months in a Moscow hospital. The physicians there noticed his generalized lymphadenopathy and proposed a diagnosis of Crohn's disease, a form of chronic inflammatory bowel disorder. No one thought of AIDS. The patient returned to his hometown and, between summer 1983 and 1986, indulged in homosexual relationships with twenty-two partners. In 1984 he had a bout of chronic pneumonia and two crops of shingles; toward the end of 1985 he manifested Kaposi's sarcoma. The diagnosis of AIDS was not made until toward the end of 1986, whereupon the public health authorities undertook, in January 1987, a rigorous epidemiologic inquiry.

K's twenty-two partners were tracked down. They all denied having had homosexual relationships outside of those with "Patient Zero," but admitted heterosexual contacts. They were young men eighteen to twenty years old. None considered himself homosexual and, until January 1987, none had ever heard of AIDS. Tests showed that five of these twenty-two partners were seropositive. Each of them had had heterosexual contacts with several women, on the average five. Only two had transmitted the infection to their partners, the first to a single woman, the second to two. The latter, though only weakly seropositive, sparked a tragic chain reaction: on the one hand, his blood was used to transfuse six recipients, of whom five became seropositive; on the other hand, one of the women he infected gave birth to a sick infant while the other gave blood for the treatment of a hemophiliac (who remained negative eleven months after the transfusion). From an epidemiologic as well as a sociocultural point of view, it is interesting to note that one of the seropositives had anal sex with two women who desired thereby to retain their virginity; neither of these women was infected.[31]

The infant just mentioned, a victim of intrauterine infection, died in Odessa in 1987, between the fourth and fifth month of life. Another case of pediatric posttransfusion AIDS had been known since 1985 but was kept secret until 1987. The first death in the Soviet Union of an adult attributed to AIDS dates from September 5, 1988: it was that of a twenty-nine-year-old woman, Olga G., a Leningrad prostitute who would have been infected through sex with foreigners arriving from Africa. Officially there were at the beginning of 1989 seven patients with overt AIDS in the Soviet Union. We lack information about the number of seropositives.

In November 1988 the Moscow AIDS prevention laboratory was informed of the HIV infection of a woman and infant who were unrelated but resided in the same city, Elista, capital of the Soviet Kalmyk Republic. The woman's husband and the child's parents were all seronegative. But the epidemiologic team led by Valentin V. Pokrovsky, president of the Soviet Academy of Medicine, found that the infected woman had a recently deceased infant, and that the latter had been hospitalized in the same facility as the infected infant. Screening of the patients in this pediatric hospital in Elista in the course of December 1988–January 1989 led to the discovery of a horrible tragedy, unique down to that time in the history of AIDS: twenty-nine small children (average age around two years) and six mothers had been infected during their hospitalization. It seems that the infection was introduced into the hospital by one of the parents. The fulminant propagation of the agent resulted from serious negligence in instrument sterilization. The children were infected by contaminated syringes, a particularly deplorable event that should never have occurred on a medical service. If one of the mothers could have been infected before her child, the infection probably followed the opposite path among the others.

The Irrepressible Spread of AIDS, 1985–1988

The total number of AIDS cases in the world reported to the World Health Organization increased from a little more than 12,000 at the beginning of 1985 to 26,700 in December of that same year; then to 53,000 in 1986; to 96,500 in 1987; and to about 145,000 at the end of 1988. These figures represented only a fraction of the real numbers, as was the case in preceding years. According to the estimates of Jonathan Mann, director of the World Program to Combat AIDS, there were about 200,000 patients worldwide with overt AIDS and about five million seropositives. By the end of December 1988 the total number of infected persons had probably reached ten million. These global indications give a good idea of the rapidity with which this disease can spread, but get at neither its geographic expansion nor its impact in particular populations and epidemiologic situations.[32]

The United States is still the most heavily affected part of the world. The total number of AIDS cases reported to the CDC went from 20,000 at the end of 1985 to 37,000 in 1986, 61,000 in 1987, and close to 86,000 in 1988, about half representing deaths. Certain trends begun before 1985 accelerated. The increase among white homosexuals slowed, but took on frightening proportions among drug addicts and their families. For the most part these patients were young and black or Hispanic. The relative number of homosexuals dropped to 63 percent while that of drug addicts increased to 19 percent. In those with overt AIDS the infection resulted from heterosexual contacts in only 5 percent of cases. The spread of the disease has now become more rapid in children than in adults: more than 1,000 pediatric cases were reported between the beginning of the epidemic and July 1988, half in the last twelve months of that period. The cumulative prevalence of cases of AIDS is on the order of magnitude of 30 per 100,000 inhabitants. In April 1988, systematic screening of active-duty military personnel (to wit about two million people) demonstrated a 0.13 percent rate of seropositivity. The overall prevalence of HIV infection in civilian applicants for U.S. military service (routinely tested since October 1985) is now 0.15 percent. Blacks and Hispanics respectively showed 3.6 and 2.5 times the average American rate of positivity. For the entire United States population, public health authorities estimate the number of seropositives at close to two million.[33]

In all the European nations together, the number of cases went from 880 reported to December 1984 to 2,200 in 1985, then exceeding 5,900 cases in 1986 and 12,000 in 1987, finally attaining about 20,000 in 1988. France holds first place in Europe for absolute numbers of cases (about a third of European AIDS patients), while Switzerland surpasses it for overall concentration (7.6 per 100,000 inhabitants).[34] The situation in Switzerland illustrates nicely how the initial stage, in which AIDS is a disease of foreigners (or at least only contracted from foreigners), advances to a situation in which local sources of infection predominate.[35]

The number of cases reported in France went from 400 in the middle of 1985, to 1,900 in December 1986, surpassing 3,700 in December 1987, reaching exactly 4,211 cases on June 30, 1988, and, according to the updated report, passing 5,600 at the end of that year. In 1988 about 3 percent of cases were pediatric. Among adults men predominated by a 6.5:1 ratio, corresponding to the preponderance of homosexual transmission (60 percent). Drug addicts represented about 14 percent, transfusion recipients 7 percent, and hemophilia patients 1 percent. Heterosexual transmission was implicated in about 10 percent of the cases described, with a trend toward a relative decrease in homosexual transmission and a discrete increase in heterosexual transmission. AIDS in France continues to spread selectively: 52 percent of the accumulated cases were reported in the Paris region and 14 percent in the area surrounding and including the Riviera.[36] More than 90 percent of death certificates reporting AIDS as a cause of death come from university hospitals.[37] Of the people dying in this group and in hospitals of certain traditionalist departments of France, an unusual number of leukemia cases was reported. Undoubtedly some of these reports were falsified at the request of patients' families. Medical demographers believe that the number of patients in France is underreported by about 20 to 30 percent, and that as of the end of 1988 there are about 250,000 seropositives in France.

Italy went from 650 patients in 1986, to 1,630 in 1987, and to more than 3,000 in 1988. AIDS has spread there with particular intensity among the addict population, such that about 70 percent of current Italian AIDS patients are drug addicts.[38] To simplify, one might say that northern Europe has been struck by AIDS primarily among homosexuals and southern Europe among drug addicts, with France encompassing both types of propagation.

The HIV-2 virus today has overrun Africa and is expanding in Europe, especially in Portugal. The first case of infection by a virus of this type in the United States was diagnosed in a patient originally from West Africa who came to New Jersey in 1987. He had consulted a physician in December 1987 for weight loss of three months and for the recent onset of neurologic symptoms.[39]

For the African continent as a whole, official WHO statistics comprise 100 AIDS patients in 1984, 700 in 1985, 3,900 in 1986, 12,000 in 1987, and 23,000 in 1988. These figures bear no relationship to reality. Suffice it to say that, according to Zairian political authorities, in this country, in the eye of the hurricane, the last word was 335 patients.

We are currently looking at a veritable explosion of the epidemic in Mexico and South America, notably Brazil, where at the end of 1988 there were more than 6,000 AIDS patients. The continent at risk is Asia: AIDS arrived there late, but in certain Asian nations the conditions are particularly propitious for its expansion. In Bangkok, for example, no drug addict had yet been infected in 1985; in 1987 this had risen to one percent seropositives, but during the first three months of 1988 the figures precipitously increased to 16 percent. The virus had just penetrated into the great southeast Asian reservoirs of male and female prostitution. At least one-half percent of Bangkok's prostitutes are already infected.

The Menace and the Hope

Around the world in the next five years, a million people in their prime will become gravely ill. It will be the main cause of death for persons under age fifty. The cost for these patients will be greater than for any other disease. We can multiply such forecasts to our heart's content, each more somber than the last. Even if today we were to arrest all possibility of new infection, or to protect the entire planet with an effective vaccine (which does not yet exist), we could not forestall the avalanche of problems that await us in the immediate future.

The epidemic's spread is exponential, justifying cataclysmic predictions. But the doubling time is very different from one country to another. It depends on several factors, notably the predominant mode of transmission and the length of time since the local onset of the epidemic. We may expect a slow-down in the epidemic's exponential growth. At first it will be transitory but will become definitive when the majority of subjects exhibiting high-risk behavior are already infected.[40] A saturation effect will come into play and cause the growth curve to fall off. AIDS does not in fact attack all the inhabitants of a country in the same way: the epidemic in the general population is the result of a series of superimposed epidemics in several different subpopulations. In contrast to what happens with certain other pandemic diseases such as influenza or plague, the routes of transmission of AIDS are in large part controllable.

The current pandemic occurred because radical changes in human behavior interrupted the long-standing equilibrium between host and parasite. Even if no vaccine or drug is found to stop the pandemic, a new equilibrium will be established between humans and virus. However, that can only happen in the long run, and at an exorbitant price in suffering and human life.

Natural selection will see to it that the virus adapts to the human host: it moves from a progressive exacerbation of its virulence (the present phase of the pandemic, still on the ascending limb), then begins to attenuate. Human beings affect their natural environment, bending it to their will; to the extent they do not succeed, they are changed in turn at the whim of unpitying mechanisms of the survival of the fittest. It is probable that genetic factors are able to facilitate or to inhibit the pathogenic effects of the AIDS virus. Recent English observations suggest that the gene coding for the Gc protein ("group-specific complement") is associated with differences in sensitivity or resistance of the HIV carrier, that is, influences the risk of infection at time of exposure as well as progression to the successive stages of disease and the severity of symptoms.[41]

A natural experiment is currently under way in Trinidad. This island in the Lesser Antilles includes about 1.3 million inhabitants, of whom 40 percent are of African origin, 40 percent Indian, and 20 percent Chinese, European, or mestizo. This population was infected quite some time ago by the HTLV-I virus. In 1983 several cases of AIDS were diagnosed there. HIV-1 infection then began spreading explosively among the island's homosexuals. According to a study by Port-of-Spain physician Courtenay Bartholomew, in a cohort of one hundred Trinidad homosexuals, forty were seropositive. More precisely, there were 44 percent African seropositives against 30 percent Indian seropositives, with homosexual practices distributed more or less equally between the two groups. The distribution of overt clinical disease between the two groups is astonishing: fifty-four black, four mestizo, one white and not a single Indian case. Bartholomew concluded from this that a genetic factor may be necessary for the appearance of AIDS: the Indians of Trinidad either lack that factor or perhaps possess another, protective genetic factor.[42]

In *The War of the Worlds* (1898), Herbert George Wells recounted how Martian invaders defied the apparently powerful weapons of men only to succumb to pathogenic microbes. Poetic intuition combined with a profound knowledge of reality and a perfect understanding of scientific theory to show Wells that survival on this Earth was possible only by slowly and painfully integrating every being into its milieu and its biocenosis:

> These germs of disease have taken toll of humanity since the beginning of things—taken toll of our prehuman ancestors since life began here. But by virtue of this natural selection of our kind we have developed resisting-power; to no germs do we succumb without a struggle, and to many—those

that cause putrefaction in dead matter, for instance—our living frames are altogether immune. . . . By the toll of a billion deaths, man has bought his birthright of the earth. . . . For neither do men live nor die in vain.[43]

We should not presume that humankind is done with this blood tribute once and for all. Heavy burdens still await us as the price of our actions, disturbing the dynamic equilibria between humans, their physical surroundings, and the totality of living beings.

Notes

Chapter 1

1. Leibowitch (1984).
2. CDC (1981a and 1986d); Black (1986), pp. 36–48; Connor and Kingman (1988), pp. 12–14.
3. CDC (1981a and 1986d); Gottlieb, Schroff, Schanker, et al. (1981).
4. CDC (1981a), p. 252.
5. Lemaire (1987), p. 372.
6. Black (1986), pp. 35–36; Shilts (1987), pp. 25–29, 40–41, 45, 53.
7. Shilts (1987), pp. 54, 61, 66.
8. Hymes, Greene, Marcus, et al. (1981).
9. Shilts (1987), p. 50.
10. Shilts (1987), pp. 60, 64, 65; cf. Drew, Conant, Miner, et al. (1982).
11. CDC (1981b); Hymes, Greene, Marcus, et al. (1981); Friedman-Kien (1981); Friedman-Kien, Laubenstein, Rubinstein, et al. (1982); Friedman-Kien and Laubenstein (1984).
12. CDC (1981b); Siegal, Lopez, Hammer, et al. (1981).
13. CDC (1981b), p. 308.
14. Altman (1981).
15. Black (1986), p. 52.
16. CDC (1981c).
17. Gottlieb, Ragaz, Vogel, et al. (1981).
18. Hymes, Greene, Marcus, et al. (1981).
19. Shilts (1987), pp. 83, 87.
20. Brennan and Durack (1981).
21. Masur, Michelis, Greene, et al. (1981).
22. Siegal, Lopez, Hammer, et al. (1981); cf. Siegal and Siegal (1983).
23. Gottlieb, Schroff, Schanker, et al. (1981).
24. Ibid., p. 1425.

Chapter 2

1. Carey (1985); cf. Dabis (1988).
2. Langmuir (1980); Dabis (1988).
3. CDC (1985b).
4. Neustadt and Fineberg (1983).
5. CDC (1986d); Koch (1987), pp. 204–206; Panem (1988).
6. Durack (1981), pp. 1466–1467.
7. Clark and Gonnell (1981); Durack (1981); Jorgenson and Lawesson (1982); Goedert, Neuland, Walle, et al. (1982).
8. Marmor, Friedman-Kien, Laubenstein, et al. (1982).
9. Leibowitch (1984), p. 22.

10. Neumann (1982).

11. Clark and Gonnell (1981).

12. Navarro and Hagstrom (1982).

13. Shearer and Hurtenbach (1982); Marx (1982); Shearer and Rabson (1984); Black (1986), pp. 95–99.

14. Clark and Gonnell (1981); Friedman-Kien, Laubenstein, and Rubinstein (1982).

15. Rogers, Morens, Stewart, et al. (1983).

16. CDC (1982k); cf. Haverkos and Curran (1982); Shilts (1987), pp. 80–82.

17. Jaffe, Choi, Thomas, et al. (1983).

18 CDC (1982a).

19. Jaffe, Choi, Thomas, et al. (1983), p. 148.

20. CDC (1981c); Masur, Michelis, Wormser, et al. (1982).

21. CDC (1982d).

22. Marx (1982); Auerbach, Darrow, Jaffe, and Curran (1984).

23. CDC (1982d); Shilts (1987).

24. Leibowitch (1984), p. 65.

25. Shilts (1987), pp. 147, 165 and 200.

26. Blattner, *Scientific American* 259 (1988): 149.

27. Shilts (1987), p. 3.

Chapter 3

1. Altman (1981).

2. Gerstoft, Malchow-Moller, Bygbjerg, et al. (1982).

3. Thomsen, Jacobsen, and Malchow-Moller (1981); Gerstoft, Malchow-Moller, Bygbjerg, et al. (1982).

4. Jensen, Mouridsen, and Petersen (1982); Clemmesen (1982).

5. Du Bois, Branthwaite, Mikhail, and Batten (1981).

6. Vilaseca, Arnau, Bacardi, et al. (1982).

7. Francioli, Vogt, Schädelin, et al. (1982).

8. Helm, Bergmann, and Nerger (1982); Koch, L'age-Stehr, and Weise (1983); L'age-Stehr, Kunze, and Koch (1983); Koch (1987), p. 195.

9. Rezza, Ippolito, Marasca, and Greco (1984).

10. Lazzarin, Crocchiolo, Galli, et al. (1987).

11. Cf. Franceschi, Tirelli, Vaccher, et al. (1986).

12. Rozenbaum, Coulaud, and Saimot (1982); Rozenbaum, Klatzmann, Mayaud, et al. (1983); Chauvet (1983), pp. 24–27; Salbaing (1983), pp. 29–31; Rozenbaum, Seux, and Kouchner (1984), pp. 18–19, 25–28.

13. Leibowitch (1984); Shilts (1987), p. 102.

14. Leibowitch (1984), p. 17.

15. Groupe de Travail Français sur le SIDA (1982, 1983a, 1983b); Rozenbaum, Seux, and Kouchner (1984), pp. 19–25; Leibowitch (1984), pp. 23–24.

16. Brunet, Bouvet, Leibowitch, et al. (1983); cf. Salbaing (1983).

17. Rozenbaum, Klatzmann, Mayaud, et al. (1983).

18. Dournon, Penalba, Saimot, et al. (1983); Salbaing (1983).

19. Andreani, Modigliani, Le Charpentier, et al. (1983).

20. Leibowitch (1984), pp. 59–60.

21. Ibid., p. 55.

22. Gorin, Picard, Laroche, et al. (1982); Laroche, Gorin, Bach, and Hewitt (1982); Picard, Gorin, Leibowitch, et al. (1982).

23. Leibowitch (1984), pp. 47–48; Saimot, Coulaud, Mechali, et al. (1987); Shilts (1987), pp. 36–37.

24. Brenky and Zémor (1985), p. 30.

25. Brunet, Bouvet, Leibowitch, et al. (1983); Leibowitch (1984), p. 48.

26. Bygbjerg (1983); Shilts (1987), pp. 3–7, 277.

27. Brunet, Klatzmann, Cavaille-Coll, and Picard (1984).

28. Vandepitte, Verwilghen, and Zachee (1983).

29. Offenstadt, Pinta, Hericord, et al. (1983).

30. Clumeck, Mascart-Lemone, De Maubege, et al. (1983); Sonnet and De Bruyere (1983).

31. Lamey and Melameka (1982).

32. Sonnet, Michaux, Zech, et al. (1987).

Chapter 4

1. CDC (1982g, 1982h, 1983a); cf. Marx (1982).

2. Black (1986), p. 60.

3. Goldsmith (1988).

4. Direction Générale de la Santé (1982b).

5. CDC (1983a).

6. CDC (1985a and 1987b).

7. Payet (1986).

8. CDC (1982e); Pitchenik, Fischl, Dickinson, et al. (1983); Moskowitz, Kory, Chan, et al. (1983).

9. CDC (1982e); Vieiria, Franck, Spora, et al. (1983); Luft, Conley, and Remington (1983).

10. Liautaud, Laroche, Duvivier, et al. (1982, 1983).

11. Malebranche, Arnoux, Guérin, et al. (1983); Pape, Liautaud, Thomas, et al. (1983).

12. Andreani, Modigliani, Le Charpentier, et al. (1983).

13. Leonidas and Hyppolite (1983); cf. Moses and Moses (1983); Greco (1983); Greenfield (1986).

14. Compas (1983); cf. Pape, Liautaud, Thomas, et al. (1986).

15. CDC (1982f); Curran (1983).

16. CDC (1982h, 1983f); White and Lesesne (1983); Desforges (1983); Evatt, Ramsey, Lawrence, et al. (1984).

17. Elliott, Hoppes, Platt, et al. (1983).

18. Davis, Horsburgh, Hasiba, et al. (1983).

19. Poon, Landay, Prasthofer, et al. (1983).

20. Ragni, Lewis, Spero, et al. (1983).

21. Goldsmith, Moseley, Monick, et al. (1983); White and Lesesne (1983).

22. Marx (1982).

23. CDC (1982i); Amman, Cowan, Wara, et al. (1983).

24. Jett, Kuritsky, Katzmann, et al. (1983).

25. Andreani, Modigliani, Le Charpentier, et al. (1983); Deresinski, Cooney, Auerbach, et al. (1984); Curran, Lawrence, Jaffe, et al. (1984); Kleinman, Yust, Maayan, et al. (1986); Habibi (1986a, 1986b).

26. Curran, Lawrence, Jaffe, et al. (1984); Haverkos (1987).

27. CDC (1983b); Harris, Small, Klein, et al. (1983); Salbaing (1983), pp. 29–31.

28. Pitchenik, Shafron, Glasser, et al. (1984).

29. CDC (1985c); Redfield, Markham, Salahuddin, et al. (1985b).

30. Van de Perre, Clumeck, Carael, et al. (1985).

31. Guinan and Hardy (1987).

32. CDC (1982j); Rubinstein, Sicklick, Gupta, et al. (1983); Joncas, Delage, Chad, et al. (1983).

33. Oleske, et al. (1983); cf. Shilts (1987), p. 299.

34. CDC (1983e); Wormser, Krupp, Hanrahan, et al. (1983); cf. Beylot, Benezech, Lacoste, et al. (1988).

35. Black (1986), p. 29.

36. Solé (1983); Curran (1983).

37. Cf. Leibowitch (1984), pp. 124–127.

38. Weiss (1988).

39. Henig (1983).

40. Allen (1984).

41. May and Anderson (1987).

42. CDC (1983e, 1984); Curran (1983); Jaffe, Bergman, and Selik (1983); Selik, Haverkos, and Curran (1984); Allen (1984); Fauci, Macher, Congo, et al. (1984).

43. *Ann. Int. Med.* 99 (1983): 216.

44. CDC (1984); Brunet and Bouvet (1984).

45. *Lancet* 1 (1983): 162–164; Curran (1983); CDC (1984, etc.).

46. Luft, Conley, and Remington (1983).

47. Soave, Danner, Honig, et al. (1984).

48. May and Anderson (1987); Downs, Ancelle, Jager, and Brunet (1987).

49. Brunet (1984).

50. Ibid.; Brunet and Bouvet (1984); WHO (1985).

51. Groupe de Travail Français (1983); Direction Générale de la Santé (1984, 1985); Brunet and Bouvet (1984).

52. Messiah, Mary, Brunet, et al. (1987); Messiah (1987).

53. Aiuti, Sirianni, Pana, et al. (1984); Gabrielli, Nortilli, Mezzelani, et al. (1984); Rezza, Ippolito, Marasca, and Greco (1984); Lazzarin, Orlando, Privitera, et al. (1986).

54. Van de Perre, Rouvroy, Lepage, et al. (1984); Piot, Quinn, Taelman, et al. (1984).

Chapter 5

1. Koch (1987), p. 204.

2. CDC (1982f).

3. Francis, Curran, and Essex (1983).

4. Giraldo, Beth, and Hagenau (1972); Giraldo, Beth, and Huang (1980).

5. Gottlieb, Schroff, Schanker, et al. (1981); Du Bois, Branthwaite, Mikhail, and Batten (1981).

6. Masur, Michelis, Greene, et al. (1981); Drew, Conant, Miner, et al. (1982); Brun-Vézinet, Klatzmann, and Rouzioux (1984); Rozenbaum, Seux, and Kouchner (1984).

7. Ravenholt (1983); McDonald, Hamilton, and Durack (1983); Brun-Vézinet, Klatzmann, and Rouzioux (1984); Rozenbaum, Seux, and Kouchner (1984).

8. Ziegler, Drew, Miner, et al. (1982); Brun-Vézinet, Klatzmann, and Rouzioux (1984).

9. Teas (1983); Leibowitch (1984), p. 114; Connor and Kingman (1988), pp. 27–28.

10. Colaert, Desmyter, Goudsmit, et al. (1983).

11. Beldekas, Teas and Herbert (1986).

12. Shilts (1987), pp. 73, 107.

13. Vallée and Carré (1904).

14. Roux (1903).

15. Boivin (1941); Burnet (1955); Lwoff (1958); Cairns, Stent, and Watson (1966); Lwoff (1969); Stanier and Lwoff (1973); Hughes (1977); Baltimore (1977); Waterson and Wilkinson (1978); Galperin (1987); Scott (1987); Fenner and Gibbs (1988).

16. Sigurdsson, Palsson, and Grimsson (1957).

17. Gajdusek and Zigas (1957).

18. Gajdusek and Gibbs (1971); Gajdusek (1977).

19. Gajdusek (1967); Faris and Martinez (1972); Haase (1986).

20. Lwoff (1953 and 1969); Galperin (1987); Scott (1987).

21. Ellermann and Bang (1908); Rous (1910–1911); Bittner (1936); Gross (1983).

22. Gross (1951); Bessis (1976); Gross (1985).

23. Burkitt (1958–1959, 1963).

24. Epstein and Barr (1964).

25. Epstein (1980); Henle, Henle, and Diehl (1968); De Thé (1984).

26. Huebner and Todaro (1969).

27. Jarrett (1966); Jarrett, Jarrett, Mackey, et al. (1973); Essex (1982); Gross (1983).

28. Crick (1957).

29. Judson (1979), p. 337.

30. Temin and Mizutani (1970); Baltimore (1970).

31. Gallo (1986).

32. Morgan, Ruscetti, and Gallo (1976).

33. Poiesz, Ruscetti, Mier, et al. (1980).

34. Gallo (1986).

35. Poiesz, Ruscetti, Gazdar, et al. (1980); Poiesz, Ruscetti, Reitz, et al. (1981).

36. Kalyanaraman, Sarngadharan, Robert-Guroff, et al. (1982).

37. Chen, McLaughlin, Gasson, et al. (1983).

38. Yoshida, Miyoshi, and Hinuma (1982); Watanabe, Seiki, and Yoshida (1983); cf. Koch (1987), p. 88.

39. Popovic, Sarin, Robert-Guroff, et al. (1983); Gallo (1984); Gallo, Essex, and Gross (1984); Robert-Guroff, Markham, Popovic, and Gallo (1985); Wong-Staal and Gallo (1985a, b).

40. Koch (1987), p. 204.

41. Essex, McLane, Lee, et al. (1983).

42. CDC (1983d).

43. Gallo (1987).

44. Gallo, Sarin, Gelmann, et al. (1983).

45. Gelmann, Popovic, Blayney, et al. (1983).

46. Montagnier (1986), p. 57.

47. Maurice (1983b); Connor (1987).

48. Arya, Gallo, Hahn, et al. (1984).

49. Leibowitch (1984).

Chapter 6

1. Delaunay (1962).

2. Lwoff (1953); Jacob and Wollman (1953); Galperin (1987); Girard (1988).

3. Montagnier (1986), p. 34.

4. Lessana-Leibowitch, Leibowitch, Frances, et al. (1984).

5. Rozenbaum, Seux, and Kouchner (1984), p. 82; Shilts (1987), p. 193.

6. Rozenbaum (1984); Rozenbaum, Seux, and Kouchner (1984), pp. 82–84; Montagnier (1986), p. 35; Gallo and Montagnier (1988).

7. Barré-Sinoussi, Chermann, Rey, et al. (1983).

8. Montagnier (1986), pp. 52–54; cf. Biagi (1987), p. 228.

9. Barré-Sinoussi, Chermann, and Rozenbaum (1987), pp. 104–113; Connor and Kingman (1988), p. 30.

10. Montagnier (1986), p. 56.

11. Ibid., p. 58.

12. Barré-Sinoussi, Chermann, Rey, et al. (1983).

13. Chermann, Barré, and Montagnier (1984); Montagnier (1986), pp. 60–63.

14. Gallo (1987).

15. Maurice (1983a, 1983b).

16. Leibowitch (1984), p. 115.

17. Gallo, Essex, and Gross (1984); Montagnier (1986), pp. 66–67; *Nature* (1987), p. 435.

18. Montagnier, Dauguet, Axler, et al. (1984).

19. Vilmer, Barré-Sinoussi, Rouzioux, et al. (1984).

20. Karpas (1983); Karpas, Gillson, Oates, et al. (1985); cf. Koch (1987), pp. 59, 66.

21. Gallo, Essex, and Gross (1984).

22. Black (1986), pp. 120–122; Shilts (1987), pp. 450–452; Connor and Kingman (1988), pp. 39–40.

23. Gallo (1987).

24. Popovic, Sarngadharan, Read, and Gallo (1984).

25. Gallo, Salahuddin, Popovic, et al. (1984); cf. Salahuddin, Markham, Popovic, et al. (1985).

26. Sarngadharan, Popovic, Bruch, et al. (1984); Schüpbach, Popovic, Gilden, et al. (1984).

27. Altmann, *New York Times*, April 21, 1984; Kalyanaraman, Montagnier, Francis, et al. (1984); Norman (1985); Shilts (1987).

28. Montagnier (1984, 1986); cf. Koch (1987), p. 96.

29. Coffin, Haase, Levy, et al. (1986); Marx (1986).

Chapter 7

1. Montagnier (1986), p. 69.

2. Brun-Vézinet, Rouzioux, Barré-Sinoussi, et al. (1984); Montagnier (1986), pp. 68–69.

3. Beardsley (1984); Montagnier (1984); Norman (1985).

4. Kalyanaraman, Montagnier, Francis, et al. (1984).

5. Safai, Gallo, Popovic, et al. (1984).

6. Montagnier, Gruest, Chamaret, et al. (1984).

7. Joyce and Sattaur (1985); *La Recherche* 174 (February 1986); Gallo, Sarin, Kramarsky, et al. (1986); *Nature* 326 (1987): 425; Connor and Kingman (1988), pp. 47–50.

8. Shilts (1987), p. 461; Connor and Kingman (1988), pp. 41–42.

9. Arya, Gallo, Hahn, et al. (1984).

10. Montagnier (1986), p. 74.

11. Cheingsong-Popov, Weiss, et al. (1984).

12. Karpas (1983); Levy, Hoffmann, Kramer, et al. (1984); Rossi, Verani, Macchi, et al. (1987).

13. Hahn, Shaw, Arya, et al. (1984).

14. Alizon, Sonigo, Barré-Sinoussi, et al. (1984).

15. Wain-Hobson, Sonigo, Danos, et al. (1985).

16. Ratner, Haseltine, Patarca, et al. (1985).

17. Sanchez-Pescador, Power, Barr, et al. (1985).

18. Muesing, Smith, Cabradilla, et al. (1985).

19. Rabson and Martin (1985); Benn, Routledge, Folks, et al. (1985); cf. Koch (1987), pp. 97–98, 103; Connor and Kingman (1988), pp. 45, 48.

20. Norman (1985); Connor and Kingman (1988), p. 47.

21. Gilden, Gonda, Sarngadharan, et al. (1986); Norman (1986a); cf. Beardsley (1986) and Gallo, Sarin, Kramarsky, et al. (1986).

22. Schüpbach (1986).

23. Connor (1987); Koch (1987), p. 95; Connor and Kingman (1988), pp. 49–50, 58–59.

24. Palca (1987); Connor and Kingman (1988), pp. 60–63.

25. Gallo and Montagnier (1987).

26. Gonda, Wong-Staal, Gallo, et al. (1985); Sonigo, Alizon, Staskus, et al. (1985); Chiu, Yaniv, Dalberg, et al. (1985).

27. Montagnier (1985); Brun-Vézinet and Rouzioux (1986); Gallo (1987); Montagnier (1987); Girard, De Thé, and Valette (1987); Girard and Valette (1988); Fauci (1988); Gallo and Wong-Staal (1988); Gonda (1988); Gonda, Boyd, Nagashima, and Gilden (1988).

28. Sodroski, Rosen, Wong-Staal, et al. (1985); Haseltine and Wong-Staal (1988).

29. Allan, Coligan, Barin, et al. (1985); Montagnier, Krust, Clavel, et al. (1985). M. Essex and T. H. Lee obtained the U.S. Patent for the medical use of this protein; cf. *Nature* 331 (1988): 649.

30. Dalgleish, Beverley, Clapham, et al. (1984); Klatzmann, Champagne, Chamaret, et al. (1984).

31. Matthews, Weinhold, Lyerly, et al. (1987); Girard and Valette (1988); Haseltine and Wong-Staal (1988).

32. Gartner, Markovits, Markovitz, et al. (1986a); Ho, Rota, and Hirsch (1986); Maddon, Dalgleish, McDougal, et al. (1986).

33. Koenig, Gendelman, Orenstein, et al. (1986); Sharer, Epstein, Cho, et al. (1986); Barnes (1986b); Vazeux, Brousse, Jarry, et al. (1987); Streicher and Joynt (1986); Price, Brew, Sidtis, et al. (1988).

34. Zagury, Bernard, Leibowitch, et al. (1984); Ho, Schooley, Rota, et al. (1984).

35. Groopman, Salahuddin, Sarngadharan, et al. (1984).

36. Zagury, Fouchard, Vol, et al. (1985).

37. Vogt, Witt, Craven, et al. (1986); Wofsy, Cohen, Hauer, et al. (1986); Vogt, et al. (1987).

38. Levy, Hollander, Shimabukuro, et al. (1985); Tervo, Lahdevirta, Vaheri, et al. (1986); Thiry, Sprecher-Goldberger, Jonkheer, et al. (1985).

39. Shaw, Harper, Hahn, et al. (1985); Gartner, Markovits, Markovitz, et al. (1986b); Stoler, Eskin, Benn, et al. (1986); Vazeux, Brousse, Jarry, et al. (1987); cf. Rosenblum, Levy, and Bredeson (1988).

40. Tschachler, Groh, Popovic, et al. (1987); Schmitt and Thivolet (1988).

41. Becker, Hazan, Nugeyre, et al. (1986).

42. Clavel, Guétard, Brun-Vézinet, et al. (1986); Clavel (1987).

43. Clavel, Guétard, Brun-Vézinet, et al. (1986); Blanc (1986); Brun-Vézinet, Rey, Katlama, et al. (1987); Clavel (1987).

44. Clavel, Guyader, Guétard, et al. (1986); Guyader, Emerman, Sonigo, et al. (1987).

45. Daniel, Letvin, King, et al. (1985).

46. Kanki, Kurth, Becker, et al. (1985).

47. Kanki, Alroy, and Essex (1985).

48. Fultz, McClure, Anderson, et al. (1986); Lowenstine, Pedersen, Higgins, et al. (1986).

49. Barin, M'Boup, Denis, et al. (1985).

50. Kanki, Barin, M'Boup, et al. (1986).

51. Kornfeld, Riedel, Viglianti, et al. (1987); Newmark (1987); Desrosiers, Daniel, Letvin, et al. (1987); Mulder (1988).

52. Duesberg (1987, 1988); see also *New Scientist*, 117, no. 1602 (1987): 34; Ward (1988); Rubin (1988) and particularly Blattner, Gallo, and Temin (1988).

Chapter 8

1. Klein (1986); Rozenbaum and Gharakhanian (1986); Gottlieb, et al. (1987); Wormser, Stahl, and Bottone (1987); Broder (1987); Curran, Jaffe, Hardy, et al. (1988); Fauci (1988); Redfield and Burke (1988); Lifson, Rutherford, and Jaffe (1988).

2. Brun-Vézinet, Rouzioux, Barré-Sinoussi, et al. (1984); Mathez, Leibowitch, Matheron, et al. (1984); Aiuti, Sirianni, Pana, et al. (1984).

3. Safai, Gallo, Popovic, et al. (1984).

4. Cheingsong-Popov, Weiss, Dalgleish, et al. (1984).

5. Feldman and Johnson (1986); Dalton and Burris (1987); Walters (1988); Fineberg (1988); Martin (1988).

6. Abb (1986); Barr, Dow, Arnott, et al. (1986); Deinhardt, Eberle, and Görtler (1987); Meyer and Paulker (1987); Schwartz, Dans, and Kinosian (1988).

7. Kwok, Mack, Mullis, et al. (1987); Ou, Kwok, Mitchell, et al. (1988); Loche and Mach (1988); Laure, Courgnaud, Rou-zioux, et al. (1988); Murakawa, Zaia, Spallone, et al. (1988); Hart, Schochetman, Spira, et al. (1988).

8. Peterman and Curran (1986); Levy (1988b).

9. Darrow, Echenberg, Jaffe, et al. (1987); Curran, Jaffe, Hardy, et al. (1988).

10. CDC (1985c); Redfield, Markham, Salahuddin, et al. (1985a, 1985b).

11. Fultz, McClure, Daugharty, et al. (1986).

12. Padian, Marquis, Francis, et al. (1987); Levy (1988b); Adachi, Koenig, Gendelman, et al. (1987).

13. Stewart, et al. (1985); Brenky and Zémor (1985), pp. 132–133.

14. Piot, Quinn, Taelman, et al. (1984); Van de Perre, Rouvroy, Lepage, et al. (1984); Kreiss, Koech, Plummer, et al. (1986); Piot, Plummer, Mhalu, et al. (1988)

15. Padian (1987); Levy (1988a).

16. Fultz (1986).

17. Mayer and DeGruttola (1987); Rozenbaum, Gharakhanian, Cardon, et al. (1988).

18. Marmor, Weiss, Lyden, et al. (1986).

19. Curran, Jaffe, Hardy, et al. (1988).

20. L'age-Stehr, Schwarz, Offermann, et al. (1985).

21. Kumar, Pearson, Martin, et al. (1987); Bierling, Cordonnier, Duedari, et al. (1986); Antin, Smith, Ewenstein, et al. (1986); O'Day (1986); Habibi and Girard (1988).

22. Neisson-Vernant, Arfi, Mathez, et al. (1986); Oksenhendler, Harzic, Le Roux, et al. (1986).

23. CDC (1987c); cf. also CDC (1988c).

24. Weiss, Goedert, Gartner, et al. (1988).

25. Curran, Jaffe, Hardy, et al. (1988); cf. Tovo, De Martino, et al. (1988).

26. Masters, Johnson, and Kolodny (1988).

27. Henderson, Saah, Zak, et al. (1986); Fauci (1988); cf. also CDC (1988b).

28. Fischl, Dickinson, Scott, et al. (1987); Lifson (1988).

29. Cooper, Gold, Maclean, et al. (1985); Piette, Tusseau, and Chapman (1987).

30. Fuchs, Hausen, Reibnegger, et al. (1988).

31. Streicher and Joynt (1986); Gartner, Markovits, Markovitz, et al. (1986a); Pauza (1988).

32. Medley, Anderson, Cox, et al. (1987); Ranki, Valle, Krohn, et al. (1987).

33. Redfield, Wright, and Tramont (1986); CDC (1986b).

34. Ostrow, Solomon, Mayer, and Haverkos (1987).

35. Rozenbaum and Gharakhanian (1986); Kernbaum and Saimot (1986); Redfield and Burke (1988).

36. Curran, Jaffe, Hardy, et al. (1988); Chavanet (1987); Kaplan, Spira, Fishbein, et al. (1988); Kernbaum (1988); Moss (1988).

37. Fribourg-Blanc (1988).

38. Blanche, Fischer, Le Deist, et al. (1986); Auger, Thomas, DeGruttola, et al. (1988); Tovo, De Martino, et al. (1988).

39. Ammann (1985); Rogers (1985); Sharer, Epstein, Cho, et al. (1986); Barnes (1986a).

40. Barnes (1986b); Vazeux, Brousse, Jarry, et al. (1987); Streicher and Joynt (1986); Price, Brew, Sidtis, et al. (1988).

41. Levy, Hollander, Shimabukuro, et al. (1985); Shaw, Harper, Hahn, et al. (1985); Wiley, Schrier, Nelson, et al. (1986).

42. Navia, Cho, Petito, et al. (1986); Gressentis (1986); Vazeux, Brousse, Jarry, et al. (1987); Grant, Atkinson, Hesselink, et al. (1987); Ostrow (1987); Rosenblum, Levy, Bredesen, et al. (1988); Price, Brew, Sidtis, et al. (1988).

43. Salbaing (1983); Rozenbaum, Klatzmann, Mayaud, et al. (1983).

Chapter 9

1. Grmek (1987).

2. Nicolle (1930); Henschen (1962); Ackerknecht (1963); Hudson (1977); Hudson (1983).

3. Cockburn (1963).

4. Grmek (1983), p. 151.

5. Lwoff (1958); Lwoff (1969); Hughes (1977).

6. Burnet (1955); Black (1975).

7. Grmek (1983), pp. 221–222.

8. Langmuir, et al. (1985); Langmuir and Ray (1987).

9. Dan (1987).

10. Zinsser (1935); Page (1953); MacArthur (1958).

11. Gourevitch (1984); Rippinger (1987).

12. Grmek (1983), pp. 244–255.

13. Mugler (1967); Grmek (1983), p. 252.

14. Biagi (1987), p. 198; cf. Crick (1981).

15. Politzer (1954); Biraben (1975–1976); McNeill (1976).

16. Rosquist, Skurnik, and Wolf-Watz (1988); Lenski (1988).

17. Roberts (1965); Brossolet (1974); Wylie (1981).

18. Guerra (1978); Grmek (1983), pp. 199–226; Quetel (1986).

19. Smith (1986); Vachon (1987); Brandt (1987, 1988a, 1988b); Krech (1988).

20. Fribourg-Blanc, Niel, and Mollaret (1966); Fribourg-Blanc and Mollaret (1968).

21. Oriel and Cockburn (1974); Grmek (1983), pp. 206–207.

22. Stearn and Stearn (1945); Hopkins (1983).

23. Grmek (1966); Guerra (1987).

24. Gessain (1983).

25. Stevenson (1965).

26. McNicoll and Doetsch (1983).

27. Watson (1928); Greenough and Davis (1983).

28. Mollaret (1987).

29. McDade, et al. (1977); Lattimer and Ormsbee (1981); Fleurette (1983); Winn (1988).

30. Martini and Siegert (1971); Brès (1978).

31. Frame, Baldwin, Gocke, et al. (1970); Monath (1975).

32. Brès (1978).

33. Ibid., p. 3009.

Chapter 10

1. Ablin, Gonder, and Immerman (1985).

2. Jonckheere (1944); Grapow (1956), pp. 60, 65.

3. Montagnier (1986), p. 131.

4. Numbers 25; cf. Preuss (1923), pp. 586–588, and Grmek (1983), p. 212.

5. André (1987).

6. Grmek (1983), pp. 208–210.

7. Appelboom and Rouffin (1986); Appelboom, Rouffin, Van Herweghem, et al. (1987); cf. Werthemann (1930); Cole (1952).

8. Gerlo (1980).

9. Lesky (1965), pp. 345–349; Holubar and Frankl (1981); Gottlieb and Ackerman (1988).

10. Kaposi (1872); cf. Rothman (1962a) and Shiels (1986).

11. Kaposi (1872), p. 269.

12. Breimer (1984), p. 157.

13. De Amicis (1882); cf. Ronchese (1958).

14. Philippson (1902); Mariani (1909); Dalla Favera (1911); cf. Katner and Pankey (1987), p. 1069.

15. Bluefarb (1957); Rothman (1962b); Safai and Good (1980); Gottlieb and Ackerman (1988).

16. Hallenberg (1914).

17. Smith and Elmes (1934).

18. Dupont, Chabeuf, and Vanbreuseghem (1948); Dupont (1951).

19. Gigase (1984), p. 554; cf. Oettle (1963), pp. 28–29, and Hutt (1981), p. 6.

20. Murray (1952); Thijs (1957); Quenum (1957); Quenum and Camain (1958).

21. Coulaud, Vilde, and Regnier (1984).

22. Hansemann (1905); Stoddard and Cutler (1916); cf. Ainsworth (1986).

23. Wolf and Cowen (1937); Thalhammer (1957); Hentsch (1971).

24. Grmek (1983), pp. 307–354.

25. Van der Meer and Brug (1942); Hamperl (1956); Gajdusek (1976).

26. Wyatt, Saxton, et al. (1950); Smith (1956); Diosi and David (1968).

27. Wyatt, Simon, Trumbull, and Evans (1953); cf. Hamperl (1956).

28. Sunderam, McDonald, Manialtis, et al. (1986); CDC (1986a, 1987a); Pinching (1987); Goldman (1987).

29. Predöhl (1888); Flick (1925); Jedlicka (1932); Coury (1972); Dubos and Dubos (1987).

Chapter 11

1. Jaffe, Bergman, and Selik (1983); Selik, Haverkos, and Curran (1984).

2. Sterry, Marmor, Konrads, et al. (1983).

3. Nicolle (1930); cf. Lemaire (1985).

4. CDC (1983a).

5. CDC (1985a) and CDC (1987b); cf. Ostrow, Solomon, Mayer, and Haverkos (1987).

6. Cf. Huminer, Rosenfeld, and Pitlik (1987); Katner and Pankey (1987).

7. Wyatt, Simon, Trumbull, et al. (1953).

8. Hamperl (1956).

9. Nichols (1982).

10. Wyatt, Simon, Trumbull, et al. (1953), p. 358.

11. Contreras (1957); cf. Katner and Pankey (1987).

12. Tedeschi (1958); Cox and Helwig (1959).

13. Anderson and Barrie (1960).

14. Hennigar, Vinijchaikul, Roque, and Lyons (1961); Lyons, Vinijckaikul, and Hennigar (1961); cf. Selik, Haverkos, and Curran (1984); Gorman, Dorfman, and Kramer (1987).

15. Watanabe, Chinchinian, Weitz, et al. (1965).

16. Faris and Martinez (1972); Stemmermann, Hayashi, Glober, et al. (1980); Weinstein, Edelstein, Madara, et al. (1981); cf. Huminer, Rosenfeld, and Pitlik (1987); Katner and Pankey (1987).

17. Elvin-Lewis, Witte, Witte, et al. (1973).

18. Witte, Witte, Winnich, et al. (1984); Clark and Shapiro (1987); Gorman, Dorfman, and Kramer (1987); Shoumatoff (1988), pp. 161–162; Garry, Witte, Gottlieb, et al. (1988).

19. Leibowitch (1984), p. 38.

20. Madden, Tzan, Roman, et al. (1987).

21. Evatt, Gomperts, McDougal, et al. (1985).

22. Moore, Cone, and Alexander (1985).

23. Rodriquez, Dewhurst, Sinangil, et al. (1985).

24. Volsky, Wu, Stevenson, et al. (1986).

25. Shumatoff (1988), p. 150.

26. Galvao-Castro and Pereira (1986).

Chapter 12

1. Brunet, Bouvet, Leibowitch, et al. (1983); Huminer, Rosenfeld, and Pitlik (1987); Katner and Pankey (1987); Froland, Jenum, Lindboe, et al. (1988).

2. Seagrave (1948).

3. Williams, Stretton, and Leonard (1960, 1983); cf. Nichols (1982).

4. Schonell, Crofton, Stuart, et al. (1968); Hagmar, Kutti, Lundin, et al. (1969); cf. Huminer, Rosenfeld, and Pitlik (1987).

5. Bygbjerg (1983); Brunet, Bouvet, Leibowitch, et al. (1983); Vandepitte, Verwilghen, and Zachee (1983); Shilts (1987).

6. Brunet, Bouvet, Leibowitch, et al. (1983); Thomsen, Jacobsen, and Malchow-Moller (1981); Du Bois, Branthwaite, Mikhail, et al. (1981).

7. Sterry, Konrads, and Laaser (1979); Konrads and Sterry (1983); Sterry, Marmor, Konrads, and Steigleder (1983).

8. Bültmann, Flad, Kaiserling, et al. (1982); cf. Huminer, Rosenfeld, and Pitlik (1987).

9. Flatau, Resnitzky, Grishkan, et al. (1977); cf. Huminer (1985).

10. Lindboe, Froland, Wefring, et al. (1986).

11. Froland, Jenum, Lindboe, et al. (1988).

12. Madhok, Melbye, Lowe, et al. (1985).

13. Bryceson, Tomkins, Ridley, et al. (1988).

14. Guyader, Emerman, Sonigo, et al. (1987).

15. Quenum (1957); Quenum and Camain (1958); Oettle (1963); Gigase (1984); Shiels (1986).

16. Ackerman and Murray (1963); Olweny, Hutt, and Owor (1981).

17. Oettle (1963); Hutt (1981); Gigase (1984).

18. Quenum and Caiman (1958); Davies (1963); Taylor, Smith, Bull, et al. (1971); Kyalwazi (1981); Basset (1984) and particularly Gigase (1984).

19. Kyalwazi (1969).

20. Master, Taylor, Kyalwazi, et al. (1970); Taylor (1973); cf. Downing, Elgin, and Bayley (1984).

21. Biggar, Melbye, Kestems, et al. (1984).

22. Bayley, Downing, Cheinsong-Popov, et al. (1985); cf. Clumeck, Hermans, and De Wit (1987).

23. Otu (1986).

24. Bayley (1984).

25. Giraldo, Beth, and Haguenau (1972); Giraldo, Beth, and Huang (1980).

26. Ziegler, Templeton, and Vogel (1984).

27. Weber (1984); De Cock (1984).

28. Vandepitte, Verwilghen, and Zachee (1983); Jonckheer, et al. (1985); Rogan, Jewell, Mielke, et al. (1987).

29. Ravisse, Reynaud, Depoux, and Salles (1959).

30. Ibid.; Lamey and Melameka (1982); cf. Piot, Quinn, Taelman, et al. (1984).

31. Nahmias, Weiss, Yao, et al. (1986).

32. Desmyter, Goubau, Chamaret, and Montagnier (1986).

33. Montagnier (1986), p. 93.

34. Epstein, Moffitt, and Mayner (1985).

35. Forthal, Getchell, and Mann (1986); Getchel, Hicks, Srinivasan, et al. (1987); Myers, Josephs, Rabson, et al. (1987); Smith, Srinivasan, Schochetman, et al. (1988).

36. Saxinger, Levine, Dean, et al. (1985); Saxinger, Levine, Lange-Wantzin, and Gallo (1985).

37. Levy, Pan, Beth-Giraldo, et al. (1986); Wendler, Schneider, Gras, et al. (1986); Neppert, Gohring, Schneider, et al. (1986).

38. Carswell, Sewankambo, Lloyd, et al. (1986).

39. Hancock and Carim (1986), p. 119.

40. Biggar, Gigase, Melbye, et al. (1985).

41. Biggar (1986); Desmyter, Surmont, Goubau, et al. (1986); Biggar, Saxinger, Sarin, et al. (1986).

Chapter 13

1. Henrickson, Maul, Osborn, et al. (1983).

2. London, Sever, Madden, et al. (1983).

3. Marx, Maul, Osborn, et al. (1984).

4. Daniel, Letvin, King, et al. (1985).

5. Murray, in Girard and Valette (1988).

6. For HIV-1 infection, see Francis, Feorino, Broderson, et al. (1984); Alter, Eichberg, Masur, et al. (1984); Gajdusek, Amyx, Gibbs, et al. (1985); Fultz, McClure, Swenson, et al. (1986); Fultz, McClure, Daugharty, et al. (1986); for HIV-2 infection, see Clavel (1987).

7. Essex and Kanki (1988).

8. Lowenstine, Pedersen, Higgins, et al. (1986); Ohta, Masuda, Tsujimoto, et al. (1988); Fukasawa, Miura, Hasegawa, et al. (1988).

9. Miyoshi, Yoshimoto, Fujishita, et al. (1982); Yamamoto, Hinuma, Zur Hausen, et al. (1983).

10. Kimura (1981, 1983); Nei (1987).

11. McClure, Johnson, Feng, et al. (1988).

12. Yokoyama and Gojobori (1987); Yokoyama, Moriyama, and Gojobori (1987); Yokoyama, Chung, and Gojobori (1988).

13. Gonda, Boyd, Nagashima, and Gilden (1988).

14. Temin (1980, 1984, 1988); Varmus (1988).

15. Sonigo, Alizon, Staskus, et al. (1985); Gonda, Wong-Staal, Gallo, et al. (1985).

16. Chiu, Yaniv, Dalberg, et al. (1985); Stephens, Casey, and Rice (1986); McClure and Weiss (1987).

17. Gonda, Braun, Carter, et al. (1987).

18. Pedersen, Ho, and Brown (1987).

19. Guyader, Emerman, Sonigo, et al. (1987).

20. Smith, Srinivasan, Schochetman, et al. (1988); Sharp and Li (1988); Yokoyama, Chung, and Gojobori (1988); Li, Tanimura, and Sharp (1988).

21. Chakrabarti, Guyader, Alizon, et al. (1987); Franchini, Gurgo, Guo, et al. (1987).

22. Kappes, Morrow, Lee, et al. (1988).

23. Fukasawa, Miura, Hasegawa, et al. (1988); Hirsch, Riedel and Mullins (1988); Gonda, Boyd, Nagashima, et al. (1988); Sharp and Li (1988).

24. Desrosiers (1986); Penny (1988).

25. Yokoyama, Chung, and Gojobori (1988); cf. Benn, Rutledge, Folks, et al. (1985); Hahn, Shaw, Taylor, et al. (1986); Alizon and Montagnier (1987).

26. Gallo and Montagnier (1988).

27. Ohta, Masuda, Tsujimoto, et al. (1988).

28. Kashamura (1973), p. 137; cf. Noireau (1987).

29. Giunta and Groppa (1987).

30. Kanki, Barin, M'Boup, et al. (1986); Kanki, Barin, M'Boup, and Essex (1987); Montagnier (1986), p. 97; Murphey-Corb, Martin, Rangan, et al. (1986); Kanki, Hopper, and Essex (1987); Essex and Kanki (1988).

31. Gallo (1987), at 56.

32. Fukasawa, Miura, Hasegawa, et al. (1988); Mulder (1988).

33. Montagnier (1985), pp. 98, 101–102; cf. Desrosiers (1986); Gallo and Montagnier (1988).

34. De Thé, in Hirsch (1987), p. 76.

35. Hancock and Carim (1986), p. 73.

36. Brun-Vézinet, Jaeger, Rouzioux, et al. (1986); Gonzalez, Georges-Courbot, Martin, et al. (1987).

37. Biggar, Melbye, Kestens, et al. (1985); Biggar, Johnson, Oster, et al. (1985); Hancock and Carim (1986), p. 117; Biggar (1986).

38. Rodriquez, Dewhurst, Sinangil, et al. (1985); Shumatoff (1988), p. 150.

39. Weber (1983); cf. Lacey and Waugh (1984).

40. De Cock (1984).

41. Colebunders, Taelman, and Piot (1984).

42. Miyoshi, Yoshimoto, Fujishita, et al. (1982, 1983); Gallo and Wong-Staal (1982); Wong-Staal and Gallo (1985b); Weiss, in Weiss, Teich, Varmus, and Coffin (1985), pp. 409–414.

43. Fleming (1983, 1984); Hunsmann, Schneider, Schmitt, and Yamamoto (1983); Klingholz, in Burkel (1988), pp. 16–17.

44. Gallo, Sliski, and Wong-Staal (1983); Gallo, Sliski, and De Noronha (1986); cf. Gallo (1988).

45. Gallo (1986), at 95.

46. Taguchi (1986).

47. Watanabe, Seiki, Hirayama, and Yoshida (1986).

48. Wong-Staal and Gallo (1985b).

49. Leibowitch (1984); Seligmann, Hager, and Seward (1984).

50. Hancock and Carim (1986), p. 117. For the opinion that new infectious diseases are always coming out of Africa, see Kiple (1987).

51. Hancock and Carim (1986), p. 116.

52. Katner and Pankey (1987); Huminer, Rosenfeld, and Pitlik (1987).

53. Zapevalov (1985); cf. Revel, in Mérieux (1987), pp. 33–38; Revel (1987).

54. Seale (1985).

55. Medvedev (1986); Seale and Medvedev (1987); Seale (1988).

56. Girard (1987), pp. 80, 96, 112, 124, 129; cf. Hancock and Carim (1986), p. 72; Biagi (1987), pp. 167, 195–200.

57. Gallo (1987), at 56.

58. Liautaud, Laroche, Duvivier, et al. (1983); Pape, Liautaud, Thomas, et al. (1983).

59. Gazzolo, Gessain, Robin, et al. (1984); Koch (1987), p. 2.

60. Moses and Moses (1983); Seligmann, Hager, and Seward (1984); Gallo (1987); Gallo, Robert-Guroff, Wong-Staal, et al. (1987); Kéraly (1987), pp. 50–51; Koch (1987), p. 2.

61. Gurgo, Guo, Franchini, et al. (1988).

62. Barry, Mellors, and Bia (1984).

63. Shumatoff (1988), p. 163; cf. De Cock (1984).

64. Leibowitch (1984), pp. 113–114.

65. Shumatoff (1988).

66. Girard (1987), p. 223.

Chapter 14

1. Holland, Spindler, Horodyski, et al. (1982); Clark and Mak (1984).

2. Eigen and Schuster (1977).

3. Eigen (1988), pp. 119–121; Haseltine and Wong-Staal (1988).

4. Hahn, Shaw, Taylor, et al. (1986); Alizon and Montagnier (1987); Evans, McHugh, Stites, et al. (1987); Saag, Hahn, Gibbons, et al. (1988); Fisher, Ensoli, Looney, et al. (1988); Fenyö, Morfeldt-Mansson, Chiodi, et al. (1988); Wain-Hobson, Colloque ''Cent-Gardes'' (1988).

5. Lenski (1988).

6. Durack (1981).

7. Grmek (1969a, 1969b).

8. Cf. Sonea and Panisset (1983); Margulis and Sagan (1986).

9. Grmek (1969b, 1983, 1987); cf. Galzigna (1987).

10. Dubos (1963).

11. Kjeldsen (1975).

12. Coury (1972); Jenicek and Cléroux (1982); Guillaume (1986); Dubos and Dubos (1987).

13. De Cock (1984).

14. Wilkes, Fortin, Felix, et al. (1988).

15. Raymond (1987); Quinn, Piot, McCormick, et al. (1987).

16. CDC (1986a); Bricaire, Haas, and Patri (1986); Sunderam, McDonald, Maniatis, et al. (1986); Mann, Snider, Francis, et al. (1986); Goldman (1987); Pinching (1987).

17. Gordon, Valentine, Holzman, et al. (1984); cf. Koch (1987), p. 205.

18. Bove (1984); cf. Shilts (1987), pp. 220–223, 249, 344–345.

19. Greenwalt (1984).

20. Black (1986), p. 75.

21. Melief and Goudsmit (1986); Habibi (1986b).

22. Klein and Alter (1987).

23. CDC (1986c); Ranki, Valle, Krohn, et al. (1987); Ward, Holmberg, Allen, et al. (1988); Masters, Johnson, and Kolodny (1988).

24. Laga and Piot (1988); Kohlhof and Flessenkämper (1988).

25. Ingram (1976); Egli (1981); Aronson (1983).

26. Curran (1983).

27. Machin, McVerry, Chiengsong-Popov, et al. (1985); Madhok, Melbye, Lowe, et al. (1985); Evatt, Gomperts, McDougal, and Ramsey (1985).

28. Ragni, Lewis, Spero, et al. (1983).

29. CDC (1982f); Curran (1983).

30. CDC (1982h, 1983f); White and Lesesne (1983).

31. Desforges (1983).

32. *Lancet*, 1 (1983): 745.

33. Melbye, Biggar, Chermann, et al. (1984); Ramsey, Palmer, McDougal, et al. (1984).

34. Kitchen, Barin, Sullivan, et al. (1984).

35. Evatt, Gomperts, McDougall, and Ramsey (1985).

36. Rouzioux, Brun-Vézinet, Couroucé, et al. (1985).

37. Mathez, Leibowitch, Sultan, et al. (1986).

38. Allain (1986).

39. Elliott, Hoppes, Platt, et al. (1983); Davis, Horsburgh, Hasiba, et al. (1983); Poon, Landay, Prasthofer, et al. (1983).

40. Lissen, Wichmann, Jimenez, et al. (1983); Papaevangelou, Economidou, Kallikinos, et al. (1984); Melbye, Froebel, Mahdok, et al. (1984); Giudizzi, Biagotti, Almerignogna, et al. (1986); Dal Bo Zanon, Vicarioto, Girolami, et al. (1986); Haverkos (1987).

41. Casteret (1987).

42. Haverkos (1987); Klein and Alter (1987).

43. Apfelbaum and Gelfand (1934); Ashley (1972); Rublowsky (1974); Stimmel (1975); Trebach (1982); Koch (1987), pp. 202, 210, 226.

44. Jaffe, Seehaus, Wagner, et al. (1988).

45. Reynes, Quaranta, Pesce, et al. (1985); Angarano, Pastore, Monno, et al. (1985); Franceschi, Tirelli, Vaccher, et al. (1986); Lazzarin, Crocchiolo, Galli, et al. (1987).

46. Lowenstein, Le Jeune, Dormont, et al. (1986).

47. Franck (1987).

48. Hancock and Carim (1986), p. 102.

49. Marotta (1981); Moss, Bacchetti, Gorman, et al. (1983); Black (1986); Shilts (1987); Katner and Pankey (1987).

50. Kingsley, Detels, Kaslow, et al. (1987).

51. Trichopoulos, Sparos, and Petridou (1988).

52. Dritz (1980); Darrow, Barret, Jay, and Young (1981); Moss, Bacchetti, Gorman, et al. (1983); Shilts (1987).

53. Escande, in Rémy and Bardèche (1986), ''Préface.''

54. Cavailhès, Dutey, and Bach-Ignasse (1984); Brenky and Zémor (1985), pp. 45–81; Pollak (1988).

55. Mollaret (1987); Bolling and Voeller (1988); Brown and Primm (1988).

Chapter 15

1. Piot, Plummer, Mhalu, et al. (1988).

2. Biggar (1986); Pinching (1986); Clumeck, Hermans, and De Wit (1987); Anderson, May, McLean, et al. (1988).

3. Castro, Lieb, Jaffe, et al. (1988).

4. Biggar (1986); Melbye, Njelesani, Bayley, et al. (1986); Koch (1987); Giraldo, Beth-Giraldo, Clumeck, Gharbi, and Kyalwazi (1988).

5. Koch (1987), p. 3.

6. Colebunders, Francis, Mann, et al. (1987).

7. Piot, Quinn, Taelman, et al. (1984).

8. Bayley (1984); Downing, Elgin, and Bayley (1984).

9. Van de Perre, Rouvroy, Lepage, et al. (1984).

10. Serwadda, Mugerwa, Sewankambo, et al. (1985).

11. Quinn, Mann, Curran, and Piot (1986); Newmark (1986).

12. Brun-Vézinet, Rouzioux, Montagnier, et al. (1984); Wendler, Schneider, Gras, et al. (1986); Giraldo, Beth-Giraldo, Clumeck, Gharbi, and Kyalwazi (1988).

13. Biggar (1986); Clumeck, Hermans, and De Wit (1987).

14. Quinn, Piot, McCormick, et al. (1987); Marlink and Essex (1987).

15. Clavel (1987); Molbak, Lauritzen, Fernandes, et al. (1986); Affres, Christoforov, Reigneau, et al. (1986); Biberfeld, Böttiger, Bredberg-Radén, et al. (1986); Newmark (1986); Denis, Barin, Gershy-Damet, et al. (1987).

16. Clavel, Brun-Vézinet, Guétard, et al. (1987); Clavel, Guétard, Brun-Vézinet, et al. (1987); Clavel (1987); Blanc (1986); Brun-Vézinet, Rey, Katlama, et al. (1987); *Lancet* 1 (1988): 1027–1028.

17. Saimot, Coulaud, Mechali, et al. (1987).

18. Shoumatoff (1988), pp. 136, 142–143.

19. Brun-Vézinet, Rey, Katlama, et al. (1987); *Concours Méd.*, December 26, 1987; Kong, Shei-Wen, Kappes, et al. (1988); Dufoort, Couroucé, Ancelle-Park, et al. (1988).

20. Rey, Salaun, Lesbordes, et al. (1986).

21. De Thé, in Girard and Valette (1988), pp. 51–54.

22. Rey, Girard, Harzic, et al. (1987); De Thé, in Girard and Valette (1988), pp. 51–54; Evans, Moreau, Odehouri, et al. (1988).

23. Barin, M'Boup, Denis, et al. (1985).

24. Shoumatoff (1988), p. XII.

25. Mollaret (1987); Shoumatoff (1988).

26. Cf. Kashamura (1973).

27. Carael, in Hirsch (1987), pp. 55–58.

28. Mann, Francis, Quinn, et al. (1986); Quinn, Mann, Curran, and Piot (1986); cf. Biagi (1987), pp. 170–180.

29. Van de Perre, Clumeck, Carael, et al. (1985); cf. Hirsch (1987), pp. 54–56.

30. Kreiss, Koech, Plummer, et al. (1986); Hancock and Carim (1986), p. 124; Koch (1987), p. 174.

31. Biggar, Melbye, Kestems, et al. (1985); Biggar, Johnson, Oster, et al. (1985).

32. Van de Perre, Le Polain, Carael, et al. (1987); Piot, Plummer, Mhalu, et al. (1988).

33. Shoumatoff (1988), pp. 131–134; Caputo (1988).

34. Serwadda, Mugerwa, Sewankambo, et al. (1985); Shoumatoff (1988).

35. Serwadda, Mugerwa, Sewankambo, et al. (1985).

36. CDC (1987b).

37. Caputo (1988).

38. Shoumatoff (1988), p. 132.

39. Carswell, Sewankambo, Lloyd, et al. (1986).

40. Burton (1986); Hrdy (1987); Shoumatoff (1988), p. 148.

41. Iliffe (1987).

42. Biggar (1986); Hrdy (1987).

43. Montagnier (1986), p. 118; Hancock and Carim (1986), p. 128; Hrdy (1987).

44. Biggar (1986).

45. Mertens, ''Mission d'évaluation de la situation endémo-épidémiques de la peste au Zaïre,'' *Rapport à l'OMS*, April 1987; cf. Mollaret (1987).

46. *Bull. Epid. Hebd. de l'OMS* 40 (1986): 309–311.

47. *The Times*, May 11, 1987, *Le Monde*, May 13, 1987, and *Concours Méd.*, September 19, 1987 p. 2769.

48. Greenberg, Nguyen-Dinh, Mann, et al. (1988).

Chapter 16

1. Mann (1988); Fleming (1988).

2. Jossay and Donadieu (1986); Kaplan, Wofsy, and Volberding (1987); Bolognesi (1988).

3. Brenky and Zémor (1985), pp. 105–108; Montagnier (1986), pp. 180–181; Andrieu, Even, Venet, et al. (1988).

4. Fauci, Macher, Congo, et al. (1984); Jossay and Donadieu (1987); Broder (1987); Tastemain (1987); Vittecoq (1987); Kaplan, Wofsy and Volberding (1987); Bolognesi (1988).

5. Rozenbaum, Dormont, Spire, et al. (1985).

6. Cf. Davidson and Hudson (1986).

7. Mitsuya and Broder (1986).

8. Yarchoan, Weinhold, and Lyerly (1986).

9. Fischl, Richman, Grieco, et al. (1987); Tastemain (1987); Connor and Kingman (1988), pp. 142–144.

10. Dournon, Matheron, Rozenbaum, et al. (1988); Creagh-Kirk, Doi, Andrews, et al. (1988).

11. Pert, Hill, Ruff, et al. (1986); Mitsuya and Broder (1987); Yarchoan, Mitsuya, and Broder (1988); Broder and Fauci (1988); Deen, McDougal, Inacker, et al. (1988);

Connor and Kingman (1988), pp. 133–159; Bartlett (1988); Fisher, Bertonis, Meier, et al. (1988).

12. Dalgleish (1986); Barnes (1986c); Plata and Wain-Hobson (1987); Matthews and Bolognesi (1988); Koff and Hoth (1988).

13. Zagury, Léonard, Fouchard, et al. (1987); Zagury, Bernard, Cheynier, et al. (1988).

14. Mertz (1987); Koff and Hoth (1988); Connor and Kingman (1988), pp. 160–184.

15. Baltimore (1987).

16. Conant, Hardy, Sernatinger, et al. (1986); cf. Goldsmith (1987).

17. Rozenbaum, Seux, and Kouchner (1984), pp. 113–154; Bernex (1985); Brenky and Zémor (1985); Nungasser (1986); Black (1986); Feldman and Johnson (1986); Velimirovic (1987); Kübler-Ross (1987); Mérieux (1987); Koch (1987), pp. 21–23, 194–245; Martin (1988); Henrion (1988); Fineberg (1988); Panem (1988); Presidential Commission (1988); Burkel (1988); Fee and Fox (1988).

18. Herzlich, in Hirsch (1987); Sournia (1987); Herzlich and Pierret (1988).

19. CDC (1985e); Ide (1986); Bayer, Fox, and Willis (1986); Franck (1987).

20. Brunet, Gluckman, Habibi, and Rozenbaum (1985); Zuger and Miles (1987).

21. Hardy, Rauch, Echenberg, et al. (1986); Berk (1988).

22. Bayer, Fox, and Willis (1986); Dalton and Burris (1987); Walters (1988); Kim and Perfect (1988).

23. Benezech, Rager, and Beylot (1987); Beylot, Benezech, Lacoste, et al. (1988).

24. Kramer (1985); Laygues (1985); Simonin (1986); Peabody (1986); Fernandez (1987); Dreuilhe (1987); Juliette (1987); Hocquenghem (1987); Sontag (1988); cf. Biagi (1987).

25. Davidson and Hudson (1986); Aron (1988); cf. Biagi (1987).

26. Gessain, Barin, Vernant, et al. (1985); Vernant, Gessain, Gout, et al. (1986); Jacobson, Raine, Mingioli, et al. (1988).

27. Wong-Staal and Gallo (1985b); Weiss, in Weiss, Teich, Varmus, and Coffin (1985), pp. 409–414; Tubiana, Lejeune, Lecaer, et al. (1985).

28. Manzari, Fazio, Martinotti, et al. (1984).

29. Manzari, Grandilone, Barillari, et al. (1985).

30. Pandolfi, Manzari, De Rossi, et al. (1985).

31. Pokrovsky, Yankina, and Pokrovsky (1987).

32. Biggar (1987); Chavanet (1987); Piot, Plummer, Mhgalu, et al. (1988); Mann, Chin, Piot, et al. (1988); WHO, Global Program on AIDS, Update 1988.

33. Curran, Morgan, Hardy, et al. (1985); Koop (1986); Curran, Jaffé, Hardy, et al. (1988); Heyward and Curran (1988); CDC (1988a–1988d); Burke, Brundage, Redfield, et al. (1988); *J. Amer. Med. Ass.* 260 (1988): 1205–1206.

34. CDC (1985d); Brunet, Ancelle, and Foulon (1986); Downs, Ancelle, Jager, and Brunet (1987); WHO, Global Program on AIDS, Update 1988.

35. Somaini (1986).

36. Direction Générale de la Santé (1985 and 1988); *Bull. Epidém. Hebd.* 33 (1988).

37. Hatton, Maguin, Nicaud, et al. (1986).

38. Luzzi, Aiuti, Rezza, et al. (1987).

39. CDC (1988a).
40. Koch (1987); May and Anderson (1987); Anderson and May (1988).
41. Diamond (1987).
42. Bartholomew, Saxinger, Clark, et al. (1987).
43. Wells (1898).

Bibliography

Abb, J. "Determination of antibodies against LAV/HTLV-III: Comparative evaluation of four different commercial test kits." *AIDS Res.* 2 (1986):93–97.

Ablin, R. J., Gonder, M. J., and Immerman, R. S. "AIDS: A disease of ancient Egypt?" *New York St. J. Med.* 85 (1985):200–201.

Abrams, E. J., and Patrias, K. *AIDS Bibliography, 1986–1987*. Bethesda, Md., National Institutes of Health, 1987.

Ackerknecht, E. H. *Geschichte und Geographie der wichtigsten Krankheiten*. Stuttgart, Enke, 1963.

Ackerman, L., and Murray, J. F., eds. *Symposium on Kaposi's Sarcoma*. Basel-New York, Karger, 1963.

Adachi, A., Koenig, S., Gendelman, H., et al. "Productive, persistent infection of human colorectal cell lines with HIV." *J. Virol.* 61 (1987):209.

Affres, H., Christoforov, B., Reigneau, O., et al., "Un cas de SIDA à virus LAV-II au Mali." *Presse Méd.* 15 (1986):2211–2212.

Ainsworth, G. C. *Introduction to the History of Medical and Veterinary Mycology*. Cambridge, Eng., Cambridge University Press, 1986.

Aiuti, F., Sirianni, M. C., Pana, A., et al. "Immunological and virological studies in a risk population for AIDS in Rome (Italy)." *Ann. N.Y. Acad. Sci.* 437 (1984):554–558.

Alizon, M. and Montagnier, L. "Genetic variability in human immunodeficiency viruses." *Ann. N.Y. Acad. Sci.* 511 (1987):376–384.

Alizon, M., Sonigo, P., Barré-Sinoussi, F., et al. "Molecular cloning of the lymphadenopathy associated virus." *Nature* (Lond.) 312 (1984):757–760.

Alizon, M., Wain-Hobson, S., Montagnier, L., and Sonigo, P. "Genetic variability of the AIDS virus: Nucleotide sequence analysis of two isolates from African patients." *Cell* 46 (1986):63–74.

Allain, J. P. "Prevalence of HTLV-III/LAV antibodies in patients with hemophilia and in their sexual partners in France." *New Engl. J. Med.* 315 (1986):517–518.

Allan, J., Coligan, J. E., Barin, F., et al. "Major glycoprotein antigen that induce antibodies in AIDS patients are encoded by HTLV-III." *Science* (Wash.) 226 (1985):1091–1094.

Allen, J. R. "Epidemiology of the acquired immunodeficiency syndrome (AIDS) in the United States." *Semin. Oncol.* 11 (1984):4–11.

Alter, H. J., Eichberg, J. W., Masur, H., et al. "Transmission of HTLV-III infection from human plasma to chimpanzees: An animal model for AIDS." *Science* (Wash.) 226 (1984):549–552.

Altman, D. *AIDS in the Mind of America*. Garden City, N.Y., Anchor Press, 1986.

Altman, L. K. "Rare cancer seen in 41 homosexuals." *New York Times*, July 3, 1981, p. 20.

Ammann, A. J. "The acquired immunodeficiency syndrome in infants and children." *Ann. Intern. Med.* 103 (1985):734–737.

Ammann, A. J., Cowan, M. J., Wara, D. W., et al. "Acquired immunodeficiency in an infant: Possible transmission by means of blood products." *Lancet*, 1 (1983): 956–958.

Anderson, C.D. and Barrie, H.J., "Fatal pneumocystis pneumonia in an adult: Report of a case." *Amer. J. Clin. Path.* 34 (1960):365–370.

Anderson, R. M., and May, R. M., "Epidemiological parameters of HIV transmission." *Nature* (Lond.) 333 (1988):514–519.

Anderson, R. M., May, R. M., and McLean, A. R. "Possible demographic consequences of AIDS in developing countries." *Nature* (Lond.) 332 (1988):228–234.

André, L. J. "Le S.I.D.A. a-t-il existé?" *Méd. Trop.* (Marseille) 47 (1987):229–230.

Andreani, T., Modigliani, R., Le Charpentier, Y., et al. "Acquired immunodeficiency with intestinal cryptosporidiosis: Possible transmission by Haitian whole blood." *Lancet* 1 (1983):1187–1190.

Andrieu, J. M., Even, P., Venet, A., et al. "Effects of cyclosporin on T-cell subset in human immunodeficiency virus disease." *Clin. Immun. Immunopath.* 47 (1988): 181–198.

Angarano, G., Pastore, G., Monno, L., et al. "Rapid spread of HTLV-III infection among drug addicts in Italy." *Lancet* 2 (1985):1302.

Antin, J. H., Smith, B. R., Ewenstein, B. M., et al. "HTLV-III infection after bone marrow transplantation." *Blood* 67 (1986):160–163.

Apfelbaum, E., and Gelfand, B. B. "The artificial transmission of malaria among intravenous diacetylmorphine addicts." *J. Amer. Med. Ass.* 102 (1934):1664.

Appelboom, T., and Rouffin, C. "Can a diagnosis be made in retrospect? The case of Desiderius Erasmus." *J. Rheumatol.* 13 (1986):1181–1184.

Appelboom, T., Rouffin, C., Van Herweghem, J. L., et al. "The historical autopsy of Erasmus Roterodamus (c.1466–1536)." In T. Appelboom, ed., *Art, History and Antiquity of Rheumatic Diseases*, pp. 76–77. Brussels, Elsevier, 1987.

Aron, J.-P. *Mon sida*. Paris, Bourgois, 1988.

Aronson, D. L. "Pneumonia death in haemophiliacs." *Lancet* 2 (1983):1023.

Arya, S. K., Gallo, R. C., Hahn, B. H., et al. "Homology of genome of AIDS-associated virus with genomes of human T-cell leukemia viruses." *Science* (Wash.) 225 (1984):927–930.

Ashley, R. *Heroin, the Myth and the Facts*. London, St. James Press, 1972.

Auerbach, D. M., Darrow, W. W., Jaffe, H. W., and Curran, J. W. "Cluster of cases of the acquired immune deficiency syndrome. Patients linked by sexual contacts." *Amer. J. Med.* 76 (1984):487–492.

Auger, I., Thomas, P., DeGruttola, V., et al. "Incubation periods for pediatric AIDS patients." *Nature* (Lond.) 336 (1988):575–577.

Baltimore, D. "Viral RNA-dependent DNA polymerase in virions of RNA tumor viruses." *Nature* (Lond.) 226 (1970):1209–1211.

Baltimore, D., ed. *Nobel Lectures in Molecular Biology. New York, Elsevier, 1977.*

Baltimore, D. "Why is AIDS virus so special?" in C. Mérieux, ed., *SIDA: Epidémies et sociétés. Compte rendu de la réunion organisée aux Pensières, Annecy*, pp. 48–53. Lyon, Mérieux, 1987.

Baltimore, D., and Wolf, S., eds. *Confronting AIDS: Directions for Public Health, Health Care and Research*. Washington, D.C., National Academy Press, 1986.

Barin, F., M'Boup, S., Denis, F., et al. "Serological evidence for virus related to simian T-lymphotropic retrovirus III in residents of West Africa." *Lancet* 2 (1985): 1387–1389.

Barnes, D. M. "Brain function decline in children with AIDS." *Science* (Wash.) 232 (1986a):1196.

Barnes, D. M. "Brain endothelial cells infected by AIDS virus." *Science* (Wash.) 233 (1986b):418–419.

Barnes, D. M. "Strategies for an AIDS vaccine." *Nature* (Lond.) 233 (1986c):1149–1153.

Barr, A., Dow, B. C., Arnott, J., et al. "Anti-HTLV-*III* screening specificity and sensitivity." *Lancet* 1 (1986):1032.

Barré-Sinoussi, F., Chermann, J.-C., Rey, F., Nugeyre, M. T., Chamaret, S., Gruest, J., Dauguet, C., Exler-Blin, C., Vézinet–Brun, F., Rouzioux, C., Rozenbaum, W., and Montagnier, L. "Isolation of a T-lymphotropic retrovirus from a patient at risk for acquired immune deficiency syndrome (AIDS)." *Science* (Wash.) 220 (1983): 868–871.

Barré-Sinoussi, F., Chermann, J.-C., and Rozenbaum, W. *Le SIDA en question*. Paris, Plon, 1987.

Barry, M., Mellors, J., and Bia, F. "Haiti and the AIDS connection." *J. Chron. Dis.* 37 (1984):593–595.

Bartholomew, C., Saxinger, W. C., Clark, J. W., et al. "Transmission of HTLV-I and HIV among homosexual men in Trinidad." *J. Amer. Med. Ass.* 257 (1987):2604–2608.

Bartlett, J. A. "HIV therapeutics: An emerging science." *J. Amer. Med. Ass.* 260 (1988):3051–3052.

Basset, A. "Aspects cliniques de la maladie de Kaposi." *Bull. Soc. Path. Exot.* 77 (1984):529–532.

Bayer, R., Fox, D. M., and Willis, D. P. *AIDS: The Public Context of an Epidemic. The Milbank Quarterly*, vol. 64, suppl. 1. New York, Milbank Memorial Fund, 1986.

Bayley, A. C. "Aggressive Kaposi's sarcoma in Zambia, 1983." *Lancet* 1 (1984): 1318–1320.

Bayley, A. C., Downing, R. G., Cheingsong-Popov, R., et al. "HTLV-III serology distinguishes atypical and endemic Kaposi's sarcoma in Africa." *Lancet* 1 (1985): 359–361.

Beardsley, T. "Dispute over AIDS patent priority." *Nature* (Lond.) 310 (1984):174.

Beardsley, T. "French virus in the picture." *Nature* (Lond.) 320 (1986):563.

Becker, J. L., Hazan, U., Nugeyre, M. T., et al. "Infection de cellules d'insectes en culture par le virus HIV, agent du SIDA, et mise en évidence d'insectes d'origine africaine contaminés par ce virus." *C.R. Acad. Sci. Paris* (3d series) 303 (1986): 303–306.

Beldekas, J., Teas, J., and Hebert, J. R. "African swine fever and AIDS." *Lancet* 1 (1986):564–565.

Benezech, M., Rager, P., and Beylot, J. "SIDA et hépatite B dans la population carcérale: Une réalité épidémiologique incontournable." *Bull. Acad. Nat. Méd.* 171 (1987):215–218.

Benn, S., Rutledge, R., Folks, T., et al. "Genomic heterogeneity of AIDS retroviral isolates from North America and Zaire." *Science* (Wash.) 230 (1985):949–951.

Berk, R. A., ed. *The Social Impact of AIDS in the USA*. Cambridge, Mass., Abt, 1988.

Berken, A. "AIDS, neither new nor transmissible?" *New York St. J. Med.* 84 (1984): 440–441.

Bernex, R. *SIDA. Nous sommes tous concernés*. Paris, Atlas, 1985.

Bessis, M. "How the mouse leukemia virus was discovered: A talk with Ludwik Gross." *Nouv. Rev. Franç. Hématol.* 16 (1976):287–304.

Beveridge, W.I.B. *Influenza, the Last Great Plague*. New York, Prodist, 1977.

Beylot, J., Benezech, M., Lacoste, D., et al. "Les maladies infectieuses à HBV et à HIV en milieu carcéral." *Concours Méd.* 110 (1988):775–783.

Biagi, E. *Il sole malato. Viaggio nella paura dell'AIDS*. Milan, Mondadori, 1987.

Biberfeld, G., Böttiger, B., Bredberg-Radén , U., et al. "Findings in four HTLV-IV seropositive women from West Africa." *Lancet* 2 (1986):1330.

Bierling, P., Cordonnier, C., Duedari, N., et al. "LAV/HTLV type III in allogenic bone marrow transplantation." *Ann. Int. Med.* 104 (1986):131–132.

Biggar, R. J. "The AIDS problem in Africa." *Lancet* 1 (1986):79–83.

Biggar, R. J. "AIDS and HIV infection: Estimates of the magnitude of the problem worldwide in 1985/1986." *Clin. Immunol. Immunopathol.* 45 (1987):297–309.

Biggar, R. J., Gigase, P. L., Melbye, M., et al. "ELISA HTLV antibody reactivity associated with malaria and immune complexes in healthy Africans." *Lancet* 2 (1985):520–523.

Biggar, R. J., Johnson, B. K., Oster, C., et al. "Regional variation in prevalence of antibody against human T-lymphotropic virus types I and III in Kenya." *Intern. J. Cancer* 35 (1985):763–767.

Biggar, R. J., Melbye, M., Kestems, L., et al. "Kaposi's sarcoma in Zaire is not associated with HTLV-III infection." *New Engl. J. Med.* 311 (1984):1051–1052.

Biggar, R. J., Melbye, M., Kestems, L., et al. "Seroepidemiology of HTLV-III antibodies in a remote population ef Eastern Zaire." *Brit. Med. J.* 290 (1985):808–810.

Biggar, R. J., Saxinger, C., Sarin, P., et al. "Non-specificity of HTLV-III reactivity in sera from rural Kenya and eastern Zaire." *East Afr. Med. J.* 63 (1986):683–684.

Biraben, J.-N. *Les hommes et la peste dans les pays européens et méditerranéens*. Vol. I: *La peste dans l'histoire*. Vol. II: *Les hommes face à la peste*. Paris, Mouton, 1975–1976.

Bittner, J. J. "Some possible effects of nursing on the mammary gland tumor incidence in mice." *Science* (Wash.) 84 (1936):162.

Black, D. *The Plague Years. A Chronicle of AIDS, the Epidemic of Our Times*. New York, Simon and Schuster, 1986.

Black, F. L. "Infectious diseases in primitive societies." *Science* (Wash.) 187 (1975): 515–518.

Blanc, M. "L'autre virus du sida." *Recherche* 17, no. 179 (1986):974–976.

Blanche, S., Fischer, A., Le Deist, F., et al. "Infections à LAV et syndrome immunodéficitaire acquis (SIDA) chez le nourrisson." *Arch. Franç. Pédiatr.* 43 (1986): 87–92.

Blattner, W., Gallo, R. C., and Temin, H. M. "HIV causes AIDS." *Science* (Wash.) 241 (1988):514–517.

Bloom, A. L. "Acquired immunodeficiency syndrome and other possible immunological disorders in European haemophiliacs." *Lancet.* 1 (1984):1452–1455.

Bloom, A. L. "AIDS in haemophiliacs and homosexuals." *Lancet* 1 (1986):36.

Blouin, C., Chimot, E., and Launière, J. *Sida Story.* Paris, Editions Universitaires-Begedis, 1986.

Bluefarb, S. M. *Kaposi's Sarcoma: Multiple Idiopathic Haemorrhagic Sarcoma.* Springfield, Thomas, 1957.

Boivin, A. F. *Constitution chimique et nature biologique des virus.* Paris, Masson, 1941.

Bolling, D. R., and Voeller, B. "SIDA et rapport anal hétérosexuel." *J. Amer. Med. Ass.* (French ed.) 13 (1988):642.

Bolognesi, D., ed. *Human Retroviruses, Cancer and AIDS: Approaches to Prevention and Therapy.*, New York, Liss, 1988.

Bouvet, E., Leibowitch, J., Mayaud, C., et al. "Acquired immunodeficiency syndrome in France." *Lancet* 1 (1983):700–701.

Bove, J. R. "Transfusion-associated AIDS: A cause for concern." *New Engl. J. Med.* 310 (1984):115–116.

Brandt, A. M. *No Magic Bullet: A Social History of Venereal Disease in the United States since 1800. With a New Chapter on AIDS.* 2d ed. New York and Oxford, Oxford University Press, 1987.

Brandt, A. M. "The syphilis epidemic and its relation to AIDS." *Science* (Wash.) 239 (1988a):375–380.

Brandt, A. M. "AIDS in historical perspective: Four lessons from the history of sexually transmitted diseases." *Amer. J. Publ. Health* 78 (1988b):367–371.

Breimer, L. H. "Did Moritz Kaposi describe AIDS in 1872?" *Clio Medica* 19 (1984):156–159.

Brenky, D., and Zémor, O. *La route du Sida. Enquête sur une grande peur.* Paris, Londreys, 1985.

Brennan, R. O., and Durack, D. T. "Gay compromise syndrome." *Lancet* 2 (1981): 1338–1339.

Bres, P. "Les virus Lassa, Marburg et Ebola, nouveaux venus en pathologie tropicale." *Presse Méd.* 7 (1978):2921–2926, 3007—3012.

Bricaire, F., Haas, C. and Patri, B. "La tuberculose chez l'immunodéprimé." *Ann. Méd. Int.* 137 (1986):338–341.

Broder, S., ed. *AIDS: Modern Concepts and Therapeutic Challenges.* New York, Dekker, 1987.

Broder, S., and Fauci, A. S. "Progress in drug therapy for HIV infection." *Public Health Rep.* 103 (1988):224–229.

Broder, S., and Gallo, R. C. "A pathogenic retrovirus (HTLV-III) linked to AIDS." *New Engl. J. Med.* 311 (1984):1292–1297.

Brossolet, J. "Expansion européenne de la suette anglaise." In *Proc. 23d Intern. Congr. Hist. Med.* (1972), t. I, pp. 595–600. London, 1974.

Brown, L. S., and Primm, B. J. "Sexual contacts of intravenous drug abusers: Implications for the next spread of the AIDS epidemics.'' *J. Natl. Med. Ass.* 80 (1988): 651–656.

Brun-Vézinet, F., and Rouzioux, C. ''Etiologie virale du SIDA.'' *Concours Méd.* 108 (1986):2071–2079.

Brun-Vézinet, F., Jaeger, G., Rouzioux, C., et al. ''Lack of evidence for human or simian T-lymphotropic virus type III infection in Pygmies.'' *Lancet* 2 (1986):854.

Brun-Vézinet, F., Klatzmann, D., and Rouzioux, C. R. ''Principales hypothèses étiologiques du SIDA.'' *Concours Méd.* 106 (1984):785–791.

Brun-Vézinet, F., Rey, M. A., Katlama, C., et al. ''Lymphadenopathy-associated virus type 2 in AIDS and AIDS-related complex. Clinical and virological features in four patients.'' *Lancet* 1 (1987):128–132.

Brun-Vézinet, F., Rouzioux, C., Barré-Sinoussi, F., et al. ''Detection of IgG antibodies to lymphadenopathy associated virus (LAV) by ELISA, in patients with AIDS.'' *Lancet* 1 (1984):1253—1256.

Brun-Vézinet, F., Rouzioux, C., Montagnier, L., et al. ''Prevalence of antibodies to lymphadenopathy-associated virus in African patients with AIDS.'' *Science* (Wash.) 226 (1984):453–456.

Brunet, J. B. ''Géographie du SIDA.'' *Concours Méd.* 106 (1984):729–734.

Brunet, J. B., and Bouvet, E. ''Le syndrome d'immunodépression acquise: Données épidémiologiques en France et dans le monde.'' *Bull. Acad. Nat. Méd.* 168 (1984): 278–281.

Brunet, J. B., Ancelle, R., and Foulon, G. ''La surveillance du SIDA en Europe.'' *Rev. Épid. Santé Publ.* 34 (1986):126–133.

Brunet, J. B., Bouvet, E., Leibowitch, J., et al. ''Acquired immunodeficiency syndrome in France.'' *Lancet* 1 (1983):700–701.

Brunet, J. B., Gluckman, J. C., Habibi, B., and Rozenbaum, W. *Le praticien et le SIDA*. Paris, Secrétariat d'Etat chargé de la santé, 1985.

Brunet, J. B., Klatzmann, D., Cavaille-Coll, M., and Picard, O. ''AIDS in France: The African hypothesis in the epidemic of Kaposi's sarcoma and opportunistic infections in homosexual men.'' In A. E. Friedman-Kien and L. J. Laubenstein, eds., *AIDS*, pp. 318–321. New York, Masson, 1984.

Bryceson, A., Tomkins, A., Ridley, D., et al. ''HIV-2-associated AIDS in the 1970s.'' *Lancet* 2 (1988):221.

Bültmann, B. D., Flad, H. D., Kaiserling, E., et al. ''Disseminated mycobacterial histiocytosis due to M. fortuitum associated with helper T-lymphocyte immune deficiency.'' *Virchows Arch.* 395 (1982):217–225.

Burke, D. S., Brundage, J. F., Redfield, R. R., et al. ''Measurement of the false positive rate in screening program for human immunodeficiency virus infection.'' *New Engl. J. Med.* 319 (1988):961–964.

Burkel, E., ed. *Der AIDS-Komplex. Dimensionen einer Bedrohung*. Frankfurt, Ullstein, 1988.

Burkitt, D. ''A sarcoma involving the jaws in African children.'' *Brit. J. Surg.* 46 (1958–1959):218–223.

Burkitt, D. ''A lymphoma syndrome in tropical Africa.'' *Intern. Rev. Exp. Pathol.* 2 (1963):67–138.

Burnet, M. *Viruses and Man*. Harmondsworth, Penguin Books, 1955.

Burton, M. "AIDS and female circumcision." *Science* (Wash.) 231 (1986):1236.

Bygbjerg, I. C. "AIDS in a Danish surgeon (Zaire 1976)." *Lancet* 1 (1983):925.

Cairns, J., Stent, G. S., and Watson, J. D., eds. *Phage and the Origin of Molecular Biology*. New York, Cold Spring Harbor Laboratory, 1966.

Cantwell, A., Jr. *AIDS, the Mystery and Solution*. Los Angeles, Aries Rising Press, 1986.

Caputo, R. "Uganda, land beyond sorrow." *Natl. Geogr. Mag.* 173 (1988):468–491.

Carey, J. "How medical sleuths track killer diseases." *US News and World Report*, October 14, 1985, pp. 69–70.

Carne, C. A., Weller, I.V.D., Johnson, A. M., et al. "Prevalence of antibodies to human immunodeficiency virus, gonorrhoea rates and changed social behaviour in homosexual men in London." *Lancet* 1 (1987):656–658.

Carswell, J. W., Sewankambo, N., Lloyd, G., et al. "How long has the AIDS virus been in Uganda?" *Lancet* 1 (1986):1217.

Casteret, A. M. "La tragédie des hémophiles." *Express*, December 4, 1987, pp. 31–32.

Castro, K. G., Lieb, S., Jaffe, H. W., et al. "Transmission of HIV in Belle Glade, Florida: Lessons for other communities in the United States." *Science* (Wash.) 239 (1988):193–197.

Cavailhès, J., Dutey, P., and Bach-Ignasse, G. *Rapport Gai. Enquête sur les modes de vie des homosexuels*. Paris, Persona, 1984.

CDC (Centers for Disease Control). "Pneumocystis pneumonia—Los Angeles." *Morb. Mortal. Weekly Rep.* 30 (1981a):250–252.

CDC. "Kaposi's sarcoma and pneumocystis pneumonia among homosexual men— New York City and California." *Morb. Mortal. Weekly Rep.* 30 (1981b):305–308.

CDC. "Follow-up on Kaposi's sarcoma and Pneumocystis pneumonia." *Morb. Mortal. Weekly Rep.* 30 (1981c):409–410.

CDC. "Persistent, generalized lymphadenopathy among homosexual males." *Morb. Mortal. Weekly Rep.* 31 (1982a):249–251.

CDC. "Diffuse, undifferentiated non-Hodgkins lymphoma among homosexual males—United States." *Morb. Mortal. Weekly Rep.* 31 (1982b):277–279.

CDC. "Update on Kaposi's sarcoma and opportunistic infections in previously healthy persons—United States." *Morb. Mortal. Weekly Rep.* 31 (1982c):295–301.

CDC. "A cluster of Kaposi's sarcoma and Pneumocystis carinii pneumonia among homosexual residents of Los Angeles and Orange counties, California." *Morb. Mortal. Weekly Rep.* 31 (1982d):305–307.

CDC. "Opportunistic infections and Kaposi's sarcoma among Haitians in the United States" *Morb. Mortal. Weekly Rep.* 31 (1982e):353–354, 360–361.

CDC. "Pneumocystis carinii pneumonia among persons with hemophilia A." *Morb. Mortal. Weekly Rep.* 31 (1982f):365–367.

CDC. "Update on acquired immune deficiency syndrome (AIDS)." *Morb. Mortal. Weekly Rep.* 31 (1982g):507–514.

CDC. "Update on acquired immunodeficiency syndrome (AIDS) among patients with hemophilia A." *Morb. Mortal. Weekly Rep.* 31 (1982h):644–646.

CDC. "Possible transfusion-associated acquired immune deficiency syndrome (AIDS) in California." *Morb. Mortal. Weekly Rep.* 31 (1982i):652–654.

CDC. "Unexplained immunodeficiency and opportunistic infections in infants—New York, New Jersey, California." *Morb. Mortal. Weekly Rep.* 31 (1982j):665–667.

CDC. "Epidemiologic aspects of the current outbreak of Kaposi's sarcoma and opportunistic infection." *New Engl. J. Med.* 306 (1982k):248–252.

CDC. *Case Definitions of AIDS Used by CDC for Epidemiology Surveillance.* Atlanta, CDC. 1983a.

CDC. "Immunodeficiency among female sexual partners of males with acquired immune deficiency syndrome (AIDS)—New York." *Morb. Mortal. Weekly Rep.* 31 (1983b):697–698.

CDC. "Acquired immunodeficiency syndrome (AIDS) in prison inmates—New York, New Jersey." *Morb. Mortal. Weekly Rep.* 31 (1983c):700–701.

CDC. "Human T-cell leukemia infection in patients with acquired immunodeficiency syndrome. Preliminary observations." *Morb. Mortal. Weekly Rep.* 32 (1983d):233–234.

CDC. "Update: Acquired immunodeficiency syndrome (AIDS)—United States." *Morb. Mortal. Weekly Rep.* 32 (1983e):465–467.

CDC. "Update: Acquired immunodeficiency syndrome (AIDS) among patients with hemophilia." *Morb. Mortal. Weekly Rep.* 32 (1983f):613–615.

CDC. "Update: Acquired immunodeficiency syndrome (AIDS)—United States." *Morb. Mortal. Weekly Rep.* 33 (1984):661–664.

CDC. "Revision of the case definition of acquired immunodeficiency syndrome for national reporting—United States." *Morb. Mortal. Weekly Rep.* 34 (1985a):373–375.

CDC. *Organization, Mission and Functions.* Atlanta, CDC. 1985b.

CDC. "Heterosexual transmission of HTLV-III/LAV." *J. Amer. Med. Ass.* 254 (1985c):373–375.

CDC. "Acquired immunodeficiency syndrome—Europe." *J. Amer. Med. Ass.* 254 (1985d):2052–2054.

CDC. "Results of a Gallup poll on acquired immunodeficiency syndrome—New York City, United States, 1985." *Morb. Mortal. Weekly Rep.* 34 (1985e):513–514.

CDC. "Tuberculosis—United States, 1985—and the possible impact of human T-lymphotropic virus type III/lymphadenopathy associated virus infection." *Morb. Mortal. Weekly Rep.* 35 (1986a):74–76.

CDC. "Classification system for human T-lymphotropic virus type III/lymphadenopathy associated virus infections." *Morb. Mortal. Weekly Rep.* 35 (1986b):334–339.

CDC. "Transfusion-associated human T-lymphotropic virus type III/lymphadenopathy associated virus infection from a seronegative donor." *Morb. Mortal. Weekly Rep.* 35 (1986c):389–391.

CDC. Reports on AIDS, published in the *MMWR* June 1981–May 1986. Atlanta, CDC. 1986d.

CDC. "Diagnosis and management of mycobacterial infection and disease of persons with human immunodeficiency virus infection." *Ann. Int. Med.* 106 (1987a):254–256.

CDC. "Revision of the CDC surveillance case definition for acquired immunodeficiency syndrome." *Morb. Mortal. Weekly Rep.* 36, supp. 1 (1987b):3–15.

CDC. "Human immunodeficiency virus infections in health-care workers exposed to blood of infected patients." *Morb. Mortal. Weekly Rep.* 36 (1987c):285–289.

CDC. "Human immunodeficiency virus infection in the United States: A review of current knowledge." *Morb. Mortal. Weekly Rep.* 36, supp. (1987d).

CDC. "AIDS due to HIV-2 infection—New Jersey." *Morb. Mortal. Weekly Rep.* 87 (1988a):33–35.

CDC. "AIDS and HIV update; Infection among health care workers." *Morb. Mortal. Weekly Rep.* 37 (1988b):229–239.

CDC. "Update: Acquired immune deficiency syndrome (AIDS)." *Morb. Mortal. Weekly Rep.* 37 (1988c):286–295.

DC. "Increase in pneumonia mortality among young adults and the HIV epidemic—New York City." *Morb. Mortal. Weekly Rep.* 37 (1988d):593–596.

Chakrabarti, L., Guyader, M., Alizon, M., et al. "Sequence of simian immunodeficiency virus from macaque and its relationship to other human and simian retroviruses." *Nature* (Lond.) 328 (1987):543–547.

Chauvet, J.-F. "Le SIDA, syndrome d'immunodéficience acquise. A propos de 4 cas cliniques observés à l'hôpital Claude Bernard." Thèse de Médecine, Paris, 1983.

Chavanet, P. "Le SIDA dans le monde." *Lettre de l'Infectiologue* 2 (1987):409–415.

Cheingsong-Popov, R., Weiss, R., Dalgleish, A., et al. "Prevalence of antibody to human T-lymphotropic virus type III in AIDS and AIDS-risk patients in Britain." *Lancet* 2 (1984):477–480.

Chen, I.S.Y., McLaughlin, J., Gasson, J. C., et al. "Molecular characterization of genome of a novel human T-cell leukaemia virus." *Nature* (Lond.) 305 (1983):502–505.

Chermann, J.-C., Barré, F., and Montagnier, L. "Rétrovirus et syndrome d'immunodéficience acquise (SIDA)." *Bull. Acad. Nat. Méd.* 168 (1984):288–295.

Chiu, I., Yaniv, A., Dahlberg, J. E., et al. "Nucleotide sequence evidence for relationship of AIDS retrovirus to lentiviruses." *Nature* (Lond.) 317 (1985):366–368.

Clark, M., and Gonnell, M. "Disease that plagues gays." *Newsweek*, December 21, 1981.

Clark, M., and Shapiro, D. "A new clue in the AIDS mystery: Evidence that the disease was around in the '60s." *Newsweek*, November 9, 1987.

Clark, S. P., and Mak, T. W. "Fluidity of a retrovirus genome." *J. Virol.* 50 (1984): 759–765.

Clavel, F. "HIV-2, the West African AIDS virus." *AIDS* 1 (1987):135–140.

Clavel, F., Brun-Vézinet, F., Guétard, D., et al. "LAV type II: Un second rétrovirus associé au Sida en Afrique de l'Ouest." *C.R. Acad. Sci. Paris* 302 (1986):485–488.

Clavel, F., Guétard, D., Brun-Vézinet, F., et al. "Isolation of a new human retrovirus from West African patients with AIDS." *Science* (Wash.) 233 (1986):343–346.

Clavel, F., Guyader, M., Guétard, D., et al. "Molecular cloning and polymorphism of the human immune deficiency virus type 2." *Nature* (Lond.) 324 (1986):691–695.

Clemmesen, J. "Kaposi's sarcoma in homosexual men: Is it a new disease?" *Lancet* 2 (1982):51–52.

Clumeck, N., Hermans, P., and De Wit, S. "Some epidemiological and clinical characteristics of African AIDS." *Antibiot. Chemother.* 38 (1987):41–51.

Clumeck, N., Mascart-Lemone, F., De Maubege, J., et al. "Acquired immunodeficiency syndrome in Black Africans." *Lancet* 1 (1983):642.

Clumeck, N., Sonnet, J., Taelman, H., et al. "Acquired immunodeficiency syndrome in African patients." *New Engl. J. Med* 310 (1984a):492–496.

Clumeck, N., Sonnet, J., Taelman, H., et al. "Acquired immunodeficiency syndrome in Belgium and its relation to Central Africa." *Ann. N.Y. Acad. Sci.* 437 (1984b): 264–269.

Cockburn, A. *The Evolution and Eradication of Infectious Diseases*. Baltimore, Md., Johns Hopkins University Press, 1963.

Coffin, J. M. "Genetic variation in AIDS viruses." *Cell* 46 (1986):1–4.

Coffin, J., Haase, A., Levy, J., et al. "Human immunodeficiency viruses." *Science* (Wash.) 232 (1986):697.

Colaert, J., Desmyter, J., Goudsmit, J., et al. "African swine fever virus antibody not found in AIDS patients." *Lancet* 1 (1983):1098.

Cole, H. M., and Lundberg, G. D. *AIDS: From the Beginning*. Chicago, American Medical Association, 1986.

Cole, H.N.E. "Erasmus and his diseases." *J. Amer. Med. Ass.* 148 (1952):529–531.

Colebunders, R., Francis, H., Mann, J., et al. "Slow progression of an illness occasionally occurs in HIV infected Africans." *AIDS*. 1 (1987):65.

Colebunders, R., Taelman, H., and Piot, P. "AIDS: An old disease from Africa?" *Brit. Med. J.* 289 (1984):765.

Compas, J.-C. "Pourquoi Haïti?" *Le Monde*, July 7, 1983.

Conant, M., Hardy, D., Sernatinger, J., et al. "Condoms prevent transmission of AIDS-associated retrovirus." *J. Amer. Med. Ass.* 255 (1986):1706.

Connor, S. "AIDS: Mystery of the missing data." *New Scientist*, February 12, 1987, p. 49.

Connor, S., and Kingman, S. *The Search for the Virus: The Scientific Discovery of AIDS and the Quest for a Cure*. Harmondsworth, Penguin Books, 1988.

Contreras, R. "Angiosarcoma de Kaposi primario del corazon." *Arch. Inst. Cardiol. Mex.* 27 (1957):463–479.

Cooper, D. A., Gold, J., Maclean, P., et al. "Acute AIDS retrovirus infection. Definition of a clinical illness associated with seroconversion." *Lancet* 1 (1985):537–540.

Coulaud, J.-P., Vilde, J.-L. and Regnier, B. "Les aspects cliniques du SIDA avéré." *Bull. Acad. Nat. Méd.* 168 (1984):267–270.

Coury, C. *Grandeur et déclin d'une maladie. La tuberculose au cours des âges*. Suresnes, Lepetit, 1972.

Cox, F. H., and Helwig, E. B. "Kaposi's sarcoma." *Cancer* 12 (1959):289–298.

Creagh-Kirk, T., Doi, P., Andrews, E., et al. "Survival experience among patients with AIDS receiving zidovudine." *J. Amer. Med. Ass.*" 260 (1988):3009–3015.

Crick, F.H.C. "On protein synthesis." *Symp. Soc. Exp. Biol.* 12 (1957):138–163.

Crick, F.H.C. *Life Itself: Its Origin and Nature*. New York, Simon and Schuster, 1981.

Curran, J. W. "AIDS—two years later." *New Engl. J. Med.* 309 (1983):609–611.

Curran, J. W., Evatt, B. L., and Lawrence, D. N. "The acquired immune deficiency syndrome: The past as prologue." *Ann. Int. Med.* 98 (1983):401–403.

Curran, J. W., Jaffe, H. W., Hardy, A. M., et al. "Epidemiology of HIV infection and AIDS in the United States." *Science* (Wash.) 239 (1988):610–616.

Curran, J. W., Lawrence, D. N., Jaffe, H., et al. "Acquired immunodeficiency syndrome (AIDS) associated with transfusions." *New Engl. J. Med.* 310 (1984):69–75.

Curran, J. W., Morgan, W. M., Hardy, A. M., et al. "The epidemiology of AIDS: Current status and future prospects." *Science* (Wash.) 229 (1985):1352–1357.

Dabis, F. "Les Centers for Disease Control: Mythe et réalité." *Concours Méd.* 110 (1988):1711–1719.

Dal Bo Zanon, R., Vicarioto, M., Girolami, A., et al. "First case in Italy of fatal AIDS in a hemophiliac." *Acta Haemat.* 75 (1986):34–37.

Dalgleish, A. G. "AIDS: An old disease from Africa?" *Brit. Med. J.* 289 (1984): 630.

Dalgleish, A. G. "Antiviral strategies and vaccines against HTLV-III/LAV." *J. Roy. Coll. Phys. Lond.* 20 (1986):258–267.

Dalgleish, A. G., Beverley, P. C., Clapham, P. R., et al. "The CD4 (T4) antigen is an essential component of the receptor for the AIDS retrovirus." *Nature* (Lond.) 312 (1984):763–767.

Dalla Favera, G. B. "Ueber das sogen. Sarcoma idiopathicum multiplex haemorrhagicum (Kaposi)." *Arch. Derm. Syphil.* 109 (1911):387–440.

Dalton, H. L., and Burris, S. *AIDS and the Law.* New Haven, Yale University Press, 1987.

Dan, B. B. "Toxic shock syndrome: Back to the future." *J. Amer. Med. Ass.* 257 (1987):1094–1095.

Daniel, M. D., Letvin, N. L., King, N. W., et al. "Isolation of T-cell tropic HTLV-III-like retrovirus from macaques." *Science* (Wash.) 228 (1985):1201–1204.

Daniels, V. G. *AIDS, the Acquired Immunodeficiency Syndrome.* Lancaster and Boston, MTP Press, 1987.

Darrow, W. W., Barett, D., Jay, K., and Young, A. "The gay report on sexually transmitted diseases." *Amer. J. Public Health* 71 (1981):1004–1011.

Darrow, W. W., Echenberg, D. F., Jaffe, H. W., et al. "Risk factors for human immunodeficiency virus (HIV) infections in homosexual men." *Amer. J. Public Health* 77 (1987):479–483.

Davidson, S., and Hudson, R. *Rock Hudson, His Story.* Morrow and Co., 1986.

Davies, J.N.P. "Kaposi's sarcoma, a re-evaluation based on the disease in Africans." In L. V. Ackermann and J. F. Murray, eds., *Symposium on Kaposi's Sarcoma*, pp. 59–62. New York, 1963.

Davis, K. C., Horsburgh, C. R., Hasiba, U., et al. "Acquired immunodeficiency syndrome in a patient with hemophilia." *Ann. Int. Med.* 98 (1983):284–286.

De Amicis, T. *Studio clinico ed anatomo-patologico su dodici nuove osservazioni di dermo-polimelano-sarcoma idiopatico.* Naples, Trani, 1882.

De Cock, K. M. "AIDS: An old disease from Africa?" *Brit. Med. J.* 289 (1984):306–308, 1454–1455.

Deen, K. C., McDougal, J. S., Inacker, R., et al. "A soluble form of CD4 (T4) protein inhibits AIDS virus infection." *Nature* (Lond.) 331 (1988):82–86.

Deinhardt, F., Eberle, J., and Görtler, L. "Sensitivity and specificity of eight commercial and one recombinant anti-HIV ELISA tests." *Lancet* 1 (1987):40.

Delaunay, A. *L'Institut Pasteur des origines à aujourd'hui.* Paris, France-Empire, 1962.

Denis, F., Barin, F., Gershy-Damet, G., et al. "Prevalence in human T-lymphotropic retroviruses type III (HIV) and type IV in Ivory Coast." *Lancet* 1 (1987):408–411.

Deresinski, S. C., Cooney, D.P., Auerbach, D. M., et al. "AIDS transmission via transfusion therapy." *Lancet* 1 (1984):102.

Desforges, J. F. "AIDS and the preventive treatment in hemophilia." *New Engl. J. Med.* 308 (1983):94–95.

Desmyter, J., Goubau, P., Chamaret, S., and Montagnier, L. "Anti-LAV/HTLV-III in Kinshasa mothers in 1970 and 1980." In *Program and Abstracts of the International Conference on AIDS*, p. 106. Paris, 1986.

Desmyter, J., Surmont, I., Goubau, P., et al. "Origins of AIDS." *Brit. Med. J.* 293 (1986):1308.

Desrosiers, R. C. "Origin of the human AIDS virus." *Nature* (Lond.) 319 (1986): 728.

Desrosiers, R. C., Daniel, M. D., Letvin, N. L., et al. "Origins of HTLV-4." *Nature* (Lond.) 327 (1987):107.

De Thé, G. *Sur la piste du cancer* Paris, Flammarion, 1984.

DeVita, V., Helman, S., and Rosenberg, S. A. *AIDS: Etiology, Diagnosis, Treatment and Prevention*. Philadelphia, Lippincott, 1985.

Diamond, J. M. "AIDS, infectious, genetic or both?" *Nature* (Lond.) 328 (1987): 199–200.

Diosi, P., and David, C. "Cytomegalic inclusion disease. A historical outline." *Clio Medica* 3 (1968):149–166.

Direction Générale De La Santé. "Infections opportunistes et sarcome de Kaposi chez des patients jeunes, non immunodéprimés antérieurement." *Bull. Épid. Hebd.*, no. 37 (1982a).

Direction Générale De La Santé. "Syndrome d'immuno-dépression acquise." *Bull. Épid. Hebd.*, no. 50 (1982b).

Direction Générale De La Santé. "Situation du SIDA en France au 1er janvier 1984." *Bull. Épid. Hebd.*, no. 2 (1984).

Direction Générale De La Santé. "Le point sur le SIDA." *Bull. Épid. Hebd.*, no. 34 (1985).

Direction Générale De La Santé. "Situation du SIDA en France au 30 juin 1988." *Bull. Épid. Hebd.*, no. 33 (1988).

Dournon, E., Matheron, S., Rozenbaum, W., et al. "Effects of zidovudine in 365 consecutive patients with AIDS or AIDS-related complex." *Lancet* 2 (1988):1297–1302.

Dournon, E., Penalba, C., Saimot, A. G., et al. "AIDS in a Haitian couple in Paris." *Lancet* 1 (1983):1040–1041.

Downing, R. G., Elgin, R. P., and Bayley, A. C. "African Kaposi's sarcoma and AIDS." *Lancet* 1 (1984):478–480.

Downs, A., Ancelle, R. A., Jager, H. C., and Brunet, J. B. "AIDS in Europe: Current trends and short-term predictions estimated from surveillance data, January 1981–June 1986." *AIDS* 1 (1987):53–57.

Dreuilhe, A.-E. *Corps à corps*. Paris, Gallimard, 1987.

Drew, W. L., Conant, M. D., Miner, R. C., et al. "Cytomegalovirus and Kaposi's sarcoma in young homosexual men." *Lancet* 2 (1982):125–127.

Dritz, S. K. "Medical aspects of homosexuality." *New Engl. J. Med.* 302 (1980):463–464.

Du Bois, R. M., Branthwaite, M. A., Mikhail, J. R., and Batten, J. C. "Primary Pneumocystis carinii and cytomegalovirus infections." *Lancet* 2 (1981):1339.

Dubos, R. "Infection into disease." In D. J. Ingle, ed., *Life and Disease*, pp. 100–110. New York, Basic Books, 1963.

Dubos, R., and Dubos, J. *The White Plague: Tuberculosis, Man and Society*. London, Rutgers University Press, 1987.

Duesberg, P. H. "Retroviruses as carcinogens and pathogens: Expectations and reality." *Cancer Research* 47 (1987):1199–1220.

Duesberg, P. H. "HIV is not the cause of AIDS." *Science* (Wash.) 241 (1988):514–517.

Dufoort, G., Couroucé, A. M., Ancelle-Park, R., et al. "No clinical signs 14 years after HIV-2 transmission via blood transfusion." *Lancet* 2 (1988):510.

Dupont, A. *L'angio-reticulomatose cutanée*. Louvain, Duculot et Gembloux, 1951.

Dupont, A., Chaboeuf, M., and Van Breuseghem. "Angiomatose de Kaposi chez les Noirs." *Arch. Belg. Derm. Syph.* 4 (1948):132–136.

Durack, D. T. "Opportunistic infections and Kaposi's sarcoma in homosexual men." *New Engl. J. Med.* 305 (1981):1465–1467.

Edwards, D., Harper, P. G., Pain, A. K., et al. "Kaposi's sarcoma associated with AIDS in a woman from Uganda." *Lancet* 1 (1984):631–632.

Egli, H. "The situation of the haemophiliac: Yesterday and today." *Haemostasis* 10 (1981):1–10.

Eigen, M. "La fisica dell'evoluzione molecolare." In M. Galzigna, ed., *La vita, le forme, i numeri* (*BioLogica*, vol. 1, pp. 103–124). Ancona, 1988.

Eigen, M., and Schuster, P. "The hypercycle: A principle of natural self-organization." *Naturwissenschaften* 64 (1977):541–565.

Ellermann, V., and Bang, O. "Experimentelle Leukämie bei Hühnern." *Zbl. Bakt.* 46 (1908):595–609.

Elliott, J. L., Hoppes, W. L., Platt, M. S., et al. "The acquired immunodeficiency syndrome and Mycobacterium avium-intracellulare in a patient with hemophilia." *Ann. Int. Med.* 98 (1983):290–293.

Ellrodt, A., Barré-Sinoussi, F., Le Bras, P., et al. "Isolation of human T-lymphotropic retrovirus (LAV) from Zairian married couple, one with AIDS, one with prodromes." *Lancet* 1 (1984):1383–1385.

Elvin-Lewis, M., Witte, M., Witte, C. V., et al. "Systemic chlamydial infection associated with generalized lymphedema and lymphangiosarcoma." *Lymphology* 6 (1973):113–121.

Epstein, J. S., Moffitt, A. L., Mayner, R. E. "Antibodies reactive with HTLV-III found in freezer banked sera from children in West Africa." In *Program and Abstracts of the 25th Interscience Conference on Antimicrobial Agents and Chemotherapy*, p. 130. Washington, D.C, 1985.

Epstein, M. A. "Le virus d'Epstein-Barr et les maladies humaines." *Concours Méd.* 102 (1980):4650–4660.

Epstein, M. A., and Barr, Y. M. "Cultivation in vitro of human lymphoblasts from Burkitt's malignant lymphoma." *Lancet* 1 (1964):252–253.

Essex, M. "Feline leukemia, a naturally occuring cancer of infectious origin." *Epidemiol. Rev.* 4 (1982):189–203.

Essex, M., and Kanki, P. J. "The origin of the AIDS virus." *Scient. Amer.* 259, no. 4 (1988):64–71.

Essex, M., McLane, M. F., Lee, T. H., et al. "Antibodies to cell membrane antigens associated with human T-cell leukemia virus in patients with AIDS." *Science* (Wash.) 220 (1983):859–862.

Evans, L. A., McHugh, T. M., Stites, D. P., et al. "Differential ability of human immunodeficiency virus isolates to productively infect human cells." *J. Immunol.* 138 (1987):3415–3418.

Evans, L. A., Moreau, J., Odehouri, K., et al. "Simultaneous isolation of HIV-1 and HIV-2 from an AIDS patient." *Lancet* 2 (1988):1389–1391.

Evatt, B. L., Gomperts, E. D., McDougal, J. S., and Ramsey, R. B. "Coincidental appearence of LAV/HTLV-III antibodies in hemophiliacs and the onset of the AIDS epidemics." *New Engl. J. Med.* 312 (1985):483–486.

Evatt, B. L., Ramsey, R. B., Lawrence, D. N., et al. "The acquired immunodeficiency syndrome in patients with hemophilia." *Ann. Int. Med.* 100, (1984):499–504.

Faris, A. A., and Martinez, A. J. "Primary progressive multifocal leukoencephalopathy: A central nervous system disease caused by a slow virus." *Arch. Neurol.* 27 (1972):357–360.

Farthing, C. F., et al. *A Colour Atlas of AIDS*. Chicago, Yearbook Medical Publ., 1986.

Fauci, A. S. "The human immunodeficiency virus: Infectivity and mechanisms of pathogenesis." *Science* (Wash.) 239 (1988):617–622.

Fauci, A. S., Macher, A. M., Congo, D. L., et al. "Acquired immunodeficiency syndrome: epidemiologic, clinical, immunologic and therapeutic considerations." *Ann. Int. Med.* 100 (1984):92–106.

Fee, E., and Fox, D. M., ed. *AIDS: The Burdens of History*. Berkeley, Los Angeles, and London, 1988.

Feldman, D. A., and Johnson, T. M., ed. *The Social Dimension of AIDS: Method and Theory*. New York, Praeger, 1986.

Fenner, F., and Gibbs, A., eds. *Portraits of Viruses. A History of Virology*. Basel, Karger, 1988.

Fenyö, E. M., Morfeldt-Mansson, L., Chiodi, F., et al. "Distinct replicative and cytopathic characteristics of human immunodeficiency virus isolates." *J. Virol.* 62 (1988):4414–4419.

Feorino, P. M., Kalyanaraman, V. S., Haverkos, H. W., et al. "Lymphadenopathy associated virus infection of a blood donor-recipient pair with acquired immunodeficiency syndrome." *Science* (Wash) 225 (1984):753–757.

Fernandez, D. *La gloire du paria*. Paris, Grasset, 1987.

Fettner, A. G., and Check, W. A. *The Truth about AIDS: Evolution of an Epidemic*. New York, Holt, Rinehart and Winston, 1984.

Fineberg, H. V. "The social dimensions of AIDS." *Scient. Amer.* 259, no. 4 (1988):128–134.

Fischl, M. A., Dickinson, G. M., Scott, G. B., et al. "Evaluation of heterosexual partners, children and household contacts of adults with AIDS." *J. Amer. Med. Ass.* 257 (1987):640–644.

Fischl, M. A., Richman, D. D., Grieco, M. H., et al. "The efficacy of azidothymidine (AZT) in the treatment of patients with AIDS and AIDS-related complex." *New Engl. J. Med.* 317 (1987):185–191.

Fisher, A. G., Ensoli, B., Looney, D., et al. "Biologically diverse molecular variants within a single HIV-1 isolate." *Nature* (Lond.) 334 (1988):444–447.

Fisher, R. A., Bertonis, J. M., Meier, W., et al. "HIV infection is blocked in vitro by recombinant soluble CD4." *Nature* (Lond.) 331 (1988):76–81.

Flatau, E., Resnitzky, P., Grishkan, A., and Levy, E. "Malignant evolution of Kaposi's sarcoma with impaired cellular immunity." *Harefuah* 93 (1977):242–244.

Fleming, A. F. "HTLV—try Africa." *Lancet* 1 (1983):279.

Fleming, A. F. "HTLV from Africa to Japan." *Lancet* 1 (1984):279.

Fleming, A. F., ed. *The Global Impact of AIDS.* New York, Liss, 1988.

Fleurette, J. "La maladie des légionnaires." *Recherche* 14, no. 141 (1983):146–155.

Flick, L. F. *Development of Our Knowledge of Tuberculosis.* Philadelphia, Wickersham, 1925.

Follansbee, S. E., Busch, D. F., Wofsky, C. B., et al. "An outbreak of *Pneumocystis carinii* pneumonia in homosexual men." *Ann. Int. Med.* 96 (1982):705–713.

Forthal, D. N., Getchell, J. P., and Mann, J. "Antibodies to human T-lymphotropic virus type III/lymphadenopathy-associated virus (HTLV-III/LAV) in sera collected in 1976, equator region Zaire." In *Program and Abstracts of the International Conference on AIDS,* p. 129. Paris, 1986.

Fougère, P. "Les sciences médicales: SIDA, cause nationale." *Revue des Deux Mondes* (1987):753–761.

Frame, J. D., Baldwin, J. D., Gocke, D. J., et al. "Lassa fever, a new virus disease of man from West Africa." *Amer. J. Trop. Med. Hyg.* 19 (1970):670–676.

Franceschi, S., Tirelli, U., Vaccher, E., et al. "Increased prevalence of HTLV-*III* antibody among drug addicts from Italian province with US military base." *Lancet* 1 (1986):804.

Franchini, G., Gurgo, C., Guo, H. G., et al. "Sequence of simian immunodeficiency virus and its relationship to the human immunodeficiency viruses." *Nature* (Lond.) 328 (1987):539–543.

Francioli, P., Vogt, M., Schädelin, J., et al. "Syndrome de déficience immunitaire acquise, infections opportunistes et homosexualité. Présentation de trois cas observés en Suisse." *Schweiz. Med. Wschr.* 112 (1982):1682–1687.

Francis, D. P., Curran, J. W., and Essex, M. "Epidemic acquired immune deficiency syndrome: Epidemiologic evidence for a transmissible agent." *J. Natl. Cancer Inst.* 71 (1983):1–4.

Francis, D. P., Feorino, P. M., Broderson, J.R., et al. "Infection of chimpanzees with lymphadenopathy-associated virus." *Lancet* 2 (1984):1276–1277.

Franck, M. "Sida: La psychose." *Le Point*, March 23, 1987.

Fribourg-Blanc, A. "Deux observations d'annulation spontanée d'une séropositivité HIV." *Méd. Mal. Infect.* (1988):216–218.

Fribourg-Blanc, A., and Mollaret, H. H. "Natural treponematoses of the African primate." *Primates in Medicine* 3 (1968):110–118.

Fribourg-Blanc, A., Niel, G., and Mollaret, H. H. "Confirmation sérologique et microscopique de la tréponématose du cynocéphale de Guinée." *Bull. Soc. Path. Exot.* 59 (1966):54–59.

Friedman-Kien, A. E. "Disseminated Kaposi's sarcoma syndrome in young homosexual men." *J. Amer. Acad. Dermatol.* 5 (1981):468–471.

Friedman-Kien, A. E., and Laubenstein, L. J., eds., *AIDS: The Epidemic of Kaposi's Sarcoma and Opportunistic Infections.* New York, Masson, 1984.

Friedman-Kien, A. E., Laubenstein, L. J., Rubinstein, P., et al. "Disseminated Kaposi's sarcoma in homosexual men." *Ann. Int. Med.* 96 (1982):693–700.

Froland, S. S., Jenum, P., Lindboe, C. F., et al. "HIV-1 infection in a Norwegian family before 1970." *Lancet* 1 (1988):1344–1345.

Fuchs, D., Hausen, A., Reibnegger, G., et al. "Neopterin as a marker for activated cell-mediated immunity: Application in HIV infection," *Immun. Today* 9 (1988): 150–155.

Fukasawa, M., Miura, T., Hasegawa, A., et al. "Sequence of simian immunodeficiency virus from African green monkey, a new member of the HIV/SIV group." *Nature* (Lond.) 333 (1988):457–461.

Fultz, P. N. "Components of saliva inactivate human immunodeficiency virus." *Lancet* 2 (1986):121.

Fultz, P. N., McClure, H. M., Anderson, D. C., et al. "Isolation of a T-lymphotropic retrovirus from naturally infected sooty mangabey monkeys." *Proc. Natl. Acad. Sci. USA* 83 (1986):5286–5290.

Fultz, P. N., McClure, H. M., Daugharty, H., et al. "Vaginal transmission of human immunodeficiency virus (HIV) to a chimpanzee." *J. Infect. Dis.* 154 (1986):896–900.

Fultz, P. N., McClure, H. M., Swenson, R. B., et al. "Persistent infection of chimpanzees with HTLV-III/LAV, a potential model for acquired immunodeficiency syndrome." *J. Virol.* 58 (1986):116–124.

Gabrielli, G. B., Nortilli, R., Mezzelani, P., et al. "Linfadenopatia persistente generalizzata: Pre-AIDS. Prima descrizione di un caso osservato in Italia." *Minerva Medica* 75 (1984):2653–2658.

Gajdusek, D. C. "Slow virus infection of the nervous system." *New Engl. J. Med.* 276 (1967):392–400.

Gajdusek, D. C. "Pneumocystis carinii as the cause of human disease; historical perspective and magnitude of the problem." *Natl. Canc. Inst. Monogr.* 43 (1976):1–11.

Gajdusek, D. C. "Unconventional viruses and the origin and disappearence of kuru." *Science* (Wash.) 197 (1977):943–960.

Gajdusek, D. C., Amyx, H. L., Gibbs, C. J., et al. "Transmission experiments with human T-lymphotropic retroviruses and human AIDS tissue." *Lancet* 1 (1984): 1415–1416.

Gajdusek, D. C., Amyx, H. L., Gibbs, C. J., et al. "Infection of chimpanzees by human T-lymphotropic retroviruses in brain and other tissues from AIDS patients." *Lancet* 1 (1985):1415–1416.

Gajdusek, D. C., and Gibbs, C. J. "Transmission of two subacute spongiform encephalopathies of man (kuru and Creutzfeld-Jakob disease) to New World monkeys." *Nature* (Lond.) 230 (1971):588–591.

Gajdusek, D. C., and Zigas, V. "Degenerative disease of the central nervous system in New Guinea: The endemic occurrence of kuru in the native population." *New Engl. J. Med.* 257 (1957):974–978.

Gallo, R. C. "Human T-cell leukemia-lymphoma virus and T-cell malignancies in adults." *Cancer Surv.* 3 (1984):113–159.

Gallo, R. C. "The first human retrovirus." *Scient. Amer.* 255, no. 6 (1986):88–98.

Gallo, R. C. "The AIDS virus." *Scient. Amer.* 256, no. 1 (1987):45–56.

Gallo, R. C. "Personal reflections on the origin of human leukemia." *Hämat. Bluttransfus.* 31 (1988):XXXIII–XLVII.

Gallo, R. C., and Montagnier, L., "The chronology of AIDS research." *Nature* (Lond.) 326 (1987):435–436. Commentary pp. 425–426.

Gallo, R. C., and Montagnier, L. "AIDS in 1988." *Scient. Amer.* 259, no. 4 (1988): 41–48.

Gallo, R. C., and Wong-Staal, F. "Retroviruses as etiologic agents of some animal and human leukemias and lymphomas and as tools for elucidating the molecular mechanism of leukemo-genesis." *Blood* 60 (1982):545–557.

Gallo, R. C., and Wong-Staal, F., eds. *Retrovirus Biology: An Emerging Role in Human Diseases.* New York, Dekker, 1988.

Gallo, R. C., Essex, M., and Gross, L., eds. *Human T-Cell Leukemia/Lymphoma Virus: The Family of Human T-Lymphotropic Retroviruses; Their Role in Malignancies and Association with AIDS.* New York, Cold Spring Harbor Laboratory, 1984.

Gallo, R. C., Robert-Guroff, M., Wong-Staal, F., et al. "HTLV-III/LAV and the origin and pathogenesis of AIDS." *Arch. Allergy Appl. Immun.* 82 (1987):471–475.

Gallo, R. C., Salahuddin, S. Z., Popovic, M., et al. "Frequent detection and isolation of cytopathic retrovirus (HTLV-III) from patients with AIDS and at risk for AIDS." *Science* (Wash.) 224 (1984):500–503.

Gallo, R. C., Sarin, P. S., Gelmann, E. P., et al. "Isolation of human T-cell leukemia virus in acquired immunodeficiency syndrome (AIDS)." *Science* (Wash.) 220 (1983):865–868.

Gallo, R. C., Sarin, P. S., Kramarsky, B., et al. "First isolation of HTLV-III." *Nature* (Lond.) 321 (1986):119.

Gallo, R. C., Sliski, A. H., and De Noronha, C. M. and F. "Origins of human T-lymphotropic viruses." *Nature* (Lond.) 320 (1986):219.

Gallo, R. C., Sliski, A. H., and Wong-Staal, F. "Origin of human T-cell leukemia-lymphoma virus." *Lancet* 2 (1983):962–963.

Gallo, R. C., Wong-Staal, F., Montagnier, L., et al. "HIV-HTLV gene nomenclature." *Nature* (Lond.) 333 (1988):504.

Galperin, C. "Le bactériophage, la lysogénié et son déterminisme génétique." *Hist. Phil. Life Sci.* 9 (1987):175–224.

Galvao-Castro, B., and Pereira, M. S. "HTLV-III antibody in Brazilian Indians." *Lancet* 1 (1986):976.

Galzigna, M. "Medicare la morale. La cura dei costumi, non del corpo." *Il Manifesto,* April 2, 1987.

Garoogian, R. *AIDS 1981–1983: An Annotated Bibliography.* Mineola, N.Y., Vantage Information, 1984.

Garry, R. F., Witte, M. H., Gottlieb, A., et al. "Documentation of an AIDS virus infection in the United States in 1968." *J. Amer. Med. Ass.* 260 (1988):2085–2087.

Gartner, S., Markovits, P., Markovitz, D. M., et al. "The role of mononuclear phagocytes in HTLV-III/LAV infection." *Science* (Wash.) 233 (1986a):215–219.

Gartner, S., Markovits, P., Markovitz, D. M., et al. "Virus isolation from an identification of HTLV-III/LAV producing cells in brain tissue from a patient with AIDS." *J. Amer. Med. Ass.* 256 (1986b):2365–2371.

Gazzolo, L., Gessain, A., Robin, Y., et al. "Antibodies to HTLV-III in Haitian immigrants in French Guyana." *New Engl. J. Med.* 311 (1984):1252–1253.

Gelderblom, H. R., Hausmann, E. H., Oezel, M., et al. "Fine structure of human immunodeficiency virus (HIV) and immunolocalization of structural proteins." *Virology* 156 (1987):171–176.

Gelmann, E. P., Popovic, M., Blayney, D., et al. "Proviral DNA of a retrovirus, human T-cell leukemia virus in two patients with AIDS." *Science* (Wash.) 220 (1983):862–865.

Gerlo, A. *La correspondance d'Erasme*. Brussels, Presses Universitaires, 1980.

Gerstoft, J., Malchow-Moller, A., Bygbjerg, I., et al. "Severe acquired immunodeficiency in European homosexual men." *Brit. Med. J.* 285 (1982):17–19.

Gessain, A., Barin, F., Vernant, J. C., et al. "Antibodies to human T-lymphotropic virus type I in patients with tropical spastic paraparesis." *Lancet* 2 (1985):407–410.

Gessain, R. "Conséquences tragiques d'un éternuement ou l'atchoum qui tue." *Concours Méd.* 105 (1983):1532.

Getchell, J. P., Hicks, D. R., Srinivasan, A., et al. "Human immunodeficiency virus from a serum sample collected in 1976 in Central Africa." *J. Infect. Dis.* 156 (1987):833–837.

Gigase, P. L. "Epidémiologie du sarcome de Kaposi en Afrique." *Bull. Soc. Path. Exot.* 77 (1984):546–559.

Gilden, R. V., Gonda, M. A., Sarngadharan, M. G., et al. "HTLV-III legend correction." *Science* (Wash.) 232 (1986):307.

Giraldo, G., et al., eds., *Recent Advances in AIDS and Kaposi's Sarcoma*. Basel, Karger, 1987 ("Antibiotics and Chemotherapy," vol. 38).

Giraldo, G., Beth, E., and Haguenau, F. "Herpes-type virus particles in tissue culture of Kaposi's sarcoma from different geographic regions." *J. Natl. Cancer Inst.* 49 (1972):1509–1526.

Giraldo, G., Beth, E., and Huang, E. S. "Kaposi's sarcoma and its relationship to cytomegalovirus: CMV, DNA and CMV early antigens in Kaposi's sarcoma (Senegal, Uganda, New York)." *Intern. J. Cancer* 26 (1980):23–29.

Giraldo, G., Beth-Giraldo, E., Clumeck, N., Gharbi, M. R., and Kyalwazi, S. K. *AIDS and associated cancers in Africa*. Basel, Karger, 1988.

Girard, M. "The Pasteur Institute's contributions to the field of virology." *Ann. Rev. Microbiol.* 42 (1988):745–763.

Girard, M., and Valette, L., eds. *Retroviruses of Human AIDS and Related Animal Diseases* (2e Colloque des "Cent Gardes," Marnes-la-Coquette, 1987). Lyons, Fondation Mérieux et Pasteur Vaccin, 1988.

Girard, M., De Thé, G., and Valette, L., eds. Retroviruses of human AIDS and related animal diseases. (Colloque des "Cent Gardes," Marnes-la-Coquette, 1986). Lyons, Fondation Mérieux et Pasteur Vaccin, 1987.

Girard, R. *Tristes chimères (SIDA)*. Paris, Grasset, 1987.

Giudizzi, m. G., Biagotti, R., Almerignogna, F., et al. "HTLV-III seropositivity in symptom-free Italian haemophiliacs. Correlation with consumption of commercial concentrate and abnormalities of T and B lymphocytes." *Scand. J. Haematol.* 36 (1986):198–202.

Giunta, S., and Groppa, G. "The primate trade and the origin of AIDS viruses." *Nature* (Lond.) 329 (1987):22.

Gluckman, J. C. "Physiopathologie du SIDA et l'épidémiologie de l'infection par le virus LAV." *Rev. Épid. Santé Publ.* 34 (1986):112–117.

Gluckman, J. C., Klatzmann, D., and Montagnier, L. "LAV (Lymphadenopathy Associated Virus) infection and acquired immunodeficiency syndrome." *Ann. Rev. Immun.* 4 (1986):97–117.

Gocke, D. J., Raska, K. , Polack, W., et al. "HTLV-III antibody in commercial immunoglobulin." *Lancet* 1 (1986):37–38.

Goedert, J. J., Gallo, R. C., et al. "Determinants of retrovirus (HTLV-III) antibody and immunodeficiency conditions in homosexual men." *Lancet* 2 (1984):711–716.

Goedert, J. J., Neuland, C. Y., Walle, W. C., et al. "Amyl nitrite may alter T lymphocytes in homosexual men." *Lancet* 1 (1982):412–416.

Goldman, K. P. "AIDS and tuberculosis." *Brit. Med. J.* 295 (1987):511–512.

Goldsmith, J. C., Moseley, P. L., Monick, M., et al. "T-lymphocyte subpopulation abnormalities in apparently healthy patients with hemophilia." *Ann. Int. Med.* 98 (1983):294–296.

Goldsmith, M. F. "Sex in the age of AIDS calls for common sense and 'condom sense.' " *J. Amer. Med. Ass.* 257 (1987):2261–2263, 2266.

Goldsmith, M. F. "Sex experts and medical scientists join forces against a common foe: AIDS." *J. Amer. Med. Ass.* 259 (1988):641–643.

Gonda, M. A. "Molecular genetics and structure of the human immunodeficiency virus." *J. Electron. Microsc. Tech.* 8 (1988):17–40.

Gonda, M. A., Boyd, A. L., Nagashima, K., and Gilden, R. V. "Pathobiology, molecular organization and ultrastructure of the human immunodeficiency virus." *Archives of AIDS Research* 3 (1988):1–42.

Gonda, M. A., Braun, M. J., Carter, S. G., et al. "Characterization and molecular cloning of a bovine lentivirus related to human immunodeficiency virus." *Nature* (Lond.) 330 (1987):388–391.

Gonda, M. A., Braun, M. J., Clements, J. E., et al. "Human T-cell lymphotropic virus type III shares sequence homology with a family of pathogenic lentiviruses." *Proc. Natl. Acad. Sci. USA* 83 (1986):4007–4011.

Gonda, M. A., Wong-Staal, F., Gallo, R. C., et al. "Sequence homology and morphological similarity of HTLV-III and visna virus, a pathogenic lentivirus." *Science* (Wash.) 227 (1985):173–177.

Gonzalez, J. P., Georges-Courbot, M. C., Martin, P.M.V., et al. "True HIV-1 infection in a Pygmy." *Lancet* 1 (1987):1499.

Gordon, S. M., Valentine, F. T., Holzman, R. S., et al. "Acquired immunodeficiency syndrome possibly related to transfusion in an adult without known disease-risk factors." *J. Infect. Dis.* 149 (1984):1030–1032.

Gorin, I., Picard, O., Laroche, L., et al. "Kaposi's sarcoma without the U.S. or 'popper' connection." *Lancet* 1 (1982):908.

Gorman, C., Dorfman, A., and Kramer, S. "Strange trip back to the future: The case of Robert R. spurs new questions about AIDS." *Time Magazine*, November 9, 1987, p. 75.

Gottlieb, G. J., and Ackerman, A. B. *Kaposi's Sarcoma: A Text and Atlas*. Philadelphia, Lea and Febiger, 1988.

Gottlieb, G. J., Ragaz, A., Vogel, J. V., et al. "A preliminary communication on extensively disseminated Kaposi's sarcoma in young homosexual men." *Amer. J. Dermatopath*. 3 (1981):111–114.

Gottlieb, M. S., et al., eds. *Current Topics in AIDS*. New York, Wiley, 1987.

Gottlieb, M. S., Groopman, J. E., Weinstein, W. M., et al. "The acquired immunodeficiency syndrome." *Ann. Int. Med*. 99 (1983):208–220.

Gottlieb, M. S., Schroff, R., Schanker, H. M., Weisman, J. D., Fan, P. T., Wolf, R. A., and Saxon, A. "Pneumocystis carinii pneumonia and mucosal candidiasis in previously healthy homosexual men: Evidence of a new acquired cellular immunodeficiency." *New Engl. J. Med*. 305 (1981):1425–1431.

Gourevitch, D. *Le triangle hippocratique dans le monde gréco-romain. Le malade, sa maladie et son médecin*. Rome, Ecole Française de Rome, 1984.

Grant, I., Atkinson, J. H., Hesselink, J. R., et al. "Evidence of early central nervous system involvement in the AIDS and other HIV infections: Studies with neuropsychologic testing and magnetic resonance imaging." *Ann. Intern. Med*. 107 (1987): 828–836.

Grapow, H. *Grundriss der Medizin der alten Aegypter*. Vol 3: *Kranker, Krankheiten und Arzt*. Berlin, Akademie Verlag, 1956.

Greco, R. S. "Haiti and the stigma of AIDS." *Lancet* 2 (1983):515–516.

Green, J., and Miller, D. *AIDS, the Story of a Disease*. London, Grafton, 1986.

Greenberg, A. E., Nguyen-Dinh, P., Mann, J., et al. "The association between malaria, blood transfusion and HIV seropositivity in a pediatric population in Kinshasa, Zaire." *J. Amer. Med. Ass*. 259 (1988):545–549.

Greenfield, W. R. "Night of the living death: slow virus encephalopathies and AIDS. Do necromantic zombiists transmit HTLV-III/LAV during voodooistic rituals?" *J. Amer. Med. Ass*. 256 (1986):2199–2000.

Greenough, A., and Davis, J. A. "Encephalitis lethargica: Mystery of the past or undiagnosed disease of the present?" *Lancet* 1 (1983):922–923.

Greenwalt, T. J. "Blood-product transfusion and the acquired immunodeficiency syndrome." *Ann. Int. Med*. 100 (1984):155.

Gressentis, A. "Le SIDA et le cerveau." *Recherche* 17 (1986):1272–1273.

Griscelli, C., and Hitzig, W., eds. *Déficits immunitaires congénitaux et acquis*. Paris, Doin, 1984 (*Progrès en hématologie*, vol. 5).

Grmek, M. D. "Causes de l'extinction des Indiens de Guyane française." *Annales E.S.C.* 21 (1966):899–900.

Grmek, M. D. "Discussion on medicine and culture." In F.N.L. Poynter, ed., *Medicine and Culture*, pp. 119–120. London, Wellcome Institute, 1969a.

Grmek, M. D. "Préliminaires d'une étude historique des maladies." *Annales E.S.C.* 24 (1969b):1437–1483.

Grmek, M. D. "Le role du hasard dans la genèse des découvertes scientifiques." *Medicina nei secoli* 13 (1976):277–305.

Grmek, M. D. Les maladies à l'aube de la civilisation occidentale. Paris, Payot, 1983. American edition: *Diseases in the Ancient Greek World*. Baltimore, Johns Hopkins University Press, 1989.

Grmek, M. D. "Problème des maladies nouvelles." In C. Mérieux, ed., *Sida: Epidémies et sociétés*, pp. 97–107. (Compte rendu de la réunion organisée aux Pensières, Annecy). Lyon, Fondation Mérieux, 1987.

Grmek, M. D., Cohen, R. S., and Cimino, G., eds. *On Scientific Discovery*. The Erice Lectures, 1977. Dordrecht and Boston, Reidel, 1981.

Groopman, J. E., Salahuddin, S. Z., Sarngadharan, M. G., et al. "HTLV-III in saliva of people with AIDS-related complex and healthy homosexual men at risk for AIDS." *Science* (Wash.) 226 (1984):447–449.

Gross, L. "Spontaneous leukemia developing in C3H mice following inoculation in infancy with AK-leukemia extracts or AK-embryos." *Proc. Soc. Exp. Biol. Med.* 78 (1951):27–32.

Gross, L., ed. *Oncogenic Viruses*. New York, Pergamon Press, 1983.

Gross, L. "An overview of the HTLV symposium and reflection about the past, present and future." *Cancer Research*, 45, suppl. (1985):4706–4709.

Groupe de Travail Français sur le SIDA. "Infections opportunistes et sarcomes de Kaposi survenant chez des homosexuels: Mythes ou réalités?" *Rev. Prat.* 32 (1982): 3213–3215.

Groupe de Travail Français sur le SIDA. "Sarcome de Kaposi et infections opportunistes chez des sujets jeunes sans antécédent susceptible d'entraîner une immunodépression." *Presse Méd.* 12 (1983a):2431–2434.

Groupe de Travail Français sur le SIDA. "Le syndrome d'immunodéficit acquis: Une nouvelle maladie d'origine infectieuse?" *Presse Méd.* 12 (1983b):2453–2456.

Guerra, F. "The dispute over syphilis: Europe versus America." *Clio Medica* 13 (1978):39–61.

Guerra, F. "Cause of death of the American Indians." *Nature* (Lond.) 326 (1987): 449–450.

Guillaume, P. *Du désespoir au salut: Les tuberculeux aux 19e et 20e siècles*. Paris, Auber, 1986.

Guinan, M., and Hardy, A. "Epidemiology of AIDS in women in the United States 1981 through 1986." *J. Amer. Med. Ass.* 257 (1987):2039–2042.

Gurgo, C., Guo, G., Franchini, A., et al. "Envelope sequences of two new USA HIV-1 isolates." *Virology* 164 (1988):531–536.

Guyader, M., Emerman, M., Sonigo, P., et al. "Genome organization and transactivation of the human immunodeficiency virus type 2." *Nature* (Lond.) 326 (1987):662–669.

Haase, A. T. "Pathogenesis of lentivirus infections." *Nature* (Lond.) 322 (1986):130–136.

Habibi, B. "SIDA et transfusion sanguine." *Rev. Prat.* 36 (1986a):1199–1205.

Habibi, B. "Propagation du virus du SIDA par la transfusion et les produits sanguins." *Rev. Épid. Santé Publ.* 34 (1986b):118–125.

Habibi, B., and Girard, M. "Dépistage en urgence des porteurs du VIH parmi les malades en coma dépassé, source potentielle d'organes transplantables: Fréquence élevée à Paris." *Presse Méd.* 17 (1988):1157.

Hagmar, B., Kutti, J., Lundin, P., et al. "Disseminated infection caused by Mycobacterium kansasii: Report of a case and brief review of the literature." *Acta Med. Scand.* 186 (1969):93–99.

Hahn, B. H., Shaw, G. M., Arya, S. K., et al. "Molecular cloning and characterization of the HTLV-III virus associated with AIDS." *Nature* (Lond.) 312 (1984):166–169.

Hahn, B. H., Shaw, G. M., Taylor, M. E., et al. "Genetic variation in HTLV-III/LAV over time in patients with AIDS or at risk for AIDS." *Science* (Wash.) 232 (1986):1548–1553.

Hallenberg, K. "Multiple Angiosarkome der Haut bei einem Kamerunneger." *Arch. Schiff. Trop. Hyg.* 18 (1914):647–652.

Hamperl, H. "Pneumocystis infection and cytomegaly of the lungs in the newborn and adult." *Amer. J. Path.* 32 (1956):1–8.

Hancock, G., and Carim, E. *AIDS: The deadly epidemic.* London, Gollancz, 1986.

Hansemann, D. P. "Ueber eine bisher nicht beobachtete Gehirnerkrankung durch Hefen." *Verh. Dtsch. Ges. Path.* 9 (1905):21–24.

Hardy, A. M., Allen, J. R., Morgan, W. M., and Curran, J. W. "The incidence rate of acquired immunodeficiency syndrome in selected populations." *J. Amer. Med. Ass.* 253 (1985):215–220.

Hardy, A. M., Rauch, K., Echenberg, D., et al. "The economic impact of the first 10,000 cases of acquired immunodeficiency syndrome in the United States." *J. Amer. Med. Ass.* 255 (1986):209–211.

Harris, C., Small, C. B., Klein, R. S., et al. "Immunodeficiency in female sexual partners of men with the acquired immunodeficiency syndrome." *New Engl. J. Med.* 308 (1983):1181–1184.

Hart, C., Schochetman, G., Spira, T., et al. "Direct detection of HIV RNA expression in seropositive subjects." *Lancet* 2 (1988):596–599.

Haseltine, W. A., and Wong-Staal, F. "The molecular biology of the AIDS virus." *Scient. Amer.* 259, no. 4 (1988):52–62.

Hatton, F., Maguin, P., Nicaud, V., et al. "Mortalité par SIDA en France." *Rev. Épid. Santé Publ.* 34 (1986):134–142.

Haverkos, H. W. "Epidemiology of AIDS in hemophiliacs and blood transfusion recipients." *Antibiot. Chemother.* 38 (1987):59–65.

Haverkos, H. W., and Curran, J. W. "The current outbreak of Kaposi's sarcoma and opportunistic infections." *CA—Cancer J. Clin.* 32 (1982):330–339.

Helm, E. B., Bergmann, L., and Nerger, K. "Pneumocystis-carinii-Pneumonie bei homosexuellen Männern." *Dtsch. Med. Wschr.* 107 (1982):1779–1780.

Henderson, D. K., Saah, A. J., Zak, B. J., et al. "Risk of nosocomial infection with human T-cell lymphotropic virus type III/ lymphadenopathy associated virus in a large cohort of intensively exposed health care workers." *Ann. Int. Med.* 104 (1986):644–647.

Hendry, R. M., et al. "Antibodies to simian immunodeficiency virus in African green monkeys in Africa in 1957–1962." *Lancet* 2 (1986):455.

Henig, R. M. "AIDS: A new disease's deadly Odyssey." *New York Times*, February 6, 1983, p. 28.

Henle, G., Henle, W., and Diehl, V. "Relation of Burkitt's tumor-associated herpes-type virus to infectious mononucleosis." *Proc. Natl. Acad. Sci. USA* 59 (1968):94–101.

Hennigar, G. R., Vinijchaikul, K., Roque, A. L., and Lyons, H. A. "Pneumocystis carinii pneumonia in an adult. Report of a case." *Amer. J. Clin. Path.* 35 (1961): 353–364.

Henrickson, R. V., Maul, D. H., Osborn, K. G., et al. "Epidemic of acquired immunodeficiency in a colony of macaque monkeys (California)." *Lancet* 1 (1983):388–390.

Henrion, R. *Les femmes et le sida*. Paris, Flammarion, 1988.

Henry, W. A. "The appalling saga of patient zero." *Time Magazine* (October 19, 1987), p. 42.

Henschen, F. *The History and Geography of Diseases*. New York, Delacorte Press, 1962.

Hentsch, D., ed. *Toxoplasmosis*. Bern, Huber, 1971.

Herzlich, C., and Picrret, J. "Une maladie dans l'espace public: Le sida dans six quotidiens français." *Annales E.S.C.* (1988):1109–1134.

Heyward, W. M., and Curran, J. W. "The epidemiology of AIDS in the USA." *Scient. Amer.*, 259, no. 4 (1988):72–81.

Hirsch, E. *Le SIDA. Rumeurs et faits*. Paris, Editions du Cerf, 1987.

Hirsch, V., Riedel, N., Kornfeld, H., et al. "Crossreactivity with HTLV-III/LAV and molecular cloning of simian T-lymphotropic virus type III from African green monkeys." *Proc. Natl. Acad. Sci. USA* 83 (1986):9754–9758.

Hirsch, V., Riedel, N., and Mullins, J. I. "The genome organization of STLV-3 is similar to that of the AIDS virus with a truncated transmembrane protein." *Cell* 49 (1988):307–319.

Ho, D. D., Rota, T. R., and Hirsch, M. S., "Infection of monocytes/macrophages by human T-lymphotropic virus type III." *J. Clin. Invest.* 77 (1986):1712–1715.

Ho, D. D., Schooley, R. T., Rota, T. R., et al. "HTLV-III in the semen and blood of a healthy homosexual man." *Science* (Wash.) 226 (1984):451–453.

Hocquenghem, G. *Eve*. Paris, Albin Michel, 1987.

Holland, J., Spindler, K., Horodyski, F., et al. "Rapid evolution of RNA genomes." *Science* (Wash.) 215 (1982):1577–1588.

Holubar, K., and Frankl, J. "Moritz (Kohn) Kaposi." *Amer. J. Dermatopath.* 3 (1981):349–350.

Hopkins, D. R. *Princes and Paesants: Smallpox in History*. Chicago, University of Chicago Press, 1983.

Hrdy, D. B. "Cultural practices contributing to the transmission of human immunodeficiency virus in Africa." *Rev. Infect. Dis.* 9 (1987):1109–1119.

Hudson, R. P. "How diseases birth and die." *Trans. Stud. Coll. Phys. Philadelphia* 45 (1977):18–27.

Hudson, R. P. *Disease and Its Control: The Shaping of Modern Thought*. Westport, Greenwood Press, 1983.

Huebner, R. J., and Todaro, G. J. "Oncogenes of RNA tumor viruses as determinants of cancer." *Proc. Natl. Acad. Sci. USA* 64 (1969):1087–1094.

Hughes, S. S. *The Virus: A History of the Concept*. New York, Science History Publications, 1977.

Huminer, D. "Was a case of AIDS reported in Harefuah before the first publication on the syndrome in the USA?" *Harefuah* 109 (1985):424–425.

Huminer, D., Rosenfeld, J. B., and Pitlik, S. D. "AIDS in the pre-AIDS era." *Rev. Infect. Dis.* 9 (1987):1102–1108.

Hunsmann, G., Schneider, J., Schmitt, J. and Yamamoto, N. "Detection of serum antibodies to adult T-cell leukemia virus in nonhuman primates and in people from Africa." *Int. J. Cancer.* 32 (1983):329–332.

Hutt, M.S.R. "The epidemiology of Kaposi's sarcoma." *Antibiot. Chemother.* 29 (1981):3–8.

Hymes, K. B., Greene, J. B., Marcus, A., et al. "Kaposi's sarcoma in homosexual men: A report of eight cases." *Lancet* 2 (1981):598–600.

Ide, A. F. *AIDS Hysteria*. Dallas, Monument Press, 1986.

Iliffe, J. *The African Poor*. Cambridge, Eng., Cambridge University Press, 1987.

Ingram, G. I. "The history of haemophilia." *J. Clin. Pathol.* 29 (1976):469–479.

Jacob, F., and Wollman, E. L. "Induction of phage development in lysogenic bacteria." *Cold Spring Harbor Symp. Quantit. Biol.* 8 (1953):101–121.

Jacobson, S., Raine, C. S., Mingioli, E. S., et al. "Isolation of an HTLV-1-like retrovirus from patients with tropical spastic paraparesis." *Nature* (Lond.) 331 (1988): 540–543.

Jaffe, H. W., Bergman, D. J., and Selik, R. M. "Acquired immune deficiency syndrome in the United States: The first 1,000 cases." *J. Infect. Dis.* 148 (1983):339–345.

Jaffe, H. W., Choi, K., Thomas, P. A., et al. "National case-control study of Kaposi's sarcoma and Pneumocystis carinii pneumonia in homosexual men: Part 1, Epidemiologic results." *Ann. Int. Med.* 99 (1983):145–151.

Jaffe, L. R., Seehaus, M., Wagner, C., et al. "Anal intercourse and knowledge of acquired immunodeficiency among minority-group female adolescents." *J. Pediatr.* 112 (1988):1005–1007.

Jarrett, W. F. "Experimental studies of feline and bovine leukemia." *Proc. Roy. Soc. Med.* 59 (1966):661–662.

Jarrett, W., Jarrett, O., Mackey, L., et al. "Horizontal transmission of leukemia virus and leukemia in the cat." *J. Natl. Cancer Inst.* 51 (1973):833–841.

Jedlicka, J. *Vyvoj fthiseologie*. Prague, Ceska Graf. Unie, 1932.

Jenicek, M., and Cléroux, P. D. *Epidémiologie. Principes, techniques, applications*. Paris, Maloine, 1982.

Jensen, O. M., Mouridsen, H. T., Petersen, N. S., et al. "Kaposi's sarcoma in homosexual men: Is it a new disease?" *Lancet* 1 (1982):1027.

Jett, J., Kuritsky, M. D., Katzmann, J. A., et al. "Acquired immunodeficiency syndrome associated with blood-product transfusions." *Ann. Int. Med.* 99 (1983):621–624.

Johns, D. R., Tierney, M., and Felsenstein, D. "Alteration in the natural history of neurosyphilis by concurrent infection with the human immunodeficiency virus." *New Engl. J. Med.* 316 (1987):1569–1527.

Joncas, J. H., Delage, G., Chad, Z., et al. "Acquired (or congenital) immunodeficiency syndrome in infants born of Haitian mothers." *New Engl. J. Med.* 308 (1983):842.

Jonckheer, T., et al. "A cluster of HTLV-III/LAV infection in an African family." *Lancet* 1 (1985):400–401.

Jonckheere, F. *Une maladie égyptienne. L'hématurie parasitaire.* Brussels, Fondation égyptologique reine Elisabeth, 1944.

Jorgenson, K. A., and Lawesson, S. O. "Amyl nitrite and Kaposi's sarcoma in homosexual men." *New Engl. J. Med.* 307 (1982):893–894.

Jossay, M., and Donadieu, Y. *Le sida. Etude, prévention, traitement.* Paris, Maloine, 1986.

Joyce, C., and Sattaur, O. "AIDS: French sue over who was first." *New Scient.*, December 26, 1985, p. 3.

Judson, H. F. *The Eighth Day of Creation: Makers of the Revolution in Biology.* London, Cape, 1979.

Juliette. *Pourquoi moi? Confessions d'une jeune femme d'aujourd'hui.* Paris, Laffont, 1987.

Kalyanaraman, V. S., Montagnier, L., Francis, D., et al. "Antibodies to the core protein of lymphadenopathy-associated virus (LAV) in patients with AIDS." *Science* (Wash.) 225 (1984):321–323.

Kalyanaraman, V. S., Sarngadharan, M. G., Robert-Guroff, M., et al. "A new subtype of human T-cell leukemia virus (HTLV-II) associated with a T-cell variant of hairy cell leukemia." *Science* (Wash.) 218 (1982):571.

Kanki, P. J., Alroy, J., and Essex, M. "Isolation of T-lymphotropic retrovirus related to HTLV-3/LAV from wild-caught African green monkeys." *Science* (Wash.) 230 (1985):951–954.

Kanki, P. J., Barin, F., M'Boup, S., et al. "New human T-lymphotropic retrovirus (HTLV-IV) related to simian T-lymphotropic virus type III (STLV-IIIagm)." *Science* (Wash.) 232 (1986):238–243.

Kanki, P. J., Barin, F., M'Boup, S., and Essex, M. "Relationship of simian T-lymphotropic virus type III to human retroviruses in Africa." *Antibiot. Chemother.* 38 (1987):21–27.

Kanki, P. J., Hopper, J. R., and Essex, M., "The origins of HIV-1 and HTLV-4/HIV-2." *Ann. N.Y. Acad. Sci.* 511 (1987):370–375.

Kanki, P. J., Kurth, R., Becker, W., et al. "Antibodies to simian T-lymphotropic type III in African green monkeys and recognition of STLV-III viral proteins by AIDS and related sera." *Lancet* 1 (1985):1330–1332.

Kanki, P. J., McLane, M. F., King, N. W., Jr., et al. "Serologic identification and characterization of a macaque T-lymphotropic retrovirus closely related to human HTLV-III." *Science* (Wash.) 228 (1985):1199–1201.

Kaplan, J. E., Spira, T. J., Fishbein, D. B., et al. "A six-years follow-up of HIV-infected homosexual men with lymphadenopathy. *J. Amer. Med. Ass.* 260 (1988): 2694–2697.

Kaplan, L. D., Wofsy, C. B., and Volberding, P. A. "Treatment of patients with acquired immunodeficiency syndrome and associated manifestations." *J. Amer. Med. Ass.* 257 (1987):1367–1374.

Kaposi, M. "Idiopathisches multiples Pigmentsarkom der Haut." *Arch. Derm. Syphil.* (Prague) 4 (1872):265–273. Transl. in *CA—Cancer J. Clin.* 32 (1982):343–347.

Kappes, J. C., Morrow, C. D., Lee, S. W., et al. "Identification of a novel retroviral gene unique to human immunodeficiency virus type 2 and simian immunodeficiency virus *SIV*mac." *J. Virol.* 62 (1988):3501–3505.

Karpas, A. "Unusual virus produced by cultured cells from a patient with AIDS." *Molecul. Biol. Med.* 1 (1983):457–459.

Karpas, A. "Historical overview of human lymphotropic retroviruses." *Proc. First Intern. Meeting of AVIS.* Naples, 1985.

Karpas, A. "Origin of the AIDS virus explained?" *New Scient.*, July 16, 1987, p. 67.

Karpas, A., Gillson, W., Oates, J. K., et al. "Lytic infection by a British AIDS virus and the development of a rapid cell test for viral antibodies." *Lancet* 2 (1985):695–697.

Kashamura, A. *Famille, sexualité et culture. Essai sur les moeurs sexuelles et les cultures des peuples des Grands Lacs africains.* Paris, Payot, 1973.

Katner, H. P. "Origin of AIDS." *J. Natl. Med. Ass.* 80 (1988):362.

Katner, H. P., and Pankey, G. A. "Evidence for a Euro-American origin of human immunodeficiency virus (HIV)." *J. Natl. Med. Ass.* 79 (1987):1068–1072.

Keraly, H. *Sida: La stratégie du virus.* Paris, Editions du Ranelagh, 1987.

Kernbaum, S. "Devenir des sujets infectés par le virus HIV-1." *Concours Méd.* 110 (1988):4033–4037.

Kernbaum, S., and Saimot, A. G. "Les infections opportunistes au cours du SIDA." *Concours Méd.* 108 (1986):2094–2105.

Kim, J. H., and Perfect, J. R. "To help the sick: An historical and ethical essay concerning the refusal to care for patients with AIDS." *Amer. J. Med.* 84 (1988):135–138.

Kimura, M. "Estimation of evolutionary distances between homologous nucleotide sequences." *Proc. Natl. Acad. Sci. USA* 78 (1981):454–458.

Kimura, M. *The Neutral Theory of Molecular Evolution.* Cambridge, Eng., Cambridge University Press, 1983.

Kingsley, L. A., Detels, R., Kaslow, R., et al. "Risk factors for seroconversion to human immunodeficiency virus among male homosexuals." *Lancet* 1 (1987):345–349.

Kiple, K. F. *The African Exchange: Toward a Biological History of Black People.* Durham, N.C., Duke University Press, 1987.

Kitchen, L. W., Barin, F., Sullivan, J. L., et al. "Aetiology of AIDS-antibodies to human T-cell leukaemia virus (type III) in haemophiliacs." *Nature* (Lond.) 312 (1984):367–369.

Kjeldsen, K. "Evaluation of the impact of various diseases on mortality." *Bull. W.H.O.* 52 (1975):369–375.

Klatzmann, D., Barré-Sinoussi, F., Nugeyre, M. T., et al. "Selective tropism of lymphadenopathy associated virus (LAV) for helper-inducer T-lymphocytes." *Science* (Wash.) 225 (1984):59–63.

Klatzmann, D., Champagne, E., Chamaret, S., et al. "T- lymphocyte T4 molecule behaves as the receptor for human retrovirus LAV." *Nature* (Lond.) 31 (1984):767–768.

Klein, E., ed. *Acquired Immunodeficiency Syndrome*. Basel, Karger, 1986.

Klein, H. G., and Alter, H. J. "Transfusion du sang et le sida." *J. Amer. Med. Ass.* (French edition), special number (1987):28–32.

Kleinman, Y., Yust, I., Maayan, S., et al. "Transmission of acquired immune deficiency syndrome (AIDS) by a blood transmission given in 1979 in Israel." *Isr. J. Med. Sci.* 22 (1986):404–407.

Koch, M. A., L'age-Stehr, J., and Weise, H. "Unbekannter Krankheitserreger als Ursache von tödlich verlaufenden erworbenen Immundefekten?" *Dtsch. Aerzteblatt* 7 (1983):46–49.

Koch, M. G. *Aids—vom Molekül zur Pandemie*. Heidelberg, Spektrum der Wissenschaft, 1987.

Koenig, S., Gendelman, H. E., Orenstein, J. M., et al. "Detection of AIDS virus in macrophages in brain tissue from AIDS patients with encephalopathy." *Science* (Wash.) 233 (1986):1089–1093.

Koff, W. C., and Hoth, D. F. "Development and testing of AIDS vaccines." *Science* (Wash.) 241 (1988):426–432.

Kohlhof, A., and Flessenkämper, S. "Tenth case of HIV transmission after plasma donation." *Lancet* 2 (1988):965.

Kohn, A. *False Prophets: Fraud and Error in Science and Medicine*. Oxford, Blackwell, 1988.

Kong, L. I., Shei-Wen, L., Kappes, J. C., et al. "West African HIV-2 related human retrovirus with attenuated cytopathicity." *Science* (Wash.) 240 (1988):1525–1529.

Konrads, A., and Sterry, W. "AIDS in Köln?" *Dtsch. Med. Wschr.* 108 (1983): 1336.

Koop, C. E. "Surgeon General's report on acquired immunodeficiency syndrome." *J. Amer. Med. Ass.* 256 (1986):2783–2789.

Kornfeld, H., Ridel, N., Viglianti, G. A., et al. "Cloning of HTLV-4 and its relation to simian and human immunodeficiency viruses." *Nature* (Lond.) 326 (1987):610–613.

Kramer, L. *The Normal Heart*. New York, New American Library, 1985.

Krech, T. "Syphilis and AIDS. Eine historische Parallele." *Fortschr. Med.* 106 (1988):439–442.

Kreiss, J. K., Kitchen, L. W., Prince, H. E., et al. "Human T-cell leukemia virus type III antibody, lymphadenopathy and acquired immune deficiency syndrome in haemophiliac subjects." *Amer. J. Med.* 80 (1986):345–350.

Kreiss, J. K., Koech, D., Plummer, F. A., et al. "AIDS virus infection in Nairobi prostitutes: Spread of the epidemic to East Africa." *New Engl. J. Med.* 314 (1986):414–418.

Kübler-Ross, E. *AIDS, the Ultimate Challenge*. New York, Macmillan, 1987.

Kumar, P., Pearson, J. E., Martin, D. H., et al. "Transmission of human immunodeficiency virus by transplantation of a renal allograft, with development of the acquired immunodeficiency syndrome." *Ann. Int. Med.* 106 (1987):244–245.

Kwok, S., Mack, D. H., Mullis, K. B. "Identification of human immunodeficiency virus sequences by using in vitro enzymatic amplification and oligomer cleavage.'' *J. Virol.* 61 (1987):690–694.

Kyalwazi, S. K. ''Kaposi's sarcoma (one or two diseases?)'' *East. Afr. Med. J.* 46 (1969):459–464.

Kyalwazi, S. K. ''Kaposi's sarcoma: Clinical features, experience in Uganda.'' *Antibiot. Chemother.* 29 (1981):59–67.

Lacey, C.J.N., and Waugh, M. A. ''AIDS: An old disease from Africa?'' *Brit. Med. J.* 289 (1984):496.

Laga, M., and Piot, P. ''HIV infection after plasma donation in Valencia: Yet another case.'' *Lancet* 2 (1988):905.

L'age-Stehr, J., Kunze, R., and Koch, M. A. ''AIDS in West Germany.'' *Lancet* 2 (1983):1370–1371.

L'age-Stehr, J., Schwarz, A., Offermann, G., et al. ''HTLV-III infection in kidney transplant recipients.'' *Lancet* 2 (1985):1361–1362.

Lamey, B., and Melameka, N. ''Aspects cliniques et épidémiologiques de la cryptococcose à Kinshasa. A propos de 15 cas personnels.'' *Méd. Trop.* (Marseille) 42 (1982):507–514.

Lamontagne, E. *SIDA. Vers une connaissance réelle du syndrome et de tout ce qui s'y rapporte*. Ottawa, Léméac, 1986.

Langmuir, A. D. ''The Epidemic Intelligence Service of the Centers for Disease Control.'' *Public Health Rep.* 95 (1980):570–575.

Langmuir, A. D., and Ray, C. G. ''The Thucydides syndrome.'' *J. Amer. Med. Ass.* 257 (1987):3071.

Langmuir, A. D., et al. ''The Thucydides syndrome: A new hypothesis for the cause of the plague of Athens.'' *New Engl. J. Med.* 313 (1985):1027–1030; ''Correspondence and discussion,'' ibid., 314 (1986):855–856.

Laroche, L., Gorin, I., Bach, J. W. and Hewitt, J. ''Déficit immunitaire et maladie de Kaposi chez deux jeunes homosexuels.'' *Presse Méd.* 11 (1982):1637–1638.

Lattimer, G. L., and Ormsbee, R. A. *Legionnaire's Disease*. New York, Dekker, 1981.

Laure, F., Courgnaud, V., Rouzioux, C., et al. ''Detection of HIV-1 DNA in infants and children by means of the polymerase chain reaction.'' *Lancet* 2 (1988):538–541.

Laygues, H. *Sida, témoignage sur la vie et la mort de Martin*. Paris, Hachette, 1985.

Lazzarin, A., Crocchiolo, P., Galli, M., et al. ''Milan as possible starting point of LAV/HTLV III epidemics among Italian drug addicts.'' *Boll. Ist. Sieroter. Milanese* 66 (1987):9–13.

Lazzarin, A., Orlando, G., Privitera, G., et al. ''Clinical and epidemiological aspects of the first 50 cases of AIDS in Milan.'' *Boll. Ist. Sieroter. Milanese* 65 (1986):481–486.

Leibowitch, J. *Un virus étrange venu d'ailleurs*. Paris, Grasset, 1984. American edition: *A Strange Virus of Unknown Origin*. New York, Ballantine, 1985.

Lemaire, J. F. ''Les prévisions de Charles Nicolle.'' *Le Point*, September 16, 1985, p. 85.

Lemaire, J. F. ''Naissance du SIDA.'' *Revue des Deux Mondes* (1987):372–375.

Lenski, R. E. ''Evolution of plague virulence.'' *Nature* (Lond.) 334 (1988):473–474.

Leonidas, J. L. and Hyppolite, N. "Haiti and the acquired immunodeficiency syndrome." *Ann. Int. Med.* 98 (1983):1020–1021.

Lesky, E. *Die Wiener medizinische Schule im 19. Jahrhundert.* Graz-Köln, Böhlaus Nachf., 1965.

Lessana-Leibowitch, M., Leibowitch, J., Frances, C., et al. "Lymphome T pseudomycosis fongoïde chez un Africain associé à un rétrovirus HTLV." *Ann. Derm. Vener.* 11 (1984):725–726.

Levine, A. S. "The epidemic of acquired immune dysfunction in homosexual men and its sequelae—opportunistic infections, Kaposi's sarcoma and other malignancies." *Cancer Treat. Rep.* 66 (1982):1391–1395.

Levy, J. A. "Mysteries of HIV: Challenges for therapy and prevention." *Nature* (Lond.) 333 (1988a):519–522.

Levy, J. A. "The transmission of AIDS: The case of infected cell." *J. Amer. Med. Ass.* 259 (1988b):3036–3039.

Levy, J. A., Hoffmann, A. D., Kramer, S. M., et al. "Isolation of lymphocytopathic retroviruses from San Francisco patients with AIDS." *Science* (Wash.) 225 (1984): 840–842.

Levy, J. A., Hollander, H., Shimabukuro, J., et al. "Isolation of AIDS-associated retroviruses from cerebrospinal fluid and brain of patients with neurological symptoms." *Lancet* 2 (1985):286–288.

Levy, J. A., Pan, L. Z., Beth-Giraldo, E., et al. "Absence of antibodies to the human immunodeficiency virus in sera from Africa prior to 1975." *Proc. Natl. Acad. Sci. USA* 83 (1986):7935–7937.

Li, W. H., Tanimura, M., and Sharp, P. M. "Rates and dates of divergence between AIDS virus nucleotide sequences." *Mol. Biol. Evol.* 5 (1988):313–330.

Liautaud, B., Laroche, C., Duvivier, J., et al. "Le sarcome de Kaposi (maladie de Kaposi) est-il fréquent en Haïti." 18e Congrès des Médecins Francophones de l'Hémisphère Américain (Port-au-Prince), 1982.

Liautaud, B., Laroche, C., Duvivier, J., et al. "Le sarcome de Kaposi en Haïti: Foyer méconnu ou récemment apparu?" *Ann. Derm. Ven.* 110 (1983):213–219.

Liebmann-Smith, R. *The Question of AIDS.* New York, N.Y. Academy of Sciences, 1985.

Lifson, A. R. "Do alternative modes for transmission of human immunodeficiency virus exist? A review." *J. Amer. Med. Ass.* 259 (1988):1353–1356.

Lifson, A. R., Rutherford, G. W., and Jaffe, H. W. "The natural history of human immunodeficiency virus infection." *J. Infect. Dis.* 158 (1988):1360–1367.

Lindboe, C. F., Froland, S. S., Wefring, K. W., et al. "Autopsy findings in three family members with a presumably acquired immunodeficiency syndrome of unknown origin." *Acta Path. Microb. Immun. Scand.* 94 (1986):117–123.

Lissen, E., Wichmann, I., Jimenez, J. M., et al. "AIDS in haemophilia patients in Spain." *Lancet* 1 (1983):992–993.

Loche, M., and Mach, B. "Identification of HIV-infected seronegative individuals by a direct diagnostic test based on hybridisation to amplified viral DNA." *Lancet* 2 (1988):418–421.

London, W. T., Sever, J. L., Madden, D. L., et al. "Experimental transmission of simian acquired immunodeficiency syndrome (SAIDS) and Kaposi-like skin lesions." *Lancet* 2 (1983):869–873.

Lowenstein, W., Le Jeunne, C., Dormont, D., et al. "Infection par le virus LAV chez l'héroïnomanes." *Presse Méd.* 15 (1986):1828–1829.

Lowenstine, L. J., Pedersen, N. C., Higgins, J., et al. "Seroepidemiologic survey of captive Old World primates for antibodies to human and simian retroviruses, and isolation of a lentivirus from sooty mangabeys (Cercocebus atys)." *Intern. J. Cancer* 38 (1986):563–574.

Luft, B. J., Conley, F., Remington, J. S., et al. "Outbreak of central-nervous-system toxoplasmosis in Western Europe and North America." *Lancet* 1 (1983):781–783.

Luzzi, G., Aiuti, F., Rezza, G., et al. "Italian HIV-infection updated." *Nature* (Lond.) 328 (1987):385–386.

Lwoff, A. "Lysogeny." *Bact. Rev.* 17 (1953):269–337.

Lwoff, A. "The concept of virus." *J. Gen. Microb.* 57 (1958):239–253.

Lwoff, A. *L'ordre biologique*. Paris, Laffont, 1969.

Lyons, H. A., Vinijchaikul, K., and Hennigar, G. R. "Pneumocystis carinii pneumonia unassociated with other disease." *Arch. Int. Med.* 108 (1961):929–936.

MacArthur, W. "The plague of Athens." *Bull. Hist. Med.* 32 (1958):242–246.

Machin, S. J., McVerry, B. A., Cheingsong-Popov, R., et al. "Seroconversion for HTLV-III since 1980 in British haemophiliacs." *Lancet* 1 (1985):336.

McClure, M. A., Johnson, M. S., Feng, D. F., et al. "Sequence comparisons of retroviral proteins: Relative rates of change and general phylogeny." *Proc. Natl. Acad. Sci. USA* 85 (1988):2469–2473.

McClure, M. A., and Weiss, R. A. "Human immunodeficiency virus and related viruses." *Curr. Top. AIDS.* 1 (1987):95–117.

McDade, J., et al. "Legionnaire's disease: Isolation of a bacterium and demonstration of its role in other respiratory diseases." *New Engl. J. Med.* 297 (1977):1197–1203.

McDonald, M., Hamilton, J. D., and Durack, D. T. "Hepatitis B surface antigen could harbour the infective agent of AIDS." *Lancet* 2 (1983):882–884.

McNeill, W. H. *Plagues and Peoples*. Garden City, N.Y., Anchor Press and Doubleday, 1976.

McNicol, L. A., and Doetsch, R. N. "A hypothesis accounting for the origin of pandemic cholera: A retrograde analysis." *Persp. Biol. Med.* 26 (1983):547–552.

Madden, D. L., Tzan, N. R., Roman, G. C., et al. "HIV and HTLV-I antibody studies. Pregnant women in the 1960s, patients with AIDS, homosexuals and individuals with tropical spastic paralysis." *Yale J. Biol. Med.* 60 (1987):569–574.

Maddon, P. J., Dalgleish, A. G., McDougal, S. J., et al. "The T4 gene encodes the AIDS virus receptor and is expressed in the immune system and in the brain." *Cell* 47 (1986):333–348.

Madhok, R., Melbye, M., Lowe, G.D.O., et al. "HTLV-III antibody in sequential plasma samples from haemophiliacs, 1974–1984." *Lancet* 1 (1985):524–525.

Malebranche, R., Arnoux, E., Guérin, J. M., et al. "Acquired immunodeficiency syndrome with severe gastro-intestinal manifestations in Haiti." *Lancet* 2 (1983): 873–878.

Mann, J. *Le Tableau mondial du SIDA*. Geneva, Organisation Mondiale de la Santé, 1988.

Mann, J., Chin, F., Piot, P. and Quinn, T. "The international epidemiology of AIDS." *Scient. Amer.* 259, no. 4 (1988):82–89.

Mann, J., Francis, H., Quinn, T., et al. "Surveillance for AIDS in a Central African city, Kinshasa, Zaire." *J. Amer. Med. Ass.* 255 (1986):3255–3259.

Mann, J., Kapita, B., Colebunders, R., et al. "Natural history of LAV/HTLV-III infection in Zaïre." *Lancet* 2 (1986):707–709.

Mann, J., Snider, D. E., Francis, H., et al. "Association between HTLV-III/LAV infection and tuberculosis in Zaire." *J. Amer. Med. Ass.* 256 (1986):346.

Manzari, V., Fazio, V. M., Martinotti, S., et al. "Human T-cell leukemia/lymphoma virus (HTLV-1) DNA: Detection in Italy in a lymphoma and in a Kaposi sarcoma patient." *Intern. J. Cancer* 34 (1984):891–892.

Manzari, V., Gradilone, A., Barillari, G., et al. "HTLV-I is endemic in Southern Italy: Detection of the first infectious cluster in a white population." *Int. J. Cancer* 36 (1985):557–559.

Margulis, L., and Sagan, D. *Microcosmos: Four Billion Years of Evolution from Our Microbial Ancestors.* New York, Summit Books, 1986.

Mariani, G. "Sarkomatosis Kaposi mit besonderer Berücksichtigung der viszeralen Lokalisationen." *Arch. Derm. Syphil.* 98 (1909):267–300.

Marlink, R. G., and Essex, M. "Africa and the biology of human immunodeficiency virus." *J. Amer. Med. Ass.* 257 (1987):2632–2633.

Marmor, M., Friedman-Kien, A. E., Laubenstein, L., et al. "Risk factors for Kaposi's sarcoma in homosexual men." *Lancet* 1 (1982):1083–1087.

Marmor, M., Weiss, L. R., Lyden, M., et al. "Possible female-to-female transmission of human immunodeficiency virus." *Ann. Intern. Med.* 105 (1986):969.

Marotta, T. *The Politics of Homosexuality.* Boston, Houghton Mifflin, 1981.

Martin, J., ed. *Faire face au sida.* Paris, Favre, 1988.

Martin, M. A., Bryan, T., Rasheed, S., and Khan, A. S. "Identification and cloning of endogenous retroviral sequences present in human DNA." *Proc. Natl. Acad. Sci. USA* 78 (1981).

Martini, G. A., and Siegert, R., eds. *Marburg Virus Disease.* Berlin, Springer, 1971.

Marwick, C. "AIDS-associated virus yields data to intensifying scientific study." *J. Amer. Med. Ass.* 254 (1985):2865–2870.

Marx, J. L. "New disease baffles medical community." *Science* (Wash.) 217 (1982):618–621.

Marx, J. L. "AIDS virus has new name—perhaps." *Science* (Wash.) 232 (1986):699–700.

Marx, P. A., Maul, D. H., Osborn, K. G., et al. "Simian A.I.D.S.: Isolation of a type D retrovirus and transmission of the disease." *Science* (Wash.) 223 (1984):1083–1086.

Master, S. P., Taylor, J. F., Kyalwazi, S. K., et al. "Immunological studies in Kaposi's sarcoma in Uganda." *Brit. Med. J.* 1 (1970):600–602.

Masters, W. H., Johnson, E., and Kolodny, R. C. *Crisis: Heterosexual Behavior in the Age of AIDS.* New York, Grove Press, 1988.

Masur, H., Michelis, M. A., Greene, J., et al. "An outbreak of community-acquired Pneumocystis carinii pneumonia: Initial manifestation of cellular immune dysfunction." *New Engl. J. Med.* 305 (1981):1431–1438.

Masur, H., Michelis, M. A., Wormser, G. P., et al. "Opportunistic infection in previously healthy women: Initial manifestations of a community-acquired cellular immunodeficiency." *Ann. Int. Med.* 97 (1982):533–539.

Mathez, D., Leibowitch, J., Matheron, S., et al. "Antibodies to HTLV-III associated antigens in populations exposed to AIDS virus in France." *Lancet* 2 (1984):460.

Mathez, D., Leibowitch, J., Sultan, Y., et al. "LAV/HTLV-III seroconversion and disease in haemophiliacs treated in France." *New Engl. J. Med.* 314 (1986):118–119.

Matthews, T. J., and Bolognesi, D. P. "AIDS vaccines." *Scient. American* 259, no. 4 (1988):120–127.

Matthews, T. J., Weinhoild, K. J., Lyerly, H. K., et al. "Interaction between the human T-cell lymphotropic virus type IIIB envelope glycoprotein gp120 and the surface antigen CD4." *Proc. Natl. Acad. Sci. USA* 84 (1987):5424–5428.

Maurice, J. "AIDS investigators identify second retrovirus." *J. Amer. Med. Ass.* 250 (1983a):1010–1011.

Maurice, J., "Human T-cell leukemia virus still suspected in AIDS." *J. Amer. Med. Ass.* 250 (1983b):1015 and 1021.

May, R. M., and Anderson, R. M. "Transmission dynamics of HIV infection." *Nature* (Lond.) 326 (1987):137–142.

Mayer, K. H., and DeGruttola, V. "Human immunodeficiency virus and oral intercourse." *Ann. Intern. Med.* 107 (1987):428–429.

Medley, G. F., Anderson, R. M., Cox, D. R., et al. "Incubation period of AIDS in patients infected via blood transfusion." *Nature* (Lond.) 328 (1987):719–721.

Medvedev, Zh. A. "AIDS virus infection: A Soviet view of its origin." *J. Roy. Soc. Med.* 79 (1986):494–495. With comments from J. Seale.

Melbye, M., Biggar, R. J., Chermann, J. C., and Montagnier, L. "High prevalence of lymphadenopathy virus (LAV) in European haemophiliacs." *Lancet* 2 (1984):40–41.

Melbye, M., Froebel, K. S., Mahdok, R., et al. "HTLV-III seropositivity in European hemophiliacs exposed to factor VIII concentrate imported from the USA." *Lancet* 2 (1984):1444–1446.

Melbye, M., Njelesani, E. K., Bayley, A., et al. "Evidence for heterosexual transmission and clinical manifestations of human immunodeficiency virus infection and related conditions in Lusaka, Zambia." *Lancet* 2 (1986):1113–1115.

Melief, C.J.M., and Goudsmit, J. "Transmission of lymphotropic retroviruses (HTLV-I and LAV/HTLV-III) by blood transfusion and blood products." *Vox Sang.* 50 (1986):1–11.

Mérieux, C., ed. *Sida: Epidémies et sociétés* (Compte rendu de la réunion organisée aux Pensières, Annecy). Lyons, Fondation Mérieux, 1987.

Mertz, B. "HIV vaccine approved for clinical trials." *J. Amer. Med. Ass.* 258 (1987):1433–1434.

Messiah, A. "Etude cas-témoins du S.I.D.A. chez les homosexuels masculins en France." Thèse, Paris, 1987.

Messiah, A., Mary, J. Y., Brunet, J. B., et al. "Risk factors for AIDS among homosexual men in a moderate incidence area." *Intern. J. Epidem.* 16 (1987):482–484.

Meyer, K. B., and Paulker, S. G. "Can we afford the false positive rate?" *New Engl. J. Med.* 317 (1987):238–242.

Mitsuya, H., and Broder, S. "Inhibition of the in vitro infectivity and cytopathic effect of human T-lymphotropic virus type III/lymphadenopathy associated virus (HTLV-III/LAV) by 2'3'-di-deoxynucleosides." *Proc. Natl. Acad. Sci. USA* 83 (1986): 1911.

Mitsuya, H., and Broder, S. "Strategies for antiviral therapy." *Nature* (Lond.) 325 (1987):773–775.

Miyoshi, I., Yoshimoto, S., Fujishita, M., et al. "Natural adult T-cell leukemia virus infection in African monkeys." *Lancet* 2 (1982):658.

Miyoshi, I., Yoshimoto, S., Fujishita, M., et al. "Isolation in a culture of a type C virus from a Japanese monkey seropositive to adult T-cell leukemia-associated antigens." *Gann* 74 (1983):323–326.

Molbak, K., Lauritzen, E., Fernandes, D., et al. "Antibodies to HTLV-IV associated with chronic, fatal illness resembling 'slim' disease." *Lancet* 2 (1986):1214–1215.

Mollaret, H. H. "Interprétation socio-écologique de l'apparition des maladies réellement nouvelles." In C. Mérieux, ed. *Sida: Épidémies et sociétés* (Compte rendu de la réunion organisée aux Pensières, Annecy), pp. 108–114. Lyons, Fondation Mérieux, 1987.

Monath, T. P. "Lassa fever: Review of its epidemiology and epizootiology." *Bull. WHO* 52 (1975):577–592.

Montagnier, L. "AIDS priority." *Nature* (Lond.) 310 (1984):446.

Montagnier, L. "Lymphadenopathy-associated virus: From molecular biology to pathogenicity." *Ann. Int. Med.* 103 (1985):689–693.

Montagnier, L. *Vaincre le SIDA. Entretiens avec Pierre Bourget.* Paris, Editions Cana, 1986.

Montagnier, L. "Le virus de l'immunodeficience humaine." *Rev. Prat.* 37 (1987): 2553–2558.

Montagnier, L. "Origin and evolution of HIVs and their role in AIDS pathogenesis." *J. Acq. Immun. Def. Syn.* 1 (1988):517–520.

Montagnier, L., et al. *SIDA. Des spécialistes répondent à vos questions.* Paris, Fondation intern. pour l'information scientifique, 1983.

Montagnier, L., Dauguet, C., Axler, C., et al. "A new type of retrovirus isolated from patients presenting with lymphadenopathy and acquired immune deficiency syndrome: Structural and antigenic relatedness with equine infectious anaemia virus." *Ann. Virol.* (Inst. Pasteur) 135E (1984):119–134.

Montagnier, L., Gruest, J., Chamaret, S., et al. "Adaptation of lymphadenopathy associated virus (LAV) to replication in EBV-transformed B lymphoblastoid cell lines." *Science* (Wash.) 225 (1984):63–66.

Montagnier, L., Krust, B., CLAVel, F., et al. "Identification and antigenicity of the major envelope glycoprotein of lymphadenopathy associated virus (LAV)." *Virology* 144 (1985):283–289.

Moore, J. D., Cone, E. J., and Alexander, S. S., Jr. "HTLV-III seropositivity in 1971–1972: Parenteral drug abusers—a case of false positives or evidence of viral exposure?" *New Engl. J. Med.* 314 (1985):1387–1388.

Morgan, D. A., Ruscetti, F. W., and Gallo, R. C. "Selective in vitro growth of T-lymphocytes from normal human bone marrow." *Science* (Wash.) 193 (1976): 1007–1008.

Moses, P. and Moses, J. "Haiti and the acquired immunodeficiency syndrome." *Ann. Int. Med.* 99 (1983):565.

Moskowitz, L. B., Kory, P., Chan, J. C., et al. "Unusual causes of death in Haitians residing in Miami." *J. Amer. Med. Ass.* 250 (1983):1187.

Moss, A. R. "Predicting who will progress to AIDS." *Brit. Med. J.* 297 (1988):1067–1068.

Moss, A. R., Bacchetti, P., Gorman, M., et al. "AIDS in the 'gay' areas of San Francisco." *Lancet* 1 (1983):923–924.

Moss, A. R., Osmond, D., Bacchetti, P., et al. "Risk factors for AIDS and HIV seropositivity in homosexual men." *Amer. J. Epid.* 125 (1987):1035–104.

Muesing, M. A., Smith, D. M., Cabradilla, C. D., et al. "Nucleic acid structure and expression of the human AIDS/lymphadenopathy retrovirus (ARV-2)." *Nature* (Lond.) 313 (1985):450–458.

Mugler, C. "Démocrite et le danger de l'irradiation cosmique." *Rev. Hist. Sci.* 20 (1967):221–228.

Mulder, C. "A case of mistaken non-identity." *Nature* (Lond.) 331 (1988):562–563.

Mulder, C. "Human AIDS virus not from monkeys." *Nature* (Lond.) 333 (1988):396.

Murakawa, G. J., Zaia, J. A., Spallone, P. A., et al. "Direct detection of HIV-1 RNA from AIDS and ARC patient sample." DNA 7 (1988):287–295.

Murphey-Corb, M., Martin, L. N., Rangan, S. R., et al. "Isolation of an HTLV-III related retrovirus from macaques with simian AIDS and its possible origin in asymptomatic mangabeys." *Nature* (Lond.) 321 (1986):435–437.

Murray, J. F. "Kaposi's hemangiosarcoma in the Bantu." *Leech* 22 (1952):33–36.

Myers, G., Josephs, S. S., Rabson, A. B., et al. *Human Retroviruses and AIDS 1987.* Washington, D.C., AIDS Program of the NIAID, 1987.

Nahmias, A. J., Weiss, J., Yao, X., et al. "Evidence for human infection with an HTLV-III/LAV-like virus in Central Africa, 1959." *Lancet* 1 (1986):1279–1280.

Navarro, C., and Hagstrom, J.W.C. "Opportunistic infection and Kaposi's sarcoma in homosexual men." *Lancet* 1 (1982):933.

Navia, B. A., Cho, E. S., Petito, C. K., et al. "The AIDS dementia complex." *Ann. Neurol.* 19 (1986):517–535.

Nei, M. *Molecular Evolutionary Genetics.* New York, Columbia University Press, 1987.

Neisson-Vernant, C., Arfi, S., Mathez, D., et al. "Needlestick HIV seroconversion in a nurse." *Lancet* 2 (1986):218.

Neppert, J., Gohring, S., Schneider, W., et al. "No evidence of LAV infection in the Republic of Liberia, West Africa, in the year 1973." *Blut* 53 (1986):115–117.

Neumann, H. H. "Use of steroid creams as possible cause of immunosuppression in homosexuals." *New Engl. J. Med.* 306 (1982):935.

Neustadt, R., and Fineberg, H. V. *The Epidemic That Never Was: Policy Making in the Swine Flu Scare.* New York, Vintage Books, 1983.

Newmark, P. "AIDS in an African context." *Nature* (Lond.) 324 (1986):611.

Nichols, E. K. *Mobilizing against AIDS: The Unfinished Story of a Virus.* Cambridge, Mass., Harvard University Press, 1986.

Nichols, P. W. "Letter to the Editor." *New Engl. J. Med.* 306 (1982):934–935.

Nicolle, C. *Naissance, vie et mort des maladies infectieuses*. Paris, Alcan, 1930. Revised edition: *Destin des maladies infectieuses*. Paris, 1933, and Geneva, 1961.

Noireau, F. "HIV transmission from monkey to man." *Lancet* 1 (1987):1498–1499.

Norman, C. "Patent dispute divides AIDS researchers. What is in a name. HTLV-III and LAV: Similar or identical?" *Science* (Wash.) 230 (1985):640–643.

Norman, C. "A new twist in AIDS patent fight." *Science* (Wash.) 230 (1986a):308–309.

Norman, C. "Africa and the origin of AIDS." *Science* (Wash.) 230 (1986b):1141.

Nungasser, L. G. *Epidemic of Courage: Facing AIDS in America*. New York, St. Martin's Press, 1986.

O'Day, D. M. "The risk posed by HTLV-III infected corneal donor tissue." *Amer. J. Ophthalm*. 101 (1986):246–247.

Oettle, A. G. "Geographical and racial differences in the frequency of Kaposi's sarcoma as evidence of environmental or genetic causes." *Acta Union. Intern. Contra Cancrum* 18 (1962):330–363. Also in L. V. Ackerman and J. F. Murray, *Symposium on Kaposi's Sarcoma*, pp. 17–50. New York, 1963.

Offenstadt, G., Pinta, P., Hericard, P., et al. "Multiple opportunistic infections due to AIDS in a previously healthy black woman from Zaire." *New Engl. J. Med*, 308 (1983):775.

Ohta, Y., Masuda, T., Tsujimoto, H., et al. "Isolation of simian imunodeficiency virus from African green monkeys and seroepidemiologic survey of the virus in various non-human primates." *Int. J. Cancer* 41 (1988):115–122.

Oksenhendler, E., Harzic, M., Le Roux, J. M., et al. "HIV infection with seroconversion after a superficial needlestick injury to the finger." *New Engl. J. Med*. 315 (1986):582.

Oleske, J., et al. "Acquired immunodeficiency syndrome in children." *J. Amer. Med. Ass*. 249 (1983):2345–2349.

Ollé-Goig, J. E. "Haiti and the acquired immunodeficiency syndrome." *Ann. Int. Med*. 99 (1983):565.

Olweny, C.L.M., Hutt, M.S.R., and Owor, R., eds. *Kaposi's sarcoma*. Second Kaposi's Sarcoma Symposium, Kampala, January 8–11, 1980. Basel, Karger, 1981 ("Antibiotics and Chemotherapy," vol. 29).

Oriel, J. D., and Cockburn, A. "Syphilis, where did it come from?" *Paleopath. Newsletter*, no. 6 (1974):9–12.

Ostrow, D. G. "Psychiatric consequences of AIDS: An overview." *Int. J. Neurosci*. 32 (1987):647–659.

Ostrow, D. G., Solomon, S. L., Mayer, K. H., and Haverkos, H. "Classification des manifestations cliniques de l'infection HIV chez l'adulte." *J. Amer. Med. Ass*. (French edition), special number (1987):7–20.

Otu, A. A. "Kaposi's sarcoma and HTLV-III: A study in Nigerian adult males." *J. Roy. Soc. Med*. 79 (1986):510–514.

Ou, C. Y., Kwok, S., Mitchell, S. W., et al. "DNA amplification for direct detection of HIV-1 in DNA of peripheral blood mononuclear cells." *Science* (Wash.) 239 (1988):295–297.

Owor, R., and Wamukota, W. M. "A fatal case of strongyloidiasis with Strongyloides larvae in the meninges." *Trans. Roy. Soc. Trop. Med. Hyg*. 70 (1976):497–499.

Padian, N. S. "Heterosexual transmission of acquired immunodeficiency syndrome." *Rev. Inf. Dis.* 9 (1987):947–960.

Padian, N. S., Marquis, L., Francis, D. P., et al. "Male-to-female transmission of human immunodeficiency virus." *J. Amer. Med. Ass.* 258 (1987):788–790.

Page, D. L. "Thucydides' description of the great plague of Athens." Class. Quart. 47 (1953):897–120.

Palca, J. "Settlement on AIDS finally reached between US and Pasteur." *Nature* (Lond.) 326 (1987):533.

Pandolfi, F., Manzari, V., De Rossi, G., et al. "T-helper phenotype chronic lymphocytic leukaemia and 'adult T-cell leukaemia' in Italy." *Lancet* 2 (1985):633–636.

Panem, S. *The AIDS Bureaucracy: U.S. Governement response to AIDS in First Five Years*. Cambridge, Mass., Harvard University Press, 1988.

Papaevangelou, G., Economidou, J., Kallinikos, J., et al. "Lymphadenopathy associated virus in AIDS, lymphadenopathy associated syndrome and classic Kaposi patients in Greece." *Lancet* 2 (1984):642.

Pape, J. W., Liautaud, B., Thomas, F., et al. "Characteristics of the acquired immunodeficiency syndrome in Haiti." *New Engl. J. Med.* 309 (1983):945–950.

Pape, J. W., Liautaud, B., Thomas, F., et al. "Risk factors associated with AIDS in Haiti." *Amer. J. Med. Sci.* 291 (1986):4–7.

Pauza, C. D. "HIV persistence in monocytes leads to pathogenesis and AIDS." *Cell Immunol.* 112 (1988):414–424.

Payet, M. "Les ambiguïtés du S.I.D.A." *Bull. Acad. Nat. Méd.* 170 (1986):681–688.

Peabody, B. *The Screaming Room: A Mother's Journal of Her Son's Struggle with AIDS*. San Diego, Oak Tree, 1986.

Pedersen, N. C., Ho, E., Brown, M., et al. "Isolation of a T-lymphotropic lentivirus from cats with acquired immunodeficiency." *Science* (Wash.) 235 (1987):290–293.

Penny, D. "Origins of the AIDS virus." *Nature* (Lond.) 333 (1988):494–495.

Pert, C., Hill, J. M., Ruff, M. R., et al. "Octapeptides deduced from the neuropeptide receptor-like pattern of antigen T4 in brain potently inhibit human immunodeficiency virus receptor binding and T-cell infectivity." *Proc. Natl. Acad. Sci. USA* 83 (1986): 9254–9258.

Peterman, A., and Curran, J. W. "Sexual transmission of human immunodeficiency virus." *J. Amer. Med. Ass.* 256 (1986):2222–2226.

Philippson, L. "Ueber das Sarcoma idiopathicum cutis Kaposi. Ein Beitrag zur Sarcomlehre." *Arch. Path. Anat.* 167 (1902):58–81.

Picard, O., Gorin, I., Leibowitch, J., et al. "La maladie de Kaposi. Deux observations récentes." *Presse Méd.* 45 (1982):3335–3338.

Piette, A. M., Tusseau, F., and Chapman, A. "Symptomatologie aiguë contemporaine de la primo-infection par le virus HIV." *Presse Méd.* 16 (1987):346–348.

Pinching, A. J. "AIDS and Africa: Lesson for us all." *J. Roy. Soc. Med.* 79 (1986): 501–503.

Pinching, A. J. "The acquired immune deficiency syndrome, with special reference to tuberculosis." *Tubercle* 68 (1987):65–69.

Piot, P. "Le SIDA: Un feuilleton macabre." *Rev. Épid. Santé Publ.* 34 (1986):110–111.

Piot, P., Plummer, F. A., Mhalu, F. S., et al. "AIDS: An international perspective." *Science* (Wash.) 239 (1988):573–579.

Piot, P., Plummer, F. A., Rey, M., et al. "Retrospective seroepidemiology of AIDS virus infection in Nairobi populations." In *Program and Abstracts of the International Conference on AIDS*, p. 101. Paris, 1986.

Piot, P., Quinn, T. C., Taelman, H., et al. "Acquired immunodeficiency syndrome in a heterosexual population in Zaire." *Lancet* 2 (1984):65–69.

Pitchenik, A. E., Fischl, M. A., Dickinson, G. M., et al. "Opportunistic infections and Kaposi's sarcoma among Haitians: Evidence of a new acquired immunodeficiency state." *Ann. Int. Med.* 98 (1983):277–284.

Pitchenik, A. E., Shafron, R. D., Glasser, R. M., et al. "The acquired immunodeficiency syndrome in the wife of a hemophiliac." *Ann. Int. Med.* 100 (1984):62–65.

Plata, F., and Wain-Hobson, S. "SIDA: Immunité and vaccins." *Recherche* 18 (1987):1320–1331.

Poiesz, B. J., Ruscetti, F. W., Gazdar, A. F., et al. "Detection and isolation of type C retrovirus particles from fresh and cultured lymphocytes of a patient with cutaneous T-cell lymphoma." *Proc. Natl. Acad. Sci. USA* 77 (1980):7415–7419.

Poiesz, B. J., Ruscetti, F. W., Mier, J. W., et al. "T-cell lines established from human T-lymphocytic neoplasias by direct response to T-cell growth factor." *Proc. Natl. Acad. Sci. USA* 77 (1980):6815.

Poiesz, B. J., Ruscetti, F. W., Reitz, J. S., et al. "Isolation of a new type C retrovirus (HTLV) in primary uncultured cells of a patient with Sezary T cell leukaemia." *Nature* (Lond.) 294 (1981):268–271.

Pokrovskyi, V. V., Yankina, V. I., and Pokrovskyi, V. I. "Epidemiologicheskoe rassledovanie pervogo sluchaya SPID, viyavlenogo u grazhdanina SSSR." *Zhurn. Mikrobiol. Epid. Imunolog*, no. 12 (1987):8–11.

Politzer, R. *La peste*. Geneva, O.M.S., 1954.

Pollak, M. *Les homosexuels et les sida. Sociologie d'une épidémie*. Paris, Métailié, 1988.

Poon, M. C., Landay, A., Prasthofer, E. F., et al. "Acquired immunodeficiency syndrome with Pneumocystis carinii pneumonia and Mycobacterium avium-intracellulare infection in a previously healthy patient with classical hemophilia." *Ann. Int. Med.* 98 (1983):287–290.

Popovic, M., Read-Connole, E., and Gallo, R. C. "T-4 positive neoplastic cell lines susceptible to and permissive for HTLV-III." *Lancet* 2 (1984):1472–1473.

Popovic, M., Sarin, P. S., Robert-Guroff, M., et al. "Isolation and transmission of human retrovirus (human T-cell leukemia virus)." *Science* (Wash.) 219 (1983):856–859.

Popovic, M., Sarngadharan, M. G., Read, E., and Gallo, R. C. "A method for detection, isolation and continuous production of cytopathic retroviruses (HTLV-III) from patients with AIDS and pre-AIDS." *Science* (Wash.) 224 (1984):497–500.

Predöhl, A. *Die Geschichte der Tuberkulose*. Hamburg, Voss, 1888.

Presidential Commission. Report of the Presidential Commission on the Human Immunodeficiency Virus Epidemic. Washington, D.C., 1988.

Preuss, J. *Biblisch-talmudische Medizin*. Berlin, Karger, 1913.

Price, R. W., Brew, B., Sidtis, J., et al. "The brain in AIDS: Central nervous system

HIV-1 infection and AIDS dementia complex.'' *Science* (Wash.) 239 (1988):586–592.

Quenum, A. "La maladie de Kaposi en Afrique Noire." Thèse de Médecine, Bordeaux, 1957.

Quenum, A., and Camain, R. "Les aspects africains de la maladie de Kaposi, réticulopathie maligne systématisée." *Ann. Anat. Path.* 3 (1958):337–368.

Quetel, C. *Le mal de Naples. Histoire de la syphilis.* Paris, Seghers, 1986.

Quinn, T. C., Mann, J., Curran, J. W. and Piot, P. "AIDS in Africa: An epidemiologic paradigm." *Science* (Wash.) 234 (1986):955–963.

Quinn, T. C., Piot, P., McCormick, J. B., et al. "Serologic and immunologic studies in patients with AIDS in North America and Africa: The potential role of infectious agents as cofactors in human immunodeficiency virus infection." *J. Amer. Med. Ass.* 257 (1987):2617–2621.

Rabson, A. B., and Martin, M. A. "Molecular organization of the AIDS retrovirus." *Cell* 40 (1985):45–49.

Ragni, M. V., Lewis, J. H., Spero, J. A., and Bontempo, F. A. "Acquired immunodeficiency-like syndrome in two haemophiliacs." *Lancet* 1 (1983):213–214.

Ramsey, R. B., Palmer, E. L., McDougal, J. S., et al. "Antibody to lymphadenopathy-associated virus in haemophiliacs with and without AIDS." *Lancet* 2 (1984): 397–398.

Ranki, A., Valle, S. L., Krohn, M., et al. "Long latency precedes overt seroconversion in sexually transmitted human immunodeficiency virus infection." *Lancet* 2 (1987):589–593.

Ratner, L., Haseltine, W., Patarca, R., et al. "Complete nucleotide sequence of the AIDS virus, HTLV-III." *Nature* (Lond.) 313 (1985):227–284.

Ravenholt, R. T. "Role of hepatitis B virus in acquired immunodeficiency syndrome." *Lancet* 2 (1983):885–886.

Ravisse, P., Reynaud, R., Depoux, R., and Salles, P. "Sur le premier cas de cryptococcose découvert en A.E.F." *Presse Méd.* 18 (1959):727–728.

Raymond, C. A. "Evidence mounts that other infections may trigger AIDS virus replication." *J. Amer. Med. Ass.* 257 (1987):2875.

Redfield, R. R., and Burke, D. S. "Shadow on the land: HIV infection." *Viral Immunology* 1 (1987):69–81.

Redfield, R. R. and Burke, D. S. "HIV infection: The clinical picture." *Scient. Amer.* 259, no. 4 (1988):90–98.

Redfield, R. R., Markham, P. D., Salahuddin, S. Z., et al. "Frequent transmission of HTLV-III among spouses of patients with AIDS-related complex and AIDS." *J. Amer. Med. Ass.* 253 (1985a):1571–1573.

Redfield, R. R., Markham, P. D., Salahuddin, S. Z., et al. "Heterosexually acquired HTLV-III/LAV disease (AIDS related complex and AIDS): Epidemiologic evidence for female-to-male transmision." *J. Amer. Med. Ass.* 254 (1985b):2094–2096.

Redfield, R. R., Wright, D. C., Tramont, E. C., et al. "The Walter Reed staging classification for HTLV-III/LAV infection." *New Engl. J. Med.* 314 (1986):131–132.

Reger, K.-H., and Haimhausen, P. *SIDA: Nouveau fléau du XXe siècle.* Monaco, SIP, 1986.

Rémy, F., and Bardéche, F. *Le sida. Ce que tous les parents doivent savoir.* Paris, Santé Magazine, 1986.

Revel, J. F. "Sida: Les mots meurtriers." *Le Point,* July 13, 1987, pp. 30–31.

Rey, F., Salaun, D., Lesbordes, J. L., et al. "HIV-I and HIV-II double infection in Central African Republic." *Lancet* 2 (1986):1391.

Rey, M. A., Girard, P. M., Harzic, M., et al. "HIV-1 and HIV-2 double infection in French homosexual males with AIDS-related complex (Paris, 1985)." *Lancet* 1 (1987):388–389.

Reynes, J., Quaranta, J. F., Pesce, A., et al. "Prévalence élevée des anticorps anti-LAV/HTLV-III dans une population d'héroïnomanes niçois." *Presse Méd.* 14 (1985):2348–2349.

Rezza, G., Ippolito, G., Marasca, G., and Greco, D. "AIDS in Italy." *Lancet* 2 (1984):642.

Rippinger, L. "A propos de quelques noms de maladies chez Celse et Scribonius Largus." In *Etudes de linguistique générale et de linguistique latine* (Mélanges Serbat), pp. 207–218. Paris, 1987.

Risse, G. B. "Perspectives: AIDS and history." *USCF Mag.* 9 (1986):53.

Robert-Guroff, M., Markham, P., Popovic, M., and Gallo, R. C. "Isolation, characterization and biological effects of the first human retroviruses: The human T-lymphotropic family." *Current Topics Microb. Immun.* 115 (1985):7–27.

Roberts, R. S. "A consideration of the nature of the English sweating sickness." *Med. Hist.* 9 (1965):385–389.

Rodriquez, L., Dewhurst, S., Sinangil, F., et al. "Antibodies to HTLV-III/LAV among aboriginal Amazonian Indians in Venezuela." *Lancet* 2 (1985):1098–1100.

Rogan, E., Jr., Jewell, L. D., Mielke, B. W., et al. "A case of acquired immunodeficiency syndrome before 1980." *Canad. Med. Ass. J.* 137 (1987):637–638.

Rogers, M. F. "AIDS in children: A review of the clinical, epidemiologic and public health aspects." *Pediatr. Inf. Dis.* 4 (1985):230–236.

Rogers, M. F., Morens, D. M., Stewart, J. A., et al. "National case-control study of Kaposi's sarcoma and Pneumocystis carinii pneumonia in homosexual men: Part 2, Laboratory results." *Ann. Int. Med.* 99 (1983):151–158.

Ronchese, F. "Kaposi's sarcoma. An overlooked essay of 1882." *A.M.A. Arch. Derm.* 77 (1958):542–545.

Rosenblum, M. L., Levy, R. M., and Bredesen, D. E. *AIDS and the Nervous System.* New York, Raven, 1988.

Rosquist, R., Skurnik, M., and Wolf-Watz, H. "Increased virulence of Yersinia pseudotuberculosis by two independent mutations." *Nature* (Lond.) 334 (1988):522–525.

Rossi, G. B., Verani, P., Macchi, B., et al. "Recovery of HIV-related retroviruses from Italian patients with AIDS or AIDS-related complex and from asymptomatic at-risk individuals." *Ann. N.Y. Acad. Sci.* 511 (1987):390–400.

Rothenberg, R., Woelfel, M., Stoneburner, R., et al. "Survival with the acquired immunodeficiency syndrome: Experience with 5833 cases in New York City." *New Engl. J. Med.* 317 (1987):1297–1302.

Rothman, S. "Some remarks on Moricz Kaposi and on the history of Kaposi's sarcoma." *Acta Union. Intern. Contra Cancrum* 18 (1962a):322–325. Also in L. V.

Ackerman and J. F. Murray, *Symposium on Kaposi's Sarcoma*, pp. 9–12. New York, 1963.

Rothman, S. "Remarks on sex, age and racial distribution of Kaposi's sarcoma and on possible pathogenic factors." *Acta Union. Intern. Contra Cancrum* 18 (1962b):326–329. Also in L. V. Ackerman and J. F. Murray, *Symposium on Kaposi's Sarcoma*, pp. 13–16. New York, 1963.

Rothman, S. "Some clinical aspects of Kaposi's sarcoma in the European and North American population." *Acta Union. Intern. Contra Cancrum* 18 (1962c):364–372.

Rous, F. P. "A transmissible avian neoplasma (sarcoma of the common fowl)." *J. Exp. Med.* 12 and 13 (1910, 1911): 696–705, 397–411.

Roux, E. "Sur les microbes dits invisibles." *Bull. Inst. Pasteur* 1 (1903):7–12, 49–56.

Rouzioux, C., Brun-Vézinet, F., Couroucé, A. M., et al. "Immunoglobulin G antibodies to lymphadenopathy-associated virus in differently treated French and Belgian hemophiliacs." *Ann. Int. Med.* 102 (1985):476–479.

Rozenbaum, W. "Sarcome de Kaposi et S.I.D.A." *Bull. Soc. Path. Exot.* 77 (1984): 589–591.

Rozenbaum, W., and Gharakhanian, S. "Aspects cliniques de l'infection par le virus LAV/HTLV-III." *Concours Méd.* 108 (1986):2113–2116.

Rozenbaum, W., Coulaud, J.-P., Saimot, A. G., et al. "Multiple opportunistic infection in a male homosexual in France." *Lancet* 1 (1982):572–573.

Rozenbaum, W., Dormont, D., Spire, B., et al. "Antimoniotungstate (HPA 23) treatment of three patients with AIDS and one with prodrome." *Lancet* 1 (1985):450–451.

Rozenbaum, W., Gharakhanian, S., Cardon, B., et al. "HIV transmission by oral sex." *Lancet* 1 (1988):1395.

Rozenbaum, W., Klatzmann, D., Mayaud, C., et al. "Syndrome d'immunodépression acquise chez 4 homosexuels." *Presse Méd.* 12 (1983):1149–1154.

Rozenbaum, W., Seux, D., and Kouchner, A. *Sida, réalités et fantasmes*. Paris, P.O.L., 1984.

Rubin, H. "Is HIV the causative factor in AIDS?" *Nature* (Lond.) 334 (1988):201.

Rubinstein, A., Sicklick, M., Gupta, A., et al. "Acquired immunodeficiency with reversed T4/T8 ratios in infants born to promiscuous and drug-addicted mothers." *J. Amer. Med. Ass.* 249 (1983):2350–2356.

Rublowsky, J. *The Stoned Age: A History of Drugs in America*. New York, Putnam, 1974.

Russel, W. C., and Almond, J. W. *Molecular Basis of Virus Diseases*. Cambridge, Eng., Cambridge University Press, 1987.

Saag, M. S., Hahn, G. B., Gibbons, J., et al. "Extensive variation of human immunodeficiency virus type 1 in vivo." *Nature* (Lond.) 334 (1988):440–444.

Safai, B., and Good, R. A. "Kaposi's sarcoma: A review and recent developments." *Clin. Bull.* 10 (1980):62–69.

Safai, B., Gallo, R. C., Popovic, M., et al. "Seroepidemiological studies of human T-lymphotropic retrovirus type III in acquired immunodeficiency syndrome." *Lancet* 1 (1984):1438–1440.

Saimot, A. G., Coulaud, J. P., Mechali, D., et al. "HIV-2 in a Portuguese man with AIDS (Paris, 1978) who had served in Angola in 1968–1974." *Lancet* 1 (1987):688.

Salahuddin, Z. S., Ablashi, D. V., Markham, P. D., et al. "Isolation of a new virus, HBLV, in patients with lymphoproliferative disorders." *Science* (Wash.) 234 (1986):596–601.

Salahuddin, Z. S., Markham, P. D., Popovic, M., et al. "Isolation of infectious T-cell leukemia/lymphoma virus type III (HTLV-III) from patients with acquired immunodeficiency syndrome (AIDS) or AIDS-related complex (ARC) and from healthy carriers: A study of risk groupes and tissue sources." *Proc. Natl. Acad. Sci. USA* 82 (1985):5530–5534.

Salbaing, J. "Contribution à l'étude d'immunodépression acquise (SIDA). A propos de neuf cas, en unité de soins intensifs de l'hôpital Claude Bernard." Thèse de Médecine, Paris, 1983.

Sanchez-Pescador, R., Power, M. D., Barr, P., et al. "Nucleotide sequence and expression of an AIDS-associated retrovirus (ARV-2)." *Science* (Wash.) 227 (1985): 484–492.

Sarngadharan, M. G., Popovic, M., Bruch, L., et al. "Antibodies reactive with human T-lymphotropic retroviruses (HTLV-III) in the serum of patients with AIDS." *Science* (Wash.) 224 (1984):506–508.

Saxinger, W. C., Levine, P. H., Dean, A. G., et al. "Evidence for exposure to HTLV-III in Uganda before 1973." *Science* (Wash.) 227 (1985):1036–1038.

Saxinger, W. C., Levine, P. H., Lange-Wantzin, G., and Gallo, R. C. "Unique pattern of HTLV-III (AIDS-related) antigen recognition by sera from African children in Uganda (1972)." *Cancer Research* 45, suppl. (1985):4624–4626,.

Schmidt, C. D. "The group-fantasy origins of AIDS." J. Psychohist. 12 (1984):37–78.

Schmitt, D., and Thivolet, J. "Cellules de Langerhans et VIH." *Rétrovirus* 1 (1988): 85–96.

Schonell, M. E., Crofton, J. W., Stuart, A. E., and Wallace, A. "Disseminated infection with Mycobacterium avium." *Tubercle* 49 (1968):12–30.

Schüpbach, J. "First isolation of HTLV-III." *Nature* (Lond.) 321 (1986):119–120.

Schüpbach, J., Popovic, M., Gilden, R. V., Gonda, M. A., Sarndgadharan, M. G., and Gallo, R. C. "Serological analysis of a subgroup of human T-lymphotropic retroviruses (HTLV-III) associated with AIDS." *Science* (Wash.) 224 (1984):503–505.

Schwartz, J. S., Dans, P. E., and Kinosian, B. P. "Human immunodeficiency virus test: Evaluation, performance and use." *J. Amer. Med. Ass.* 259 (1988):2574–2579.

Scott, A. *Pirates of the Cell: The Story of Viruses from Molecule to Microbe.* Oxford, Blackwell, 1987.

Seagrave, K. H. "Kaposi's disease, report of a case with unusual visceral manifestations." *Radiology* 51 (1948):248–251.

Seale, J. "AIDS virus infection: Prognosis and transmission." *J. Roy. Soc. Med.* 78 (1985):613–615.

Seale, J. R. "Origins of the AIDS viruses, HIV-1 and HIV-2: Fact or fiction?" *J. Roy. Soc. Med.* 81 (1988):537–539.

Seale, J. R., and Medvedev, Z. A. "Origin and transmission of AIDS: Multi-use hypodermics and the threat to the Soviet Union." *J. Roy. Soc. Med.* 80 (1987):301–304.

Seligmann, J., Hager, M. and Seward, D. "Tracing the origin of AIDS." *Newsweek*, May 7, 1984, pp. 62–63.

Selik, R. M., Haverkos, H. W., and Curran, J. W. "Acquired immunodeficiency syndrome (AIDS), trends in the United States, 1978–1982." *Amer. J. Med.* 76 (1984):493–500.

Selwyn, P. A. "AIDS: What is known. I. History and immunovirology." *Hosp. Pract.* 21 (1986):67–76.

Serwadda, D., Mugerwa, R. D., Sewankambo, N. K., et al. "Slim disease: A new disease in Uganda and its association with HTLV-III/LAV infection." *Lancet* 2 (1985):849–852.

Seux, D. "Les aspects psychologiques et psychiatriques du SIDA." *Concours Méd.* 106 (1984):779–782.

Sharer, L. R., Epstein, L. G., Cho, E. S., et al. "Pathologic features of AIDS encephalopathy in children: Evidence for LAV/HTLV-III infection of brain." *Hum. Pathol.* 17 (1986):271–284.

Sharp, P. M., and Li, W. H. "Understanding the origins of AIDS viruses." *Nature* (Lond.) 33 (1988):315.

Shaw, G. M., Harper, M. E., Hahn, B. H., et al. "HTLV-III infection in brains of children and adults with AIDS encephalopathy." *Science* (Wash.) 227 (1985):177–182.

Shearer, G. M., and Hurtenbach, U. "Is sperm immunosuppresive in homosexuals and vasectomized men?" *Immunol. Today* 3 (1982):153–154.

Shearer, G. M., and Rabson, A. S. "Semen and AIDS." *Nature* (Lond.) (1984):308, 230.

Sher, R., Antunes, S., Reid, B., et al. "Seroepidemiology of HIV-1 in Africa from 1970 to 1974." *New Eng. Med. J.* 317 (1987):450–457.

Shiels, R. A. "A history of Kaposi's sarcoma." *J. Roy. Soc. Med.* 75 (1986):532–534.

Shilts, R. *And the Band Played On: Politics, People and the AIDS* Epidemic. New York, St. Martin's Press, 1987.

Shoumatoff, A. *African Madness*. New York, Knopf, 1988.

Siegal, F. P., and Siegal, M. *AIDS: The Medical Mystery*. New York, Grove Press, 1983.

Siegal, F. P., Lopez, C., Hammer, G., et al. "Severe acquired immunodeficiency in male homosexuals, manifested by chronic perianal ulcerative herpes simplex lesions." *New Engl. J. Med.* 305 (1981):1439–1444.

Sigurdsson, B., Palsson, P. A., and Grimsson, H. "Visna, a demyelinating transmissible disease of sheep." *J. Neuropath. Exp. Neurol.* 16 (1957):389.

Simonin, M. *Danger de vie*. Paris, Garamont, 1986.

Smith, E. C., and Elmes, B.G.T. "Malignant disease in natives of Nigeria: An analysis of five hundred tumors." *Ann. Trop. Med. Parasit.* 28 (1934):461–513.

Smith, H. M. "AIDS—lessons from history." *MD* 30, no. 9 (1986):43–51.

Smith, M. G. "Propagation in tissue culture of a cytopathogenic virus from human salivary gland virus (SGV) disease." *Proc. Soc. Exp. Biol. Med.* 92 (1956):424–430.

Smith, T. F., Srinivasan, A., Schochetman, G., et al. "The phylogenetic history of immunodeficiency viruses." *Nature* (Lond.) 333 (1988):573–575.

Soave, R., Danner, R. L., Honig, C. L., et al. "Cryptosporidiosis in homosexual men." *Ann. Int. Med.* 100 (1984):504–511.

Sodroski, J., Rosen, C., Wong-Staal, F., et al. "Transacting transcriptional regulation of human T-cell leukemia virus type III long terminal repeat." *Science* (Wash.) 227 (1985):171–173.

Solé, R. "Croisade contre les homosexuels aux Etats-Unis." *Le Monde*, July 7, 1983.

Somaini, B. "AIDS: Eine Importkrankheit?" *Schweiz. Med. Wschr.* 116 (1986):818–821.

Sonea, S., and Panisset, M. *The New Bacteriology.* Boston, Jones and Bartlett, 1983.

Sonigo, P., Alizon, M., Staskus, K., et al. "Nucleotide sequence of the visna lentivirus: Relationship to the AIDS virus." *Cell* 42 (1985):369–382.

Sonnet, J., and De Bruyere, M. "Syndrome de déficit acquis de l'immunité—AIDS: État de la question. Données personnelles de la pathologie observée chez des Zaïrois." *Louvain Méd.* 102 (1983):297–307.

Sonnet, J., Michaux, J. L., Zech, F., et al. "Early AIDS cases originating from Zaire and Burundi (1962–1976)." *Scand. J. Infect. Dis.* 19 (1987):511–517.

Sontag, S. *Illness as Metaphor.* New York, Farrar, Strauss and Giroux, 1977.

Sontag, S. "Aids and its metaphors." *New York Rev. Books* 35 (1988):89–99.

Sournia, J. C. "Médias et SIDA." *Bull. Acad. Nat. Méd.* 171 (1987):7134–717.

Stanier, R. and Lwoff, A. "Le concept de microbe de Pasteur à nos jours." *Presse Méd.* 2 (1973):1191–1198.

Staquet, M., Hemmer, A., and Baert, A., eds. *Clinical Aspects of AIDS and AIDS-related Complex.* Proceedings of a symposium held in Brussels. Oxford-New York, Oxford University Press, 1986.

Starcic, B., Ratner, L., Josephs, S. F., et al. "Characterization of long terminal repeat sequences of HTLV-III." *Science* (Wash.) 227 (1985):538–540.

Stearn, E. W., and Stearn, A. E. *The Effect of Smallpox on the Destiny of the Amerindian.* Boston, Bruce Humphries, 1945.

Stemmerman, G. N., Hayashi, T., Glober, G. A., et al. "Cryptosporidiosis: Report of a fatal case complicated by disseminated toxoplasmosis." *Amer. J. Med.* 69 (1980): 637–642.

Stephens, r. M., Casey, J. W., and Rice, N. R. "Equine infectious anemia virus gag and pol genes: Relatedness to visna and AIDS virus." *Science* (Wash.) 231 (1986): 589–594.

Sterry, W., Konrads, A., and Laaser, U. "Kaposi-Sarkom und aplastische Panzytopenie; gleichzeitiges Auftreten bei einem Patienten." *Hautarzt* 30 (1979):540–543.

Sterry, W., Marmor, M., Konrads, A., and Steigleder, G. K. "Kaposi's sarcoma, aplastic pancytopenia and multiple infections in a homosexual (Cologne, 1976)." *Lancet* 1 (1983):924–925 5.

Stevenson, L. G. "New diseases in the seventeenth century." *Bull. Hist. Med.* 39 (1965):1–21.

Stewart, G. J., Tyler, J. P., Cunningham, A. L., et al. "Transmission of human T-cell lymphotropic virus type III (HTLV-III) by artificial insemination by donor." *Lancet* 2 (1985):581–585.

Stimmel, B. *Heroin Dependency: Medical, Economic and Social Aspects*. New York, Stratton, 1975.

Stoddard, J. L., and Cutler, E. C. "Torula infection in man." *Monogr. Rockef. Inst. Med. Res.* 6 (1916):1–98.

Stoler, M. H., Eskin, T., Benn, S., et al. "Human T-cell lymphotropic virus type III infection of the central nervous system: A preliminary in situ analysis." *J. Amer. Med. Ass.* 256 (1986):2360–2364.

Streicher, H. Z., and Joynt, R. J. "HTLV-III/LAV and the monocyte/macrophage." *J. Amer. Med. Ass.* 256 (1986):2390–2391.

Sunderam, G., McDonald, R. J., Maniatis, T., et al. "Tuberculosis as a manifestation of the acquired immunodeficiency syndrome." *J. Amer. Med. Ass.* 256 (1986):362–366.

Symmers, W.S.C. "Generalized cytomegalic inclusion-body disease associated with pneumocystis pneumonia in adults." *J. Clin. Path.* 13 (1960):1–21.

Taguchi, H. "Origin of HTLV-I virus in Japan." *Nature* (Lond.) 323 (1986):764.

Talal, N., and Shearer, G. "A clinician and a scientist look at acquired immunodeficiency syndrome (AIDS)." *Immunol. Today* 4 (1983):180–185.

Tastemain, C. "Les médicaments contre le SIDA sont-ils efficaces?" *Recherche* 18 (1987):844–846.

Taylor, J. F. "Lymphocyte transformation in Kaposi's sarcoma." *Lancet* 1 (1973): 883–884.

Taylor, J. F., Smith, V. G., Bull, D., et al. "Kaposi's sarcoma in Uganda." *Intern. J. Cancer* 8 (1971):122–135.

Teas, J. "Could AIDS agent be a new variant of African swine fever virus?" *Lancet* 1 (1983):922–923.

Tedeschi, C. G. "Some considerations concerning the nature of the so-called sarcoma of Kaposi." *Arch. Path.* 66 (1958):656–684.

Temin, H. M. "Origin of retroviruses from cellular moveable genetic elements." *Cell* 21 (1980):599–600.

Temin, H. M. "L'origine des rétrovirus." *Recherche* 15 (1984):192–203.

Temin, H. M. "Les rétrovirus et la génétique des cancers." *Rev. Prat.* 37 (1987): 2541–2551.

Temin, H. M. "Evolution of retroviruses and other retrotranscripts." In D. Bolognesi, ed., *Human Retroviruses, Cancer and AIDS*. pp. 1–28. New York, Liss, 1988.

Temin, H. M., and Mizutani, S. "RNA-dependent DNA polymerase in virions of Rous sarcoma virus." *Nature* (Lond.) 226 (1970):1211–1213.

Tervo, T., Lahdevirta, J., Vaheri, A., et al. "Recovery of HTLV-III from contact lenses." *Lancet* 1 (1986):379–380.

Thalhammer, O. "Geschichte der Toxoplasmose." In *Die Toxoplasmose bei Mensch und Tier*. Vienna, Maudrich, 1957.

Thijs, A. "L'angiosarcomatose de Kaposi au Congo Belge et au Ruanda-Urundi." *Ann. Soc. Belge Méd. Trop.* 37 (1957):295–307.

Thiry, L., Sprecher-Goldberger, S., Jonkheer, T., et al. "Isolation of AIDS virus from cell-free breast milk of three healthy virus carriers." *Lancet* 2 (1985):891–892.

Thomsen, H. K., Jacobsen, M., and Malchow-Moller, A. "Kaposi's sarcoma among homosexual men in Europe." *Lancet* 2 (1981):688.

Tovo, P. A., De Martino M., et al. "Epidemiology, clinical features, and prognostic factors of paediatric HIV infection." *Lancet* 2 (1988):1043–1046.

Trebach, A. S. *The Heroin Solution*. New Haven and London, Yale University Press, 1982.

Trichopoulos, D., Spiros, L., and Petridou, E. "Homosexual role separation and spread of AIDS." *Lancet* 2 (1988): 966.

Tschachler, E., Groh, V., Popovic, M., et al. "Epidermal Langerhans cells—a target for HTLV-III/LAV infection." *J. Invest. Dermatol.* 88 (1987):233–237.

Tubiana, N., Lejeune, C., Lecaer, F., et al. "T-lymphoma associated with HTLV-I outside the Carribean and Japan." *Lancet* 2 (1985):337.

Vachon, F. "Sida et syphilis: Un parallèle." *Méd. Malad. Infect.* 4 (1987):141–142.

Vallée, H., and Carré, H. "Nature infectieuse de l'anémie du cheval." *C. R. Acad. Sci. Paris* 139 (1904):331–333.

Van de Perre, P., Clumeck, N., Carael, M., et al. "Female prostitutes: A risk group for infection with human T-cell lymphotropic virus type III." *Lancet* 2 (1985):524–526.

Van de Perre, P., Le Polain, B., Carael, M., et al. "HIV antibodies in a remote rural area in Rwanda, Central Africa." *AIDS* 1 (1987):213–215.

Van de Perre, P., Rouvroy, D., Lepage, P., et al. "Acquired immunodeficiency syndrome in Rwanda." *Lancet* 2 (1984):62–65.

Van der Graaf, M., and Diepersloot, R. J. "Transmission of human immunodeficiency virus: A review." *Infection* 14 (1986):203–211.

Van der Meer, G., and Brug, S. L. "Infection à Pneumocystis chez l'homme et chez les animaux." *Ann. Soc. Belge Méd. Trop.* 22 (1942):301–307.

Vandepitte, J., Verwilghen, R., and Zachee, P. "AIDS and cryptococcosis (Zaïre, 1977)." *Lancet* 1 (1983):925–926.

Varmus, H. "Retroviruses." *Science* (Wash.) 240 (1988):1427–1435.

Vazeux, R., Brousse, N., Jarry, A., et al. "AIDS subacute encephalitis: Identification of HIV infected cells." *Amer. J. Path.* 126 (1987):403–410.

Velimirovic, B. "AIDS as a social phenomenon." *Soc. Sci. Med.* 25 (1987):541–542.

Vernant, J. C., Gessain, A., Gout, O., et al. "Paraparésies spastiques tropicales en Martinique. Haute prévalence d'anticorps HTLV-I." *Presse Méd.* 15 (1986):419–422.

Vieiria, J., Franck, E., Spira, T. J., et al. "Acquired immune deficiency in Haitians." *New Engl. J. Med.* 308 (1983):125–129.

Vilaseca, J., Arnau, J. M., Bacardi, R., et al. "Kaposi's sarcoma and Toxoplasma gondii brain abscess in a Spanish homosexual." *Lancet* 1 (1982):572.

Vilmer, E., Barré-Sinoussi, F., Rouzioux, C., et al. "Isolation of a new lymphotropic retrovirus from two hemophilia B siblings, one presenting with acquired immunodeficiency syndrome." *Lancet* 1 (1984):753–757.

Vittecoq, D. "Traitement des infections à HIV." *Lettre de l'Infectiologue* 2 (1987): 450–458.

Vogel, L. C., Muller, A. S., Odingo, R. S., et al., eds. *Health and Disease in Kenya*. Nairobi, East African Literature Bureau, 1974.

Vogt, M. W., et al. "Isolation patterns of the human immunodeficiency virus from cervical secretions during the menstrual cycle of women at risk for AIDS." *Ann. Int. Med.* 106 (1987):380–382.

Vogt, M. W., Witt, D. J., Craven, E. D., et al. "Isolation of HTLV-III/LAV from cervical secretions of women at risk for AIDS." *Lancet* 1 (1986):527–529.

Volsky, D. J., Wu, Y. T., Stevenson, M., et al. "Antibodies to HTLV-III/LAV in Venezuelan patients with acute malarial infections." *New Engl. J. Med.* 314 (1986): 647–648.

Wain-Hobson, S., Sonigo, P., Danos, O., et al. "Nucleotide sequence of the AIDS virus, LAV." *Cell* 40 (1985):9–17.

Wallis, C. "The deadly spread of AIDS." *Time Magazine*, September 6, 1982, p. 27.

Walters, L. "Ethical issues in the prevention and treatment of HIV infection and AIDS." *Science* (Wash.) 239 (1988):597–603.

Ward, J. W., Holmberg, S. D., Allen, J. R., et al. "Transmission of human immunodeficiency virus (HIV) by blood transfusions screened as negative for HIV antibody." *N. Engl. J. Med.* 318 (1988):473–478.

Ward, R. "Mainstream scientists confront unorthodox view of AIDS." *Nature* (Lond.) 332 (1988):574.

Watanabe, J. M., Chinchinian, H., Weitz, C., and McIlvanie, S. K. "Pneumocystis carinii pneumonia in a family." *J. Amer. Med. Ass.* 193 (1965):685–686.

Watanabe, T., Seiki, M., Hirayama, Y., and Yoshida, M. "Human T-cell leukemia virus type I is a member of the African subtype of simian viruses (STLV)." *Virology* 148 (1986):385–388.

Watanabe, T., Seiki, M., and Yoshida, M. "HTLV type I (US isolate) and ATLV (Japanese isolate) are the same species of human retrovirus." *Virology* 133 (1983): 238–241.

Waterson, A. P., and Wilkinson, L. *An Introduction to the History of Virology.* Cambridge, Cambridge University Press, 1978.

Watson, A. J. "Origin of encephalitis lethargica." *China Med. J.* 42 (1928):427–432.

Weber, J. "Is AIDS an epidemic form of African Kaposi'sarcoma?" *J. Roy. Soc. Med.* 77 (1984):572–576.

Weber, J. N. "AIDS in 1959?" *Lancet* 2 (1983):1136.

Weinstein, L., Edelstein, S. M., Madara, J. L., et al. "Intestinal cryptosporidiosis complicated by disseminated cytomegalovirus infection." *Gastroenterology* 81 (1981):584–591.

Weiss, R. A. "AIDS." *Sci. Publ. Affairs* 3 (1988):99–110.

Weiss, R. A., Clapham, P. R., Weber, J.H.N., et al. "HIV-2 antisera cross-neutralize HIV-1." *AIDS* 2 (1988):95–100.

Weiss, R. A., Teich, N., Varmus, H. E., and Coffin, J., eds. *RNA Tumor Viruses: The Molecular Biology of Tumor Viruses*, vols. 1–2. New York, Cold Spring Harbor Laboratory, 1982 and 1985.

Weiss, S. H., Goedert, J. J., Gartner, S., et al. "Risk of human immunodeficiency virus (HIV-1) infection among laboratory workers." *Science* (Wash.) 239 (1988): 68–71.

Weissmann, G. "AIDS and heat." In *The Woods Hole Cantata: Essays on Science and Society*, pp. 64–78. Boston, Houghton Mifflin, 1986.

Wells, H. G. *The War of the Worlds*, pp. 269–270. Leipzig, Tauchnitz, 1898.

Wendler, I., Schneider, J., Gras, B., et al. "Seroepidemiology of human immunodeficiency virus in Africa." *Brit. Med. J.* 293 (1986):782–785.

Werthemann, A. *Schädel und Gebeine des Erasmus von Rotterdam.* Basel, I.T., 1930.

White, G. C., and Lesesne, H. R. "Hemophilia, hepatitis and the acquired immunodeficiency syndrome." *Ann. Int. Med.* 98 (1983):403–404.

Wiley, C. A., Schrier, R. D., and Nelson, J. A. "Cellular localization of human immunodeficiency virus infection within the brains of acquired immunodeficiency syndrome patients." *Proc. Natl. Acad. Sci. USA* 83 (1986):7089–7093.

Wilkes, M. S., Fortin, A. H., and Felix, J. C. "Value of necropsy in acquired immunodeficiency syndrome." *Lancet* 2 (1988):85–88.

Williams, G., Stretton, T. B., and Leonard, J. C. "Cytomegalic inclusion disease and Pneumocystis carinii infection in adults." *Lancet* 2 (1960):951–955.

Williams, G., Stretton, T. B., and Leonard, J. C. "AIDS in 1959?" *Lancet* 2 (1983): 1136.

Winn, W. C., Jr. "Legionnaires disease: Historical perspective." *Clin. Microbiol. Rev.* 1 (1988):60–81.

Witte, M. H., Witte, C. L., Minnich, L. L., et al. "AIDS in 1968." *J. Amer. Med. Ass.* 251 (1984):2657.

Wofsy, C. B., Cohen, J. B., Hauer, L. B., et al. "Isolation of AIDS-associated retrovirus from genital secretions of women with antibodies to the virus." *Lancet* 1 (1986):527–529.

Wolf, A., and Cowen, D. "Granulomatous encephalomyelitis due to an encephalitozoon (encephalitozoitic encephalomyelitis), a new protozoon disease of man." *Bull. Neurol. Inst. N.Y.* 6 (1937):306–371.

Wong-Staal, F., and Gallo, R. C. "Human T-lymphotropic retrovirus." *Nature* (Lond.) 317 (1985a):395–403.

Wong-Staal, F., and Gallo, R. C. "The family of human T-lymphotropic leukemia viruses: HTLV-I as the cause of adult T cell leukemia and HTLV-III as the cause of acquired immunodeficiency syndrome." *Blood* 65 (1985b):253–263.

Wong-Staal, F., Shaw, G. M., Hahn, B. H., et al. "Genomic diversity of human T-lymphotropic virus type III (HTLV-III)." *Science* (Wash.) 227 (1985):759–762.

World Health Organization (WHO). "Acquired immune deficiency syndrome (AIDS): Report on the situation as of 31 December 1984." *Weekly Epidem. Record* 60 (1985):85–92.

Wormser, G. P., Krupp, L. B., Hanrahan, J. P., et al. "Acquired immunodeficiency syndrome in male prisoners: New insights into an emerging syndrome." *Ann. Int. Med.* 98 (1983):297–303.

Wormser, G. P., Stahl, R. E., and Bottone, E. J., eds. *AIDS: Acquired Immunodeficiency Syndrome and Other Manifestations of HIV Infection.* New Jersey, Noyes, 1987.

Wyatt, J. P., Saxton, J., Lee, M. S., and Pinkerton, H. "Generalized cytomegalic inclusion disease." *J. Pediatr.* 36 (1950):271.

Wyatt, J. P., Simon, T. , Trumbull, M. L., and Evans M. "Cytomegalic inclusion pneumonitis in the adult." *Amer. J. Clin. Path.* 23 (1953):353–362.

Wylie, J., and Collier, L. H. "The English sweating sickness (sudor Anglicus): A reappraisal." *J. Hist. Med.* 36 (1981):425–445.

Yamamoto, N., Hinuma, Y., Zur Hausen, H., et al. "African green monkeys are infected with adult T-cell leukaemia virus or a closely related agent." *Lancet* 1 (1983):240–241.

Yarchoan, R., Mitsuya, H., and Broder, S. "AIDS therapies." *Scient. Amer.* 259, no. 4 (1988):110–119.

Yarchoan, R., Weinhold, K. J., and Lyerly, K. H. "Administration of 3'-azido-3'-deoxythymidine, an inhibitor of HTLV-III/LAV replication, to patients with AIDS and AIDS-related complex." *Lancet* 1 (1986):575–580.

Yokoyama, S., and Gojobori, T. "Molecular evolution and phylogeny of the human AIDS viruses LAV, HTLV-III and ARV." *J. Mol. Evol.* 24 (1987):330–336.

Yokoyama, S., Chung, L., and Gojobori, T. "Molecular evolution of the human immunodeficiency and related viruses." *Mol. Biol. Evol.* 5 (1988):237–251.

Yokoyama, S., Moriyama, E. N., and Gojobori, T. "Molecular phylogeny of the human immunodeficiency and related retroviruses." *Proc. Japan. Acad.* 63 (1987): 147–150.

Yoshida, M., Miyoshi, I., and Hinuma, Y. "Isolation and characterization of retrovirus from cell lines of human adult T-cell leukemia and its implication in the disease." *Proc. Natl. Acad. Sci. USA* 79 (1982):2031–2035.

Zagury, D., Bernard, J., Cheynier, R., et al. "A group specific anamnestic immune reaction against HIV-1 induced by a candidate vaccine against AIDS." *Nature* (Lond.) 332 (1988):728–731.

Zagury, D., Bernard, J., Leibowitch, J., et al. "HTLV-III in cells cultured from semen of two patients with AIDS." *Science* (Wash.) 226 (1984):449–451.

Zagury, D., Fouchard, M., VOL, J. C., et al. "Detection of infectious HTLV-III/LAV virus in cell-free plasma from AIDS patients." *Lancet* 2 (1985):505–506.

Zagury, D., Léonard, R., Fouchard, M., et al. "Immunization against AIDS in humans." *Nature* (Lond.) 326 (1987):249–250.

Zapevalov, V. "Panic in the West, or what is behind the sensation about AIDS" (in Russian). *Literatournaya Gazeta*, October 30, 1985.

Ziegler, J. L., Beckstead, J. A., Volberding, D. I., et al. "Non-Hodgkins lymphoma in 90 homosexual men: Relation to generalized lymphadenopathy and the acquired immunodeficiency syndrome." *New Engl. J. Med.* 311 (1984):565–570.

Ziegler, J. L., Drew, W. L., Miner, R. C., et al. "Outbreak of Burkitt's-like lymphoma in homosexual men." *Lancet* 2 (1982):631–633.

Ziegler, J. L., Templeton, A. C., and Vogel, C. L. "Kaposi's sarcoma: A comparison of classical, endemic and epidemic forms." *Semin. Oncol.* 11 (1984):47–52.

Zinsser, H. *Rats, Lice and History.* Boston, Little, Brown and Co., 1935. New edition: New York, Bantam Books, 1960.

Zittoun, R., ed. *Le syndrome immunodéficitaire acquis.* Paris, Doin, 1986.

Zuger, A., and Miles, S. H. "Physicians, AIDS and occupational risk: Historic traditions and ethical obligations." *J. Amer. Med. Ass.* 258 (1987):1924–1928.

Index